HUMAN IDENTIFICATION

HUMAN IDENTIFICATION

Case Studies in
———— Forensic Anthropology ————

Edited by

TED A. RATHBUN, Ph.D.

Department of Anthropology
University of South Carolina
Columbia, South Carolina

and

JANE E. BUIKSTRA, Ph.D.

Department of Anthropology
Northwestern University
Evanston, Illinois

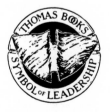

CHARLES C THOMAS • PUBLISHER
Springfield • Illinois • U.S.A.

Published and Distributed Throughout the World by

CHARLES C THOMAS • PUBLISHER
2600 South First Street
Springfield, Illinois 62717

© *1984 by* CHARLES C THOMAS • PUBLISHER
ISBN 0-398-04875-4 (cloth)
ISBN 0-398-06337-0 (paper)
Library of Congress Catalog Card Number: 83-24268

Printed in the United States of America
SC–R-3

Library of Congress Cataloging in Publication Data
Main entry under title:

Human identification.

Bibliography: p.
Includes index.
1. Forensic anthropology—Case studies. 2. Criminal
investigation—Case studies. I. Rathbun, Ted A.
II. Buikstra, Jane E.
GN69.8.H85 1984 614′.1 83-24268
ISBN 0-398-04875-4 .— ISBN 0-398-06337-0 (pbk.)

ABOUT THE AUTHORS

Editors

Jane E. Buikstra, currently a Professor of Anthropology at Northwestern University, received her graduate degrees from the University of Chicago. Her forensic interests in individuation, burned remains, and forensic archaeology derive from her osteological training in prehistoric human variation and mortuary customs. A Fellow of the American Academy of Forensic Sciences and diplomate of the American Board of Forensic Anthropology, she serves as a consultant to various law enforcement agencies in Illinois and in Indiana. Although her bio-archaeological research has centered in the North American Midwest, her studies have also taken her to South America, the Canadian Arctic, Africa, as well as other regions of the United States.

Ted A. Rathbun received his M.A. degree in 1966 and his Ph.D. in 1971, both from the University of Kansas, and is Associate Professor of Anthropology at the University of South Carolina. His academic work has concentrated on the osteology, paleopathology, and demography of prehistoric populations in Iran, Iraq, and South Carolina. Although he was appointed as consulting physical anthropologist to the Office of the Chief Medical Examiner at the Medical University of South Carolina in 1971, most of Dr. Rathbun's forensic consultations involve human identification for coroners and law enforcement agencies. He lectures on forensic anthropology to various groups and offers a yearly course on human identification in forensic anthropology to undergraduate and graduate students. He is a member of the American Academy of Forensic Sciences and is a Diplomate of the American Board of Forensic Anthropology.

Other Contributors

J. Lawrence Angel is curator of Physical Anthropology at the National Museum of Natural History, Smithsonian Institution, Washington, D.C. He received a Ph.D. at Harvard University in physical anthropology and has done field work in Greece, Turkey, and Cyprus on the social biology of culture growth. In addition to anthropology (at Berkeley, Minnesota, Harvard, and George Washington Universities) he has taught human anatomy (Jefferson

Medical College, Howard, and the U.S. Naval Hospital in Philadelphia). Dr. Angel has analyzed forensic skeletons at the Smithsonian since 1962. He is current president of the American Board of Forensic Anthropology.

William M. Bass received his first training in Forensic Anthropology under Dr. Charles E. Snow while working on his master's degree at the University of Kentucky. A desire for further training in Forensic Anthropology led Dr. Bass to the University of Pennsylvania, where he completed his Ph.D. under Dr. Wilton M. Krogman. He and Dr. Krogman worked jointly on many cases while Bass was a graduate student, and Dr. Bass has continued a tutorship program with his students at the University of Kansas (1960–1971) and the University of Tennessee (1971–present).

Richard H. Brooks received a Ph.D. from the University of Colorado and is affiliated with the University of Nevada, Las Vegas, where he is Research Professor of Anthropology, and Principal Museum Anthropologist.

Sheilagh T. Brooks was born in Tampico, Tamaulipas, Mexico and became a U.S. citizen in 1945. She received a Ph.D. in physical anthropology from the University of California, Berkeley and is Professor of Anthropology at the University of Nevada, Las Vegas, having joined the staff in 1966.

Margaret C. (Peggy) Caldwell, the daughter of a U.S. Foreign Service officer, traveled extensively with her family and as a senior in high school participated as a paleoanthropological assistant on the International Afar Research Expedition at the Hadar in the Rift Valley of Ethiopia. She was awarded a Master of Arts degree in Physical Anthropology from Arizona State University in 1981. During her graduate education she undertook several specialized projects in osteology and received additional training in forensic anthropology at the University of Arizona. Ms. Caldwell is currently a collaborator in the Department of Anthropology, Smithsonian Institution, teaches science at the Brearley School, and acts as a consultant to Dr. Gross, the New York City Medical Examiner. She is a member of the American Association of Physical Anthropologists and a trainee affiliate of the American Academy of Forensic Sciences.

Homer R. Campbell, Jr., received his D.D.S. from Baylor University School of Dentistry in 1956. He has been in private practice in Albuquerque since 1959. He has been associated with the New Mexico Medical Investigator's Office since its beginning in 1973 and is currently the Chief Forensic Odontologist. He is also Clinical Associate Professor in the Department of Pathology at the University of New Mexico School of Medicine. Dr. Campbell is a Diplomate of the American Board of Forensic Odontology, Inc., and conducts a growing practice in forensic odontological consultation. He is recognized as an innovator in the analysis of bite marks.

Michael Charney, Ph.D., was educated in anthropology at the Universities of

Texas and Colorado and at Columbia University. He is presently serving as Emeritus Professor of Anthropology at Colorado State University and is the director of the Center of Human Identification. He is a frequent consultant for law enforcement agencies in the mountain states, but has worked for other agencies from New Jersey through Canada. He has published numerous articles dealing with forensic anthropology and is probably best known for his work in casting materials and facial reconstruction techniques. He was codirector in the identification of multiple deaths in the Big Thompson flood. Dr. Charney is a fellow of the American Academy of Forensic Sciences and a Diplomate of the American Board of Forensic Anthropology.

Della Collins Cook is Associate Professor of Anthropology at Indiana University. Her interests include skeletal biology, paleopathology, and demography in North American Indian populations. She is presently evaluating population differences in dental and postcranial growth arrest indicators in prehistoric midwestern materials. She received her M.A. from the University of Chicago in 1971 and her Ph.D. in 1976.

R. C. Dailey is a consultant to the Florida Department of Law Enforcement. He has been doing forensic physical anthropology for the past 16 years and regularly lectures on methods of estimating age, sex, and racial origin as well as participating in law enforcement sponsored training programs.

Jack Duncan is currently a research and training specialist with the Florida Department of Law Enforcement. He has 17 years' experience in crime processing and was a crime laboratory analyst for 10 years.

Michael Finnegan is a Professor of Anthropology and Director of the Osteology Laboratory at Kansas State University. He is a consultant in forensic osteology and holds a Ph.D. in anthropology from the University of Colorado. He was a postdoctoral fellow at the Smithsonian Institution and is a fellow of the American Academy of Forensic Sciences, a member of the International Association for Identification, and a Diplomate of the American Board of Forensic Anthropology. Dr. Finnegan is a recipient of the Kansas Attorney General Certificate of Merit in recognition of outstanding service rendered to law enforcement in and for the State of Kansas by a private citizen. He has published numerous articles on theory, method, and application of osteological analysis in population studies and forensic application.

George W. Gill is currently an Associate Professor of Anthropology at the University of Wyoming. He received a Ph.D. from the University of Kansas. He has studied burial archaeology and human osteology in populations in western Mexico, the northwestern plains of North America, and on Easter Island. Dr. Gill has provided human skeletal identification service to the Wyoming State Crime Laboratory since 1972. In 1978 he became a Diplomate of the American Board of Forensic Anthropology and is also a member of the American Academy of Forensic Sciences. He has authored several articles and has contributed to books and special volumes.

Claire C. Gordon received her Ph.D. degree in Biological Anthropology from Northwestern University in 1982, after receiving an M.A. degree in Anthropology from Northwestern in 1977 and a B.S. degree in Biology from the University of Notre Dame in 1976. During eight years of archeological fieldwork, she has done research in Southern Illinois, the American Southwest, and Micronesia. Dr. Gordon currently holds the position of Research Anthropologist at the U.S. Army Natick Research & Development Center, where she conducts research in anthropometry, allometry, and biomechanics for application in the human engineering of personal protective clothing and equipment.

Thomas Grubbs received an M.S. degree in Mechanical Engineering from the University of Houston in 1968 and is a Professional Engineer in the State of Texas. He is currently an Aerospace Technologist with the National Aeronautics and Space Administration (NASA) at the Lyndon B. Johnson Space Center, Houston, Texas. For the past 18 years he has been responsible for mechanical design and analysis related to spacecraft, aircraft, and various specialized mechanical devices, presently working on a manned EVA task simulator for Space Shuttle 5. He has had 8 years of forensic engineering experience, mainly related to mechanical design, stability, and accident reconstruction.

Sathya V. Hanagud is Professor of Aerospace Engineering, Georgia Institute of Technology, Atlanta, Georgia. He received an M.S. Aerospace Engineering degree from the India Institute of Science in Bangalore and a Ph.D. from Stanford University in 1963, with specialization in catylization of structures, metals, and impact loading. He teaches in the field of structural engineering and materials and is a specialist in aircraft crash dynamic reconstruction. For 7 years he conducted research at Stanford Research Institute. He has written over 100 scientific papers.

Rodger Heglar is a Professor of Anthropology at SanFrancisco State University, having joined the faculty in 1967. He received his Ph.D. from the University of Michigan and has taught there (1959–1963) and at Southern Illinois University (1963–1966). He is recognized professionally in both physical anthropology and forensic anthropology. In physical (biological) anthropology his teaching and research interests are the biology of human populations, particularly in the New World, skeletal biology, paleopathology, paleoserology, and medical anthropology. In forensic anthropology (medicolegal investigation) he is Board certified and practices among the northern and Bay Area California counties. He is an Assistant Medical Examiner-Coroner in San Francisco and deputized in several neighboring counties, where his investigation and opinion in unknown person or homicide cases are desired.

J. Michael Hoffman received an M.D. degree in 1970 from the University of Maryland and M.A. and Ph.D. degrees in 1972 and 1973 from the University of Colorado. He has held teaching appointments at Northern Arizona University, the University of California-Berkeley (where he was also Curator of Human Osteology at the R. H. Lowie Museum of Anthropology), and Colorado College. His research interests include human osteology, skeletal paleopathology, and forensic physical anthropology.

Paul N. Jolly is currently Chief Deputy Coroner for the Hamilton County Coroner's Office, Cincinnati, Ohio, and Assistant Clinical Professor of Pathology at the University of Cincinnati, where he earned an M.D. degree in 1941. He has served as chief of the section of pathology for the Ohio State Medical Association, as president of the Ohio Society of Pathologists, and as counselor for Ohio for the American Society of Clinical Pathologists.

Allen M. Jones has been Forensic Pathologist, Office of the Chief Medical Examiner, Oklahoma City, since 1979. He earned M.S. and M.D. degrees from the University of Louisville and was an American Cancer Society Fellow in Surgical Pathology at Washington University. He served a residency (1975–1976) in forensic pathology, Office of the Medical Investigator, Albuquerque, New Mexico, advancing to Assistant, and Associate, Medical Investigator. He has taught at Washington University School of Medicine and the Department of Pathology at the University of New Mexico and is presently Clinical Assistant Professor of Pathology at the University of Oklahoma Health Sciences Center. Dr. Jones is certified by the National Board of Medical Examiners and the American Board of Pathology in both Anatomic Pathology and Forensic Pathology. He is a Fellow of the American Academy of Forensic Sciences.

Ellis R. Kerley was awarded an M.S. degree from the University of Michigan in 1956 and a Ph.D. degree from the University of Michigan in 1962 and has postgraduate work in Forensic Pathology and Orthopedic Pathology at the Armed Forces Institute of Pathology. His professional experience includes 3 years of research in medical genetics at the Bowman Gray School of Medicine (1950–1953); identification of the Korean War dead at Kokura, Japan (1954–1955); research in skeletal variability and age change at the Orthopedic Pathology Section of the Armed Forces Institute of Pathology (1957–1966); teaching in the Anthropology departments of the University of Kentucky, University of Kansas, and University of Maryland; and teaching in the Anatomy Department of the University of Puerto Rico Medical School. He has served as a forensic consultant for the Armed Forces, FBI, and coroners and medical examiners in various parts of the U.S. as well as the Congressional Subcommittee on the Investigation of the Assassination of President

John F. Kennedy. Dr. Kerley has held numerous professional offices and received many professional honors.

Lowell J. Levine received the D.D.S. degree from New York University in 1963. In private practice in Bayside, New York, Dr. Levine has been both on active duty and in the Naval Reserve for over 10 years. He is frequently consulted by investigative agencies around the country. He is past President and a Fellow of the American Academy of Forensic Sciences and a Diplomate of the American Board of Forensic Odontology, Inc. He is a Clinical Associate Professor in the Department of Forensic Medicine at the New York School of Medicine.

James L. Luke received his M.D. from Western Reserve University. He has served in the offices of the Chief Medical Examiner in New York and Oklahoma and became the Chief Medical Examiner of Washington, D.C. in 1971. His specialties in forensic research concern the pathology of strangulation, problems of forensic pathology and pediatrics, and blunt force injury. He is a fellow of the American Academy of Forensic Science.

William R. Maples received his Ph.D. in Anthropology from the University of Texas (Austin) in 1967. Dr. Maples spent 4 years in Kenya, where he was associated with various biomedical projects. He has taught at Western Michigan University and the University of Florida. He is currently Curator of Physical Anthropology at the Florida State Museum and Professor of Anthropology at the University of Florida. He is Head of the State Medical Museum of Florida. Dr. Maples is a Diplomate of the American Board of Forensic Anthropology and a Fellow in the American Academy of Forensic Sciences.

Patricia McFeeley is Associate Medical Investigator, Office of the Medical Investigator, New Mexico Center for Forensic and Environmental Science, Albuquerque, and Assistant Professor of Pathology, University of New Mexico, School of Medicine. Her M.D. degree was earned at the University of New Mexico in 1972, followed by 4 years of pathology residency training at the University of New Mexico and at Denver Children's Hospital and a fifth year at the University of New Mexico as a Forensic Pathology Fellow. Dr. McFeeley has conducted medical investigations in numerous aircraft accidents during the past 5 years as Assistant Medical Investigator in her present position. She is a member of the American Academy of Forensic Sciences and is certified by the American Board of Pathology in both Anatomic and Forensic Pathology.

Dan Morse is a retired physician and has held the position of Research Associate in the Department of Anthropology, Florida State University, for the past 13 years. He is certified by the American Board of Forensic Anthropology and has been a consultant to the Florida Department of Law Enforcement for the past 8 years.

Thomas T. Noguchi was Chief Medical Examiner-Coroner, Los Angeles. His recognition of the importance of forensic anthropology paved the way for the formulation of the research design for the skeletal aging study by Suchey.

Patricia A. Owings received the M.A. degree in Anthropology at California State University-Fullerton in 1981. Her M.A. thesis was based on epiphyseal union of the anterior iliac crest and medial clavicle, the research being done at the Department of the Chief Medical Examiner-Coroner, Los Angeles.

Anthony J. Perzigian is Associate Professor of Anthropology and Adjunct Associate Professor of Anatomy at the University of Cincinnati. He received a Ph.D. degree from Indiana University in 1971. His research focuses on the skeletal and dental biology of prehistoric populations. Dr. Perzigian is a Fellow of the American Anthropological Association and the Human Biology Council, a member of the American Association of Physical Anthropologists, and an associate commentator for *The Behavioral and Brain Sciences*. His forensic work has been performed for the Hamilton County Coroner's Office, Cincinnati, Ohio.

Theodore A. Reyman, M.D., Director of Laboratories at Mount Carmel Mercy Hospital, Detroit, Michigan, has held an interest in forensic pathology since his training as a resident, which included sessions at the Wayne County (Michigan) Medical Examiner's Office under Dr. Edward Zawadski. He has continued this interest through a close working relationship with Werner Spitz, M.D., the present Chief Medical Examiner. Dr. Reyman was eager to examine the tissues of Elmer McCurdy when the material was made available by Dr. Thomas Noguchi, bridging the gap between forensic pathology and the study of Egyptian and other mummified bodies that Dr. Reyman has examined in the past as part of the multidisciplinary team under the aegis of the Paleopathology Association.

J. Stanley Rhine received his Ph.D. from the University of Colorado in 1969. He taught anthropology at Colorado State University for 4 years and then assumed the post of Associate Professor at the University of New Mexico in Albuquerque. He is also Associate Curator of Physical Anthropology for the Maxwell Museum of Anthropology, and since 1974 he has been a consultant to the State Medical Investigator. He is certified by the American Board of Forensic Anthropology.

Norman J. Sauer received his Ph.D. degree in 1974 from Michigan State University, where he presently teaches. While most of his research and writing have involved Great Lakes area Native American and European skeletal samples, he has been consulting with law enforcement agencies in Michigan and nearby states for 10 years. He lectures regularly to state and local agencies about the recovery of and the information that can be gained from decomposed remains. He is a member of the American Academy of Forensic Scientists and a Diplomate of the American Board of Forensic Anthropology.

Sir Sydney A. Smith (d. 1969) received his M.D. at Edinburgh University and was Professor of Forensic Medicine there until assuming Emeritus status in 1953. Over his distinguished career he was a consultant to the Egyptian government in forensic medicine and also to the World Health Organization. He is probably best know for his *Text Book in Forensic Medicine*, first published in 1925 and now in its 10th edition, and for his popular work *Mostly Murder*, published in 1960.

Clyde C. Snow, a founding member of the American Board of Forensic Anthropology, received his M.A. in zoology from Texas Tech and his Ph.D. in physical anthropology from the University of Arizona. He served as part of the consultant team in the review of the Warren Commission investigation into the death of President John F. Kennedy. He has recently retired from the Federal Aviation Administration's Civil Aeromedical Institute, where he conducted extensive research related to aviation safety. Dr. Snow is currently a full-time consultant in forensic physical anthropology.

Richard G. Snyder has an educational background in Physical Anthropology with M.A. and Ph.D. degrees from the University of Arizona. He has done postdoctoral work in dental anthropology and in aerospace medicine at Ohio State University and the USAF School of Aerospace Medicine. He is currently Research Scientist and Head, Biomedical Department, Transportation Research Institute, Institute of Science and Technology, and Professor of Anthropology, Department of Anthropology, The University of Michigan and has held academic appointments at Michigan State University and the Universities of Oklahoma, Chicago, and Arizona. His experience also includes Manager of Biomechanics, Ford Motor Company; Chief, Physical Anthropology Laboratory, Civil Aeromedical Research Institute, Federal Aviation Administration; and Research Anthropologist, Applied Research Laboratory, College of Engineering, University of Arizona. Dr Snyder is internationally recognized as an authority on human impact tolerances; he has authored over 390 scientific papers and has received many awards. He is a member of numerous aviation, medical, and scientific biological societies, and is Board Certified in Forensic Anthropology.

T. Dale Stewart is currently Anthropologist Emeritus of the National Museum of Natural History. He identified skeletal remains for the Federal Bureau of Investigation for many years while serving as curator of Physical Anthropology at the Smithsonian Institution and has long been recognized as a distinguished scholar in forensic topics, especially age changes in young American males. Dr. Stewart received his M.D. from the Johns Hopkins Medical School and has conducted major identification seminars. He is a member of the American Anthropological Association, American Academy of Forensic Sciences, National Academy of Sciences, and is a consultant to the American Board of Forensic Anthropology.

Lucile E. St. Hoyme received her graduate education at George Washington University and Oxford University, where she was awarded the doctoral degree in 1963. Currently an emeritus curator at the Smithsonian Institution, she has been active in various phases of physical anthropological research and education. Included among her research interests are human variability, dental pathology, growth and development, and sexual dimorphism in the skeleton. This background in physical anthropology and ability to communicate clearly about the field have served Dr. St. Hoyme well in forensic anthropological consultant roles as well as in the teaching of forensic applications of physical anthropology.

James Stoutamire was a Research Associate in the Department of Anthropology, Florida State University and conducted the field training program in forensic archaeology. He is a professional archaeologist presently employed by the Florida Office of Coastal Management, Department of Environmental Regulation.

Judy Myers Suchey received an M.A. degree in Anthropology at the University of Kansas (1967) and a Ph.D. at the University of California, Riverside (1975). She is a physical anthropologist specializing in human osteology and forensic anthropology. Her major research specialty is skeletal aging. She has taught at California State University, Fullerton since 1969, currently holding the title of Professor. Dr Suchey has worked on over 200 forensic cases throughout Southern California during the past 12 years while serving on the staff of Coroner's Offices in Los Angeles, Orange, and San Bernardino counties. She is a Fellow of the American Academy of Forensic Sciences, a Diplomate of the American Board of Forensic Anthropology, and an officer of the Board of Forensic Anthropology (Treasurer).

Robert I. Sundick specialized in Physical Anthropology at the University of Toronto, receiving his M.A. degree there in 1967 and his Ph.D. in 1972. His doctoral dissertation was written on human skeletal growth as observed in American Indian populations. Between 1976 and 1978 he lived in Europe, examining Middle Ages European and prehistoric Nubian skeletons for age changes. He is currently investigating the similarities and differences seen in skeletal growth from various population groups. He has been at Western Michigan University since 1969 and is a Professor of Anthropology. He has been a member of the American Academy of Forensic Sciences since 1976 and is now a Fellow of the Academy and a Diplomate of the American Board of Forensic Anthropology.

Douglas H. Ubelaker received his Ph.D. from the University of Kansas in 1973. Since that time he has served as Curator of Physical Anthropology and currently is Chairman of the Department of Anthropology, National Museum of Natural History/Natural Museum of Man, Washington, D.C. Since 1978 he has served as consultant on forensic anthropology for the Federal Bureau of Investigation, Washington, D.C., for which he has prepared over 100 case reports. Dr. Ubelaker's research focuses primarily on problems in New World skeletal biology with special interest in prehistoric demography, bone microscopy, the prehistoric biology of Ecuador, and the excavation and interpretation of prehistoric mortuary sites.

Charles P. Warren holds M.A. degrees in anthropology from both Indiana University (1950) and the University of Chicago (1961). He is currently an Associate Professor of Anthropology in the Department of Anthropology, University of Illinois at Chicago. Professor Warren has done extensive field work in Southeast Asia, both as an ethnographer and as a physical anthropologist employed by the U.S. Department of Defense. He has been awarded a Fulbright Fellowship to the Philippines (1950–1951), a U.S. Public Health Service Grant (1958–1960), a National Science Foundation Science Faculty Fellowship (1963–1964), and the Meritorious Civilian Service Award from the Department of the Army (1975). He is a consultant to the law enforcement agencies in the Chicago Metropolitan region and to the U.S. Army Memorial Affairs Agency, Washington, D.C. He has published a book and a number of articles on the ethnography of Philippine tribal groups and has written extensively in the field of forensic anthropology. His most recent field experiences were in Southeast Asia, where he worked and did field research in Thailand, Viet Nam, and Kampuchea.

Curtis W. Wienker is Associate Professor and Director of the Graduate Program in the Department of Anthropology at the University of South Florida, Tampa. He received an M.A. and Ph.D. from the University of Arizona. He serves as a consultant to medical examiners in the greater Tampa Bay area and maintains a research interest in the population biology of living peoples.

Charles G. Wilber, Ph.D., received his graduate education at the Johns Hopkins University and later at the Air Force School of Aviation Medicine. He is Professor of Zoology and director of the Forensic Science Laboratory at Colorado State University. He has published numerous articles, technical reports, and books dealing with various aspects of forensic biology. He has particulary emphasized traumatic injuries, wound ballistics, and forensic toxicology. Dr. Wilber is qualified as an expert witness in his specialty areas, averaging 12 appearances per year in local, state, and federal courts. He is a

Fellow of the American Academy of Forensic Sciences, the New York Academy of Sciences, and is a member of the American Physiological Society. He is on the editorial board of the *American Journal of Forensic Medicine and Pathology* and edits a series of monographs dealing with environmental studies (Charles C Thomas, Publisher).

Dean V. Wiseley (deceased) was formerly Chief, Forensic Medicine Division, Department of Chief Medical Examiner-Coroner, Los Angeles. He generously gave his time in support of the skeletal age research from 1977 to 1980. In particular, he examined medical records and autopsy reports on all the females in the study.

CONTENTS

Section III
BIOLOGICAL CATEGORIES

HUMAN IDENTIFICATION

Section I
THE ROLE OF THE FORENSIC ANTHROPOLOGIST
The Case for Cooperative Research

Forensic Physical Anthropology? Probably very few people have heard of this scientific specialty. Its major focus is upon the identification of human remains in a legal context. Other specialists in the medical and legal fields are also concerned with identification, but physical anthropologists who specialize in skeletal analysis bring a particular perspective to those instances when identification cannot be made with traditional medical and legal means: fingerprints, dental and medical records, or personal recognition. We have developed special methods, skills, a documented data base, and theoretical orientations for the analysis of human remains.

Once a forensic anthropologist has become involved in the collaborative activities dealing with human remains in a legal setting, our purposes and potential contributions need to be made clear to the cooperating participants. Essentially, the forensic anthropologist provides direct physical or circumstantial information from the human remains to allow the designated authority to determine identity of the deceased and the circumstances of death. Since the anthropologist is a consultant, cooperation with law enforcement personnel—forensic pathologists, coroners or medical examiners, forensic odontologists, attorneys, and judicial officials—is essential. Communication and the establishment of responsibility are important aspects of any given case.

As the case studies in this volume illustrate, forensic physical anthropologists can provide service at the discovery site of human remains, determine if the bones are indeed human or not, provide organizational and analytical expertise at mass disasters involving multiple deaths, help to unravel the intricacies when commingling of multiple remains has occurred, and suggest possible time intervals since death. Burned remains can be especially challenging—even so, the incinerated skeleton may frequently provide clues to identity. Cause of death, although ultimately determined by a physician or the courts, may be suggested by the anthropologist from skeletal analysis. Individual identification of a decedant from the probable match with skeletal attributes such as sex, age at death, ancestry or social attribution of race, probable living height, and unique features of the skeletal structure may be made by the legal authorities. Presentation of findings and opinions as an expert witness in court may also be necessary if litigation is involved.

Anthropology, that branch of science traditionally defined as the study of humans from a holistic perspective, is characterized by the four major subdisciplines that focus on different aspects of the human condition: physical anthropology, archaeology, sociocultural anthropology, and linguistics. Physical anthropologists in general concentrate on the biological aspects of humans that have developed from a long biosocial evolution and the variation seen within our species. Osteologists, specialists in analysis of the skeleton who have further developed their expertise through training, research, and experience to render an expert opinion as to the identifiable characters of human remains, can become qualified by the court as expert witnesses. Although there are no statuatory definitions of forensic physical anthropologists, it should be clear that not all physical anthropologists or even osteologists are qualified to conduct forensic analysis.

Part of the rationale for this volume was to reduce the amount of mutual ignorance among fellow forensic scientists, medicolegal practitioners, law enforcement personnel, academic colleagues, and students concerning forensic anthropology. Although forensic physical anthropology may appear to be a relatively recent academic and forensic field, the application of anthropological data and approaches has deep historical roots as indicated by Stewart (1979). As he and Snow (1982) document, the earlier work often stemmed from forensic medicine, through which we share concerns with medicine, odontology, anatomy, and other biological sciences. Thompson (1982) also documents the role of forensic work within physical anthropology from 1930 to 1980.

The professional recognition of forensic physical anthropology as a specialty in its own right has been enhanced by the organization of those physical anthropologists interested in forensic matters into an established section of the American Academy of Forensic Sciences. Kerley (1978) and Snow (1982) chronicle the development of this group in which almost all of the contributors to this volume are members. Membership criteria incorporate the principles of forensic science and the usual basis for qualification as an "expert" witness in courts: study and practice of the application of science to legal questions through education, training, and experience. The official relations are expanded by the informal personal network and the frequent sharing of unpublished data and ideas, referrals on particular analytical problems, and in many instances cooperative analysis on an individual case. The 1983 membership directory includes 75 individuals ranging from the status of trainee affiliate through fellow. Rhine (this volume) illustrates the geographical distribution of the members in the United States and documents the uneven distribution of forensic anthropologists across the country.

Further credentials as professionals are established through certification by the American Board of Forensic Anthropologists after an arduous written and laboratory examination and review of case reports. The functions of the board include concern with standards of proficiency and training, certification, and circulation of information to potential clients. Approximately 30 individuals in the United States have received board certification.

The concept of a forensic science is also relatively obscure to many people. There are many different definitions and semantic colorings of the term, but the broad and unifying definition proposed by Matte (1970:334), "forensic science is the study and practice of the application of science to the purposes of the law," accommodates the range of activities of most of the forensic sciences. He further argues that as a profession, practitioners of a forensic science should define with scientific and semantic accuracy its data base, its purposes, and its limitations (Matte, 1970:332). These aspects are, of course, interrelated.

The data base for forensic physical anthropology is extremely broad and varied with a range of documented human skeletal collections, the most frequently referenced being the Terry collection originally developed at Washington University and presently housed at the Smithsonian Institution, and the Hamann-Todd collection at the Cleveland Museum. Other museums, medical schools, physical anthropology laboratories, and archaeological facilities have various collections that can be useful for reference in a particular case. Many physical anthropology and anatomy laboratories have as their motto "This is the place where the dead teach the living." The availability of documented skeletal materials is an essential factor in the continued refinement of accuracy in forensic activities as well as academic endeavors. The Physical Anthropology Section of the American Academy of Forensic Sciences is attempting to establish a computerized data base from the documented and positively identified skeletons analyzed by its members. This data base should allow for a continual expansion of information on contemporary populations.

Documentations of the utility and accuracy of various methods of skeletal analysis by osteologists are published regularly in the academic literature through the *American Journal of Physical Anthropology, Human Biology,* the *Journal of Human Evolution, Ossa,* and other professional journals concerned with skeletal biology. Theoretical or methodological approaches developed from analyses of prehistoric populations that may have direct application to a particular forensic case also appear in these sources. Specific references to the systematic compilation of reference data, methods, and results of forensic anthropology have appeared sporadically in the professional anthropological literature. Bass (1969,

1979), Kerley (1978), and Snow (1982) provide excellent surveys of the forensic anthropological literature.

Anthropological findings have been made available to the forensic sciences through articles in the *Journal of Forensic Science*, and more general articles also appear in the *F.B.I. Law Enforcement Bulletin* or other medical and law enforcement publications. Summary chapters of the range of forensic physical anthropological approaches to human identification are also included in some of the standard references in forensic medicine (Stewart, 1976; Kerley, 1973, 1977). Krogman's (1962) well-known text in legal medicine and the human skeleton has been expanded by the publication of works by Stewart (1970, 1979), which focus on American populations, human identification, and forensic physical anthropology.

The general purposes and range of forensic physical anthropology are illustrated by the organization of this volume and the documentation of the particular cases presented. A case study format is something of a novelty. As Stewart notes, individual cases are usually published and available to wider audiences only when they are unusual or involve celebrated characters. The cases presented here, however, were chosen to illustrate a particular aspect within the matrix of the entire identification procedure. The reprint of the early case by Smith is included to illustrate the historical perspective and the range of information to be gained by skeletal analysis.

Since forensic physical anthropology is a relatively newly recognized specialty within the forensic sciences, most of us work as consultants with other agencies in addition to our regular academic duties. Our involvement with a specific case of identification varies with local circumstances, the nature of the case, and as some of the chapters illustrate, the relations of the individual anthropologist with medical examiners, coroners, and law enforcement personnel. Rhine points out that once agencies have seen the results of the work of forensic physical anthropologists and official relationships have been established, the rate of anthropological input may rise dramatically. However, full-time employment as a forensic anthropologist is rare, and most forensic anthropology will probably continue to be conducted on a consultant basis in the near future.

Academic colleagues also are not fully aware of the range of activities in the forensic specialty. Too often they simply assume that a forensic analysis is a methodological matter without academic implications. As almost every case in this collection illustrates, however, a particular analysis is a test of the methods and skills of the analyst, and in many instances the case illustrates the need for additional documentation and stimulates scientific research with new data, improved techniques, and theoretical implications. The recognition of the forensic specialty within academic physical anthropology perhaps is best illustrated by the recent increase in regularly organized sessions of papers at the national meetings of the American Association of Physical Anthropologists. Stewart and Snow have both been "profiled" in the Newsletter of the American Anthropological Association (Profile of an anthropologist, 1979, 1982). The increasing attendance by forensic colleagues at the scientific sessions of the Physical Anthropology Section at the annual meetings of the American Academy of Forensic Sciences also indicates recognition and interest.

Colleagues in medicine and law enforcement should also realize that although forensic anthropologists deal primarily with bones, the range of knowledge and skills may articulate with many other problems dealing with human biology. Snow (1982) argues convincingly for an expansion of physical anthropology into related topics. We should remember, however, that staying within our areas of expertise is critical to the maintenance of credibility and effectiveness as forensic scientists. In some instances, our scientifically derived opinion may not be at the level of certainty hoped for by investigators. Most of our techniques, however, are accurate and valid within the range of certainty usually accepted in medicolegal matters: within reasonable medical certainty (51% and above), clear and convincing (75%), or to the exclusion of any and all reasonable doubt (95%).

Possible ambiguities of forensic anthropological analysis generally stem from the nature of scientific inquiry in the biological sciences and the nature of the data with which we deal. The human species is highly variable, and descriptive norms must take the degree of variability into account. Skeletal analyses by forensic anthropologists generally progress through a series of successively more specific diagnoses. For example, once the determination has been made that bones or other remains are from a human, then more specific determinations as to sex, age, race, etc., can be made. Population variability is recognized, and our findings are given in a range, e.g. age 17 to 22, height 5'3" to 5'6". The ultimate aim, of course, is to establish enough congruities between recovered remains and a decedent to allow "positive" or circumstantial identification.

Successful analysis may also depend upon the nature of the evidence. The information that may be established is generally proportionate to the amount of material available for analysis. When only partial specimens or skeletons are recovered, the task of identification becomes more difficult. Even when complete remains are recovered, no case of identification is really routine. Each individual is unique and, as such, each case has unique aspects. The presentations in this volume indicate some remaining areas of doubt and ambiguity in our methods and theoretical approaches.

As in all fields, diagnostic standards may be refined through additional research. Since many of the methods available to forensic anthropologists originally were developed with archaeological collections, the representativeness of the sample as well as the applicability to modern groups may indicate reservations in general applications. There is a continual need to update standards and reference groups and to refine established techniques with additional findings and often technology. Documentation of the temporal changes in populations must remain an ongoing process for both academic and applied sciences. This will enhance the degree of certainty that must be employed in applying findings from population or group studies to a specific individual in a forensic situation. Kerley (1978) indicates limits of particular methods and needs for research in the forensic field.

A current problem in the forensic application of anthropology appears to be a mutual unfamiliarity with the aims and needs of different specialists in the investigative process. Although well-established relations between agencies and particular anthropologists occur, infrequency of interaction can lead to misunderstanding and the loss of effective communication. Legal agencies may not know exactly what anthropologists can offer, and in return the anthropologist may not know the constraints or procedures of a particular investigator or agency. A successful association generally rests on cooperative good will, an explicit statement of expectations with analytical possibilities, and sufficient time for a systematic, comprehensive analysis of the material. Time and money can also be limitations. Since most anthropologists have regular employment with accompanying commitments and responsibilities, time spent on a forensic consultation can complicate regular duties. Some of the analytical methods also require time for preparation. On the other hand, investigative personnel often need and want answers or opinions in a short time, especially when a homicide is indicated.

The decision to consult a forensic physical anthropologist often depends upon the local coroner or medical examiner. Since a physical anthropologist is a professional, consultation merits recompense for time, supplies, and equipment as well as expert opinion. In some jurisdictions, sufficient funds are available for consultations, but in others, limited resources may tempt a local investigator to attempt analysis personally or to refer the material to the local physician or pathologist who may not have had experience or training with skeletal material. Several of the cases presented subsequently illustrate the unfortunate outcome when this is done.

Training specifically in forensic anthropology is rare in most departments of anthropology, and few of the current professionals received a formal training in this specialty. Expertise and forensic application of osteological findings appear to have developed through individual initiative and experiential learning. Currently, the forensic aspects of physical anthropology are emphasized in some academic departments, but formal degrees and specializations are rare. Brooks (1981) documented the range of course offerings by forensic anthropologists and found that a small number of departments offer courses specifically in forensic anthropology. Many of the courses included laboratory work with skeletal remains. The forensic aspects were occasionally included in a number of other courses. Since that survey, however, a number of individuals have instituted courses at both the graduate and undergraduate levels that examine the range of forensic anthropology rather than aiming at producing new professional forensic anthropologists. The interest in teaching forensic anthropology appears to be expanding with more course offerings and specific considerations given to problems of training and teaching at the undergraduate and graduate levels (Rathbun, 1980; Warren, 1983). Enrollments in forensic courses include majors in anthropology, biology, criminal justice, nursing, pre-medicine and dentistry, and a variety of majors who just have an interest in the topic. Graduate students from related fields appear to benefit from the materials. Forensic anthropologists also regularly participate in workshops, short courses, and seminars in the forensic sciences for medicolegal and law enforcement personnel.

The relative paucity of academic forensic offerings is also reflected by the rarity of textbooks. Krogman's (1962) basic text of skeletal material in forensic medicine was the only acceptable available work in book form until recently. Stewart's (1979) text, which emphasizes essential developments in forensics in the United States, although primarily aimed at advanced students with osteological backgrounds, is widely used. With supplemental materials, the text has also proved appropriate for use in more general undergraduate courses. Experience with students as well as nonprofessionals has indicated that text material, no matter how well based, is best illustrated with particular applications. This volume, with the emphasis on specific cases, originated from student interest and the opportunity to illustrate the involvement of forensic anthropology in the human identification process. The thematic organization suggested to each contributor included the background of the case with the individual anthropologist's circumstances of involvement; documentation of the relevant aspects for analysis; focus on a specific case that illustrates the potential problems, theoretical basis, and typical modes of analysis; and the specific considerations for the case in general as illustrated through the processual analysis. The disposition of the case is another unique feature, since examples in the literature frequently are brief and only part of the process is indicated. The bibliography for each case, in conjunction with reference to Stewart's *Essentials of Forensic Anthropology* (1979), should prove to be a useful guide to those interested in a particular analytical problem, since the typical modes of analysis as well as specialized methods are indicated.

The identification of human remains in a legal context may take many turns. The case studies in this volume document the important role of forensic physical anthropology from the time of discovery through identification and final litigation. In this first section, Stewart reviews the typical reporting of forensic cases, and the historical example by Smith reflects the traditional range of information gleaned from skeletal analysis. Rhine documents the current distribution of forensic physical anthropologists in the United States and the developments when this specialty is systematically included in cooperative forensic analysis.

Section II includes examples of anthropological expertise in determining the circumstances of death. Although individual presentations accentuate particular topics, the various phases of analysis are frequently interrelated. The anthropological perspective and the range of specialized training can be seen in these case studies, which illustrate the exhumation process, distinguishing human remains from other materials, anthropological activities and logistics with multiple individuals from mass disasters, the problems of segregating individuals when body elements from more than one person have been mingled, and estimating time since death. The significance of anthropological analysis in cooperation with other forensic specialists can be seen in the cases dealing with burned remains and establishing cause of death. Cooperative research and analysis is a theme seen in many of the presentations.

The major biological characteristics important in forensic identification are reviewed in Section III. Physical anthropologists have developed a wide range of methods and findings that are applicable to forensic diagnosis of sex, age, stature, and ancestry from human skeletal remains. The individual cases illustrate the application of academic findings to specific forensic situations. The choice of appropriate investigative techniques frequently depends upon the nature, extent, and condition of the skeletal elements. As Buikstra notes in the introduction to the section, case studies are particular examples, and although they include significant coverage of their topics and illustrate professional applications of a range of techniques, supplemental reading and training may be necessary.

In many instances, documentation of the major demographic characteristics of skeletal remains quickly leads to specific identification by the designated legal authority. Section IV provides examples of anthropological research and analysis that make identification possible from specific skeletal attributes or suggest lines of investigation that may lead to positive identification. When traditional fingerprint comparisons or medical and dental records cannot be matched with the deceased, anthropological analysis of the skeletal details or construction of facial features on the deceased's skull may develop enough circumstantial data to allow identification.

In Section V, many of the aspects of a forensic science come together in the crucible of the legal system: the Court. Through involvement in the identification process, the forensic anthropologist may be called upon as an expert witness. As in most of the other examples in this volume, anthropological activities once again occur in a collaborative context. Thorough preparation, anticipation of court procedures, and effective presentation of findings are important issues.

Forensic physical anthropology as both an academic specialty and a forensic science appears to be achieving the respect it deserves. Awareness and interest in our activities will increase in coming years. Cooperative research and integrated investigations in the legal areas will continue as mainstays in the mutual advancement of those concerned with human identification. Since learning is a process, we hope that this sampling of individual case studies by physical anthropologists will provide a base for learning for each other, students, our colleagues in academia and related forensic sciences, and law enforcement personnel.

REFERENCES

Bass, W. M. (1969). Recent developments in the identification of human skeletal material. *American Journal of Physical Anthropology, 30*:459–462.

———(1979). Developments in the identification of human skeletal material (1968–1978). *American Journal of Physical Anthropology, 51*:555–562.

Brooks, S. T. (1981). Teaching of forensic anthropology in the United States. *Journal of Forensic Sciences, 26*(4):627–631.

Kerley, E. R. (1973). Forensic anthropology. In C. H. Wecht (Ed.), *Legal Medicine Annual 1973*. New York: Appleton-Century-Crofts, pp. 161–198.

———(1977). Forensic anthropology. In C. G. Tedeschi, W. G. Eckert, and L. G. Tedeschi (Eds.), *Physical trauma*. Forensic Medicine, vol. II. Philadelphia: W. B. Saunders, pp. 1101–1115.

———(1978). Recent developments in forensic anthropology. *Yearbook of Physical Anthropology, 21*:160–173.

Krogman, W. M. (1962). *The Human Skeleton in Forensic Medicine*. Springfield: Charles C Thomas.

Matte, P. J. (1970). Forensic science: profession or trade? The search for a unifying concept. *Journal of Forensic Science, 15*(3):324–345.

Profile of an anthropologist—T. D. Stewart (1979). *Anthropology Newsletter*, September, 20(7):26.

Profile of an anthropologist: anthropometry, assassination, and aircraft disasters; a career in forensic anthropology (1982). *Anthropology Newsletter*, September, *23* (6):11–12.

Rathbun, T. A. (1980). Forensic Physical Anthropology and the Undergraduate. Paper presented at the 32nd Annual Meeting of the American Academy of Forensic Sciences, Atlanta.

Snow, C. C. (1982). Forensic anthropology. *Annual Review of Anthropology, 11*:97–131.

Stewart, T. D. (1976). Identification by the skeletal structures. In F. E. Camps (Ed.), *Gradwohl's Legal Medicine*, 3rd ed., Bristol, Great Britain: John Wright and Sons, pp. 109–135.

_____ (1979). *Essentials of Forensic Anthropology*. Springfield: Charles C Thomas.

_____ (Ed.) (1970). *Personal Identification in Mass Disasters*. Washington: National Museum of Natural History.

Thompson, D. D. (1982). Forensic anthropology. In F. Spencer (Ed.), *A History of American Physical Anthropology*. New York: Academic Press, pp. 357–369.

Warren, C. P. (1983). Teaching Forensic Anthropology to Advanced Undergraduate and Graduate Students. Paper presented at the 35th Annual Meeting of the American Academy of Forensic Sciences, Cincinnati.

Chapter 1

PERSPECTIVE ON THE REPORTING OF FORENSIC CASES

T. DALE STEWART, M.D.

This book, in which some two dozen forensic anthropology cases are described, each by the principal expert(s) involved in its solution, is a novelty. Forensic cases usually appear in print singly and have traditionally come from forensic pathologists or medical examiners. Although a case study is occasionally sufficiently sensational to run to book length, as, for instance, the Ruxton case in England (Glaister and Brash, 1937), more often each is only unusual enough to warrant a journal article, as for instance the case of J.L. in India (Culbert and Law, 1927).

The case of J.L. is not as well known as the Ruxton case. Briefly, it involved an American man who drowned in India and whose deteriorated remains were identified by his doctors in New York through comparison of a mastoid operation scar on the skull with preoperative x-rays made seven years earlier. The Ruxton case is remembered primarily because the differentiation of the skulls of the two women victims was accomplished by superimposing skull outlines on portraits from life.

The contributing experts here are forensic anthropologists, who specialize in identifying skeletal remains, and are relative newcomers to the forensic field, which adds to the novelty of the book. For the most part they are members of the American Academy of Forensic Sciences and in particular of the Section of Physical Anthropology, which was created in 1972. It was about that time that the expression "forensic anthropology" first came into use in the United States. Although one known earlier reference to it appears in the American literature (Schwidetzy, 1954), the sense in which it was used then was paternity identification, an activity in Europe necessitated by the family disruptions caused by World War II.

The available evidence points to only one other book of first-hand forensic case reports: Sir Sydney Smith's *Mostly Murder* (1960). It differs from the present work in dealing with more than just skeletal remains and in being the product of one person's forensic practice, a practice, incidentally, that extended over some 40 years in Egypt and Scotland. This rarity of published examples suggests how seldom one deals with a case unusual enough to

15

write about. Although Sir Sydney was not a physical anthropologist—in his day (he died in 1969) he was considered one of the foremost authorities in forensic medicine—his publications show him to have been remarkably astute in skeletal identification.

Sir Sydney had a knack for writing up a case in an interesting and informative manner. This appears most clearly in his 13 "Studies in Identification" published in the *Police Journal of London* between 1938 and 1942 (seven of these are included, usually with less detail, in *Mostly Murder*). For the particular audience of that journal he made each "Study" a lesson in some aspect of identification, for which the analysis of the evidence served as an illustrative case. Because it is the teaching value of an unusual case that makes it worth reporting, the writer suggested to the editors of the present book that they reprint No. 3 (1939) of Sir Sydney's "Studies in Identification" as a classic example of this kind of reporting.

Study No. 3 actually includes not one but two cases in which asymmetries in the skulls indicated to Sir Sydney the long-standing presence of wryneck in one and of eye removal in the other. Although the illustrations of the two skulls are not reprinted here, this will not handicap the reader because the anatomical descriptions make the details perfectly clear.

Whatever the means and manner of reporting unusual forensic cases, some of them end up as illustrative cases in textbooks where, in addition to instructing, they sometimes provide an oasis of interest in otherwise dry text. Also, a review of some of the well-known textbooks reveals a tendency to republish some of the good cases. For example, the "Dobkin Baptist Church Cellar" murder case in London after World War II appears in the textbooks of both Sir Sydney (1955) and Keith Simpson (1979).

The Church case got its name because the remains of a woman were found buried in the cellar of a fire-bombed church during demolition. When the skeletal features suggested that she might be the missing wife of Dobkin, the man who served as the church's fire warden during the war, a positive identification was made by her dentist from the teeth in her skull.

On this side of the Atlantic a more remarkable example of reprinting at a far earlier date should be of interest. The Becks' textbook, which by 1860 had gone through 11 editions since 1823 (with one more to come), contains in the 11th edition a section on the skeleton that ends with four illustrative cases (vol. 2, pp. 33ff). According to the Becks' editor, one of these cases was taken from an 1827 issue of the *North American Medical and Surgical Journal*, which had taken it from a British source, which in turn had taken it from a French source. Orfila and Lesueur (1831) had also included it in their book on exhumations.

What made this case so interesting was that the only thing, other than age, known about the homicide victim—a Piedmontese soldier—was that he had a sixth finger on his right hand and a sixth toe on his left foot. A Dr. Delmas, who directed the exhumation and conducted the skeletal examination, found the facets where these extra members articulated, but not the actual phalanges. Nevertheless, his observations led to a confession and a conviction.

While the forensic literature thus bears witness to the frequent use of forensic cases for illustrative purposes and that some of the cases have served this purpose overly long, innumerable other and perhaps more illustrative cases must never have been brought to the attention of general audiences. The validity of the latter statement would seem to be supported by the likelihood that not all of the cases reported in the present book would have appeared in print had it not been for the editors having solicited them.. The Academy of Forensic Sciences served to stimulate these efforts, as it also serves as a forum for the discussion of case histories and analytical procedures. In other words, a case can be made for the reporting of forensic cases being conditioned to a considerable extent by the availability of publishing media occurring in conjunction with circumstances creating interest in the subject.

A familiar set of circumstances that lends support to this generalization is the establishment of the crime laboratory in the FBI headquarters in Washington in 1932 and the creation soon thereafter (1935) of the *FBI Law Enforcement Bulletin*. The former brought the Smithsonian's physical anthropologists into the field of skeletal identification for forensic purposes, and the latter provided a convenient and accommodating publishing medium open to all for reporting unusual cases (for example, Angel, 1974; Cherry and Angel, 1977; Krogman, 1943; Stewart, 1959).

Going back in time once more, it is noteworthy that a set of circumstances somewhat like that of the FBI developed in Massachusetts in 1877. By that year, the coroner system throughout the state had fallen into disrepute, so the legislature passed a law abolishing the office of coroner and replacing it with a system of medical examiners. The latter officials were required to be members of the Massachusetts Medical Society. Also provided for was a category of Associates that, in the beginning, included such knowledgeable and public spirited men as Thomas Dwight and Oliver Wendell Holmes. These groups thereupon organized themselves into a Massachusetts Medico-Legal Society, the *Transactions* of which were intended to publicize the activities of the new system and report advances in the medicolegal field.

One result of this arrangement was that the second volume of the *Transactions* contains two reports of skeletal identifications (Abbott, 1893; Burns, 1897). Abbott's account concerns three cases that shed light on the "time since death." His third is particularly interesting, because it may be the earliest to report the finding of carrion beetles on recently skeletonized human remains. Burns's case, on the other hand, confirmed that Dwight's (1894) method of stature estimation from the skeleton yields reliable results.

These early Massachusetts case reports, taken together with the others here cited and those in the present book, make one thing very clear, namely that human skeletal remains found under circumstances requiring investigation present a great variety of details to challenge the forensic anthropologist's powers of observation and interpretation. It is little wonder, then, that when an especially unusual or complex case yields to the traditional investigative techniques, or to a new approach, and is therefore declared satisfactorily settled, one's inclination, and indeed duty, is to spread the word about what it teaches. Considering the different twists that crime continually takes as a result of cultural and technological changes, forensic anthropologists are not likely soon to run out of unusual cases to report.

REFERENCES

Abbott, S. W. (1893). Identification of the skeletons. *Trans Massachusetts Medico-Legal Soc,* *2(3)*:128–132.

Angel, J. L. (1974). Bones can fool people. *FBI Law Enf Bull, 43(1)*:17–20.

Beck, T. R., and Beck, J. B. (1860). Elements of Medical Jurisprudence, 11th ed. (2 vol.). Revised by C. R. Gilman. Philadelphia, Lippincott.

Burns, R. (1897). Identification of a human skeleton. *Trans Massachusetts Medico-Legal Soc,* *2(7)*:294–298.

Cherry, D. G., and Angel, J. L. (1977). Personality reconstruction from unidentified remains. *FBI Law Enf Bull, 46(8)*:12–15.

Culbert, W. L., and Law, F. M. (1927). Identification by comparison with roentgenograms of nasal accessory sinuses and mastoid processes. *JAMA, 88*:1634–1636.

Dwight, T. (1894). Methods of estimating the height from parts of the skeleton. *Med Rec NY, 46*:293–296.

Glaister, J., and Brash, J. C. (1937). *Medico-Legal Aspects of the Ruxton Case.* Edinburgh, E. & S. Livingstone.

Krogman, W. M. (1943). Role of the physical anthropologist in the identification of human skeletal material. *FBI Law Enf Bull, 12(5)*:12–28.

Orfila, M. J. B., and Lesueur, O. (1831). *Traité des Exhumations Juridiques, et Considerations sur les Changements Physiques que les Cadavres Eprouvent en se Pourrissant dans la Terre, dans l'Eau, dans les Fosses d'Aisance et dans le Fumier* (2 vol.) Paris.

Simpson, K. (1979). *Forensic Medicine,* 8th ed. London, Edward Arnold.

Schwidetzky, I. (1954). Forensic anthropology in Germany. *Hum Biol, 26*:1–20.

Smith, S. (1939). Studies in identification, No. 3. *Police J Lond, 12*:274–285.

Smith, Sir S. (1955). *Forensic Medicine: A Textbook for Students and Practitioners,* 10th ed. London, Churchill.

Smith, Sir S. (1960). *Mostly Murder* (With a Foreword by Earle Stanley Gardner). New York, McKay.

Stewart, T. D. (1959). Bear paw remains closely resemble human bones. *FBI Law Enf Bull, 28(11)*:18–21.

Chapter 2

STUDIES IN IDENTIFICATION, NO. 3*

SIR SYDNEY A. SMITH

It is not generally appreciated how indelibly and in what detail the record of an individual's life may be inscribed in the structure of his skeleton. The sciences of paleontology and anthropology owe their existence to man's ability to interpret form, function and habit of animals, long since dead and vanished, from fragments of their bones. In these sciences the aim has been to reconstruct species rather than individuals. The bones of man, however, may and frequently do bear the impressions of developmental abnormality, deformity, illness or injury in addition to the marks of race, sex and age, and by these peculiarities it is frequently possible to establish the individual identity of a person from an examination of his bones.

The finding of human bones in places other than recognised burial grounds invariably requires that an investigation be undertaken to learn whose bones they were, how the person died and why the body was found in such an unusual place.

One of the first facts to be established in an attempt to identify an individual from an examination of his bones is the length of time that has elapsed since death. The rate at which postmortem changes occur in bones is subject to great variation and differs according to the climate, the accessibility of the body to animals and insects, and the physical and chemical characteristics of its environment. The organic material, including the cartilage of the skeleton, is in ordinary circumstances slowly destroyed after death by the action of bacteria, insects, and drying. In hot climates, particularly if the body has remained on the surface of the ground, as much destruction of organic material can occur in a month as would require many months or even years in a temperate or cool climate. A high acidity of the soil, particularly if there is excessive moisture, is likely to result in rapid solution of even the inorganic elements of bone, so that a skeleton in such an environment may be more completely destroyed in a few years than are the skeletons in Egyptian tombs after many thousands of years. Another indica-

*From Sir Sidney Smith, Studies in identification, no 3, *Police Journal of London, 12:*274–285, 1939. Courtesy of Barry Rose Law Periodicals, Ltd.

tion of the amount of time that has elapsed since death may be gotten from the amount of mineral impregnation of the bones. In moist soils containing iron or copper, bones after many years may become densely impregnated through the salts of those minerals. The net result of these variations is that no sweeping generalisations can be made regarding the postmortem changes in bone, and it is apparent that before any estimate is made, full account must be taken of all environmental characteristics which might affect the rate of postmortem change.

The first part of the actual task of identification, particularly in communities comprising mixed races, is to establish the race of the person whose bones are being examined. The various racial characteristics of human bones constitute a highly specialised field of learning, and space does not permit more than bare mention of the fact that racial skeletal differences do exist. Europeans, Negroes, Mongolians and Egyptians are among the various members of the human family having distinctive skeletal peculiarities, especially in the conformation and proportions of the skull.

The next step in establishing identity is the estimation of the age. Beginning long before birth and continuing until death, the bones undergo continuous changes in form and structure. During periods of active growth these changes tend to occur in an orderly sequence and with such uniformity as to make an accurate estimation of age possible. After full maturity, or more particularly after the age of 25, the changes are apt to be more variable, and estimates of age based upon them are only approximations.

In the beginning, bone is formed in masses of soft tissue, and the time, the sequence and the sites in which bone is first laid down are reasonably constant phenomena. The sites of primary bone formation are called the "centres of ossification," and they continue to appear one after another well into adolescence. A bone does not form from a single centre of ossification but from the union of several different centres. The time and sequence in which these centres unite in the case of various bones provide another remarkably accurate means of estimating age. The final union of centres of ossification goes on until middle life, although in the case of the last few bones to unite there is considerable variation in the age at which union is complete. The eruption of the milk teeth, followed by the permanent teeth, provides additional and fairly reliable means of estimating the age.

The existence of highly characteristic sex differences in the skeletons of mature individuals constitutes another important means of identification. The most striking differences are those present in the pelvic bones, but sex may also be recognised from the skull, the sternum and even from the long bones of the leg and arm. The size of the individual may usually be determined by measurement of the separate long bones.

Having determined the approximate time of death and the race, age, sex and stature, the next step in identification is the recognition of individual peculiarities. In some instances this is possible because of the presence of deformities. Such deformities may represent congenital developmental faults or may have resulted from injury or disease. The acquisition of such information may be valuable not only in establishing positive identification but also in establishing exlusion. A small fragment of the skeleton may permit recognition of the fact that the individual from which it came was suffering from a particularly prominent bunion, and this alone might well be sufficient to exclude certain individuals from further consideration. The finding of evidence from the bones that an individual had a wry neck, a congenital dislocation of the hip or a club foot might be extremely valuable in the establishment of positive identification. Other developmental deformities, including clawfoot, hammer toe, extra fingers or toes, cervical rib, spina bifida, congenital angulation of tibia and so forth, likewise facilitate identification.

Many diseases leave permanent alterations in the form and structure of the skeleton, and identification may be facilitated by their recognition. Some of these diseases are primary affections of bone, whereas in cases of others the change in the bone may be secondary to systemic disease. It might be possible from an examination only of the smallest and most distal bones of the fingers to give an opinion that the deceased had suffered from chronic disease of the lungs or heart over a period of many years. In another instance where only a few of the ribs were available for examination it might be possible to say that the deceased had suffered severely from rickets in childhood. Other diseases likely to leave permanent effects in the form and structure of the skeleton include arthritis, osteomyelitis, tuberculosis, syphilis, tumours, diseases of the ductless glands and paralysis.

Information of the greatest importance regarding the cause and circumstances of death may be available from the examination of the bones. When death has occurred as the result of violence bony structures are frequently injured. Fracture of the hyoid bone is so commonly produced by manual strangulation and result so uncommonly from any other form of violence that its identification is of great importance. In the case of firearm injuries in which the bullet has passed through bone it is possible not only to identify the nature of the injury but also to approximate the calibre of the gun and the direction from which the fatal bullet was fired. Metallic traces left by the bullet in the bone may provide additional important information regarding the type of ammunition used. In the case of head injuries from assault by violence the nature of the weapon and the position of the assailant in relation to the victim may be disclosed.

It may be seen then that bones or even fragments of bone entirely devoid of soft tissue may constitute an important potential source of information in the scientific investigation of crime. The following cases give some indication of the value of such minute examination in personal identification of bones.

CASE A

A skull was found partially buried in the bank of a canal. There was no scalp or hair, no tissues of the face, and no lower jaw. A quantity of whitish, firm substance, identified as adipocere, was adherent to the base of the skull, and embedded in this substance there were four small pieces of bone. There was no history of anybody missing and no hint as to who the person could be, and the skull was sent for examination to see if any information could be elicited which might aid in the search for the missing person. In this, as in all cases, identification of the remains was of primary importance, for until the deceased person is known there is little chance of successfully investigating the case.

The examination was made on the usual lines, first to ascertain the sex, age, race, etc., then any particular features which might lead to identification, the cause of death and the length of time since the death took place.

SEX. The skull presented some difficulty in sexing owing to certain peculiarities which will be described later, but from the sharpness of the orbital margins, the poor development of the supraorbital ridges, the smooth curve at the junction of the nasal bones with the frontal bone of the skull, the shape and size of the palate and upper jaw, from the contours and shape of the forehead and skull generally, it could safely be assumed that it was the skull of a woman.

AGE. The teeth were all fully erupted except the four wisdom teeth, which had not yet made their appearance. The wisdom teeth are usually cut at about 18 years of age, but this is extremely variable, so much so that whereas the presence of wisdom teeth indicates in general an age of at least 17 to 18 years, their absence gives us no definite information about age. The sutures or joints between the individual skull bones were all open, and since a certain degree of obliteration is expected in the period between 30 and 40, we might assume that she was somewhat under that age. The hyoid bone was not ossified in its joints. From the examination of the teeth present, the sutures and articulations of the skull and the hyoid bone, it could be assumed with fair accuracy that she was a woman in the early twenties.

The capacity of the cranium was only 1,260 cubic centimetres, which is much below the average (Microcephalic).

RACE. There were certain racial characters present, and though it could readily be affirmed that the skull was not that of a Negress, the physical deformities to which I shall allude rendered it difficult to make even a guess at the race. The skull was relatively broad and low, and there was no projection of the jaw such as is found in Negroes.

On examining the face it was noticed that the two sides were not symmetrical, the right side being bigger than the left. The right forehead was fuller than the left, which was slightly flattened. The orbits were unequal. The upper jaw, or maxilla, was distinctly larger on the right side and showed the normal moulding under the orbit. The left side was shortened and free from moulding. These differences in size of the two sides gave the face a squintlike appearance which was most characteristic.

When the base of the skull was examined, the lack of symmetry was seen to be more pronounced, and two things at once struck the eye, namely the difference in size of the occipital condyles (the surfaces which form the joint between the neck and skull, and which rest on the spinal column), and the difference in size of the mastoid processes (the conelike processes to which the main rotating muscles of the neck are attached).

The left occipital condyle was much smaller than the right, depressed below the surface of the skull, and its articular surface tilted outwards. The right condyle was larger, raised above the skull surface, and showed an alignment quite different from the left. The mastoid process on the right was much more massive than normal, whereas the left process was poorly developed. The differences between right and left condyles and mastoids are well illustrated when viewed from behind.

These alterations from the normal can be readily explained and are of importance in identification.

The asymmetry of the skull is due to contraction of the left sternomastoid, the principal rotating muscle on the side of the neck, causing the head to be tilted towards the left shoulder and the chin rotated to the right. This must have occurred from a very early age and probably at or about the time of birth. As a result of this maldevelopment and faulty position, certain definite changes in growth of the bones of the head and face occurred. These changes were shown in asymmetry of the two sides of the skull, the evidence of pressure on the left condyle, which caused it to be pressed below the level of the base, and overdevelopment of the mastoid process. From this examination it was possible to decide with certainty that the deceased woman had suffered from wryneck from early infancy.

CAUSE OF DEATH. The fragments of bone embedded in the adipocere were found on examination to be the body and the two horns of the hyoid bone. The horns had not united with the body, and there was a fracture of the right horn. In the fractured ends adipocere had been deposited, showing that the fracture was present before the body or head was buried, and from its presence we may assume that strangulation was the cause of death.

TIME SINCE DEATH. From the extent of adipocere formation it was reasonable to assume that death had occurred at least six months before the body was found and that in the meantime it had been buried in damp conditions.

Conclusions

From the examination of the specimen it could reasonably be assumed (1) that the skull was that of a young woman between 20 and 30 years of age, (2) that she had suffered from birth from a condition of wryneck, causing definite physical peculiarities which must have been well known to all who knew her, (3) that death was due to manual strangulation, and (4) that the body had been buried in damp earth for several months.

As a result of this examination and report, police investigation was properly orientated, and the disappearance of a woman suffering from wryneck from a neighbouring village was ascertained. The husband of the woman was arrested, charged with murder and convicted.

CASE B

A number of bones were found in an uninhabited part of the country. They were sent for examination with a view to identification about which the police had no information. There were no clothes found with the bones. The bones were human and consisted of a skull with lower jaw, the left clavicle, the pelvis including the sacrum, the left humerus, radius and ulna, the left femur, tibia and fibula; that is to say, the head and the left upper and lower limbs with the pelvic girdle. They were in a clean, dry state, and practically free from tissues.

SEX. As I have remarked above, the sex of isolated bones can be estimated with a reasonable approach to accuracy in most cases. In this instance having the skull and pelvis as well as the long bones made the problem relatively easy.

SKULL. The articulations of the nasal bones with the frontal formed a smooth curve; the supraorbital ridges were poorly developed; the forehead was slightly bulged; the base was by no means massive; the mastoid processes were small; the lower jaw was small. The skull was definitely female in all its characters.

PELVIS. The shape of the pelvic bones and the entrance to the true pelvis, the width of the pubic arch (somewhat more than a right angle), the square shape of the pubic bone, the pinched appearance of the junction between the pubic bone and its ramus, the widely open sciatic notch, the presence of a preauricular sulcus, the width of the acetabulum (47 mm.), and the shape of the sacrum were all characteristic of the pelvis of a female.

		Averages	
Femur	Case	Female	Male
Vertical diameter of head	40.5 mm.	40.7 mm.	46.7 mm.
Vertical diameter of neck	29.0 mm.	29.5 mm.	34.3 mm.
Bicondylar width........	67.0 mm.	69.8 mm.	79.4 mm.
Height of external condyle	56.0 mm.	55.1 mm.	61.0 mm.

		Average division between	
Tibia		Males and Females	
Transverse diameter of head	65.0 mm.	71 mm.	
Humerus	Case	Female	Male
Transverse diameter of head	37.2 mm.	37.9 mm.	43.6 mm.
Clavicle			
Length.........	141 mm.	138 mm.	153 mm.

The measurements all showed definite female characters, and we could with a considerable degree of certainty decide that the skeleton was that of a female.

AGE. All epiphyses of the long bones were fused with the shafts, indicating an age of over 20 years. The secondary centres around the crest of the pelvic bones were united to the bone, although there was a line present which was somewhat deceptive. The epiphysis of the collar bone was also united, the two latter indicating an age over 24 years.

The sutures of the skull were beginning to close, suggesting an age between 30 and 40.

The dentition was complete, including the four wisdom teeth.

From the above examination we might assume the person to be middle-aged, certainly over 30 and probably not over 50 years.

STATURE. Femur.......... 41.7 cm.   Humerus........ 28.5 cm.
         Tibia............ 35.0 cm.   Radius.......... 23.6 cm.

On calculating the stature from these measurements, according to Pearson's formula, the mean of the four estimations was found to be 152.75 cm., or about 5 feet 1 inch. From the fact that the figure for each individual bone varied considerably, the average given must be considered liable to error.

RACE. The skull gave the following measurements:

Length.............. 180 mm.
Breadth .... 131 mm.
Height.............. 132 mm.
Basi-Nasal   105 mm.

$$\text{Gnathic Index} \quad \frac{\text{BA}}{\text{BN}} \times 100 = 97$$

Basi-Alveolar   102 mm.
Capacity = 1,150 cc.
Orbit (Right)   Length 35 mm.   Breadth 45.2 mm.
Orbit (Left)   Length 30 mm.   Breadth 43.7 mm.

The nasal bones were not flattened, the nasal orifice was narrow, and there was a well-marked nasal spine. There was no prognathism or jutting forward of the jaw. From the general configuration of the skull, the shape of the nasal bones and palate, and the absence of prognathism we could exclude a Negro origin. Other features, especially the height in its relationship to the breadth, together with the capacity, suggested that it was not of European origin. The gnathic index (97) lay midway between that of Europeans (94.4) and Negroes (104.4). The limb indices were as follows:

Tibio femoral index	$\dfrac{T}{F} \times 100 = 84$	Europeans . . . . below 80 Negroes . . . . over 80
Radio humeral index	$\dfrac{R}{H} \times 100 = 83$	Europeans . . . . below 75 Negroes . . . . over 80

These were peculiar and represented Negroid rather than European characters. There was a squatting facet on the lower end of the tibia suggestive of an Egyptian, Negro, Arab, or similar Eastern origin.

SPECIAL FEATURES. The teeth were covered on the right side both top and bottom with a thick layer of deposited salts. This indicated that the right side had not been used for chewing for a considerable time, no doubt on account of a gumboil or other inflammatory condition of the gum or jaw. An examination showed that the woman had a carious second molar, and this must have caused toothache and pain for a very considerable period. The condition of the teeth also indicated a want of attention to cleanliness. The state of the teeth might be expected to prove of some value in identification.

Examination of the skull disclosed a difference in the appearance of the two eye sockets; the left was smaller than the right in both diameters, and the floor seemed to bulge more inwards, giving a less roomy cavity. The opening for the optic nerve in the left orbit was extremely small, whereas in the right it was of normal size. A gelatine-zinc cast taken from the orbits brings out this difference with considerable clearness, showing not only the diminution in the size of the orbital cavity on the left but also the small size of the optic nerve and lachrymal cavity.

CAUSE OF DEATH. There was no information to be obtained from which the cause of death could be deduced.

TIME SINCE DEATH. The complete destruction of the soft parts of the body and the dry state of the bones left the question of time in a state of uncertainty. In hot climates and especially when the body is left in contact with sand, bones may become clean and dry in a few months and remain in that condition for years. In cold climates such a result could only be obtained after years of burial. When bones in such a condition are found in tropical climates no decision about the time of death can be given except in a general way to indicate that it is likely to have been at least some months before they were found.

From the above examination it could be deduced that the bones were all human and all from one person; that the missing person was a woman who was about 5 feet 1 inch in height, well developed, moderately muscular, and free from any obvious physical disability as far as the limbs were concerned.

She was probably an Egyptian, and her social standing was probably that of the peasant class. She probably had had children. She had been blind in the left eye since early childhood. The eye had either been removed or it had been atrophied since that period. Prior to her disappearance she had suffered for a prolonged period from a painful jaw or toothache on the right side which was almost certain to have been known to her friends owing to its severity. Death had occurred probably at least six months before, but no definite opinion could be given on this point or on the cause of death. Since death the body had been exposed in a warm dry place open to the attack of insects.

The presentation of the report led to the discovery that a one-eyed woman had disappeared from a neighbouring village, and her description accurately fitted that of the above.

She was a woman of 45 years of age, the wife of an agricultural labourer, and was the mother of four children. She had had her left eye removed at the age of four years by a doctor who was still practising in the neighbourhood and knew her well. She had suffered severely with a painful condition of the jaw which prevented her from sleeping. She had disappeared from the village about a year before, and it was decided at the time that she had committed suicide by drowning although the body had never been recovered.

These two cases indicate the necessity of a careful and minute examination of every particle of material in order to assist identification and also the likelihood of obtaining evidence of value even after complete destruction of the soft tissues of the body.

Chapter 3

FORENSIC ANTHROPOLOGY IN NEW MEXICO

J. STANLEY RHINE

THE FORENSIC ANTHROPOLOGIST

Forensic anthropology may be one of the most insufficiently appreciated, underrated, and underutilized of the forensic sciences in the United States. This lamentable situation exists partly because in the 1960s there were only a dozen, and as late as 1974 there were only 17, anthropologists in the United States with interest and experience in forensic science (Eckert, 1974). That is now rapidly changing, with over 40 anthropologists currently prepared to engage in forensic work (AAFS, 1980), including approximately 22 who have been certified by the American Board of Forensic Anthropologists (FSF, 1979) as possessing the expertise and opportunity for forensic work.

To date, there have been no comprehensive surveys of anthropological case loads, but Heglar's (1978) check revealed great variability both in case load and the extent to which forensic anthropologists are integrated into investigative teams. At this time New Mexico appears to be the only state in which a forensic anthropologist is considered an integral part of a forensic team effort that extends statewide.

New Mexico is one of only three (plus the territory of Guam) medicolegal investigative systems in the United States in which full statewide authority is vested (Cleveland et al., 1978). While some counties and some municipalities such as Los Angeles, San Francisco, Dallas, and New York have medicolegal investigative systems, they are empowered to operate only within the immediate area. Nor do all of those municipalities include a forensic anthropologist among their regular consultants. Elsewhere, certification of death and investigation into the nature of deaths are accomplished by local coroners and local law enforcement agencies, based upon local decisions about the circumstances of death. Many of these may make only occasional use of any trained forensic experts, and only rarely do they consider consulting a forensic anthropologist.

The forensic anthropologists are not evenly distributed through the United States (Fig. 3-1). Large sections of the country are without any routine access to forensic anthropological expertise. A third of these anthropologists are found in the more sparsely populated area west of the Mississippi and south of the Platte, while the others are spread through the Midwest and up the eastern seaboard, with a scattering in the Deep South. The Northwest and northern plains are devoid of forensic anthropologists.

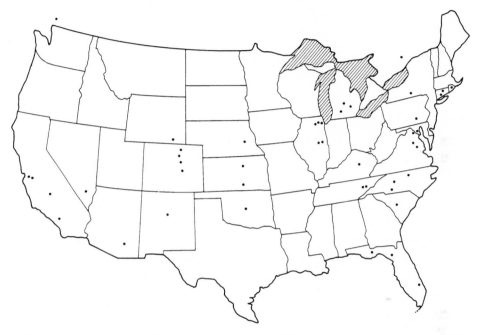

Figure 3-1. Locations of forensic anthropologists as of 1981. (Fellows, members and provisional members of the American Academy of Forensic Sciences.)

In those areas suffering a forensic anthropology vacuum, problems that would typically be addressed by the forensic anthropologist are either assessed by medical investigators, coroners, or law enforcement officials or are regarded as unsolvable. Occasionally they may be sent off to a forensic anthropologist in another state but often may not even be recognized as problems. A common but generally unproductive practice is to refer skeletal material to a physician. This is unsatisfactory, as most physicians, never seeing dried bone, are in a poor position to assess it, a limitation that they may not appreciate. Another fairly common practice has been to seek the opinion of an anthropologist in a local institution of higher learning. Indeed, until about the 1960s, archaeologists and general physical anthropologists would occasionally find themselves attempting to assess skeletal material for a sheriff or police department. In many cases, such unsophisticated handling may be adequate, but there are also many others in which critical information could slip through investigational interstices or would elude the forensically naive eye.

WHY FORENSIC ANTHROPOLOGY?

The perspective and ability of osteologically trained physical (or biological) anthropologists operating as forensic anthropologists enable them to recognize and evaluate the arcane and detailed aspects of skeletal anatomy that would elude experts in other fields. Only in the caricature world of television can one person successfully deal with the mass of data that comprises a number of forensic fields. One fact that is early learned in forensic work is that it is only at some peril that one oversteps the boundary of one's own expertise. The peril here is not only to one's own reputation—and to the field of knowledge that he or she represents—but also to endangering an innocent person's life or freedom.

Of all the scientific specialties extant today, only one deals constantly with dried human bone specimens and their interpretation: osteological anthropology. Decomposed, incinerated, and skeletonized remains readily yield pertinent information to the informed inspection of a person so trained, and the medical examiner who eschews such a consultation deprives himself of potentially important information. Indeed the forensic anthropologist would be prone to feel that the body is only the outward manifestation of the skeleton, a point of view that most forensic scientists would regard as a perversion of reality.

States fortunate enough to harbor a forensic anthropologist within their borders often call for assistance, but without a regularization of consultation procedure. Many crimes are thus left unsolved or unrecognized, and bodies are left unidentified. This is certainly not tantamount to asserting that assigning a forensic anthropologist to a case will guarantee results and that such consultation will solve all problems. Rather, it is to suggest that weaving forensic anthropology into the design of a medicolegal investigative team should reap significant dividends, allowing cross-check and feedback.

NEW MEXICO

The role of forensic anthropology in New Mexico has previously been portrayed by a summary of cases handled during a part of one year (Rhine, 1979). This paper presents a more detailed exposition. New Mexico has incorporated forensic anthropology into its normal investigative methods. Established by law in 1973, the Office of the Medical Investigator works as a branch of the School of Medicine of the University of New Mexico. Conceived by the late Chief Medical Investigator Dr. J. T. Weston as an investigative agency with a large research component, the Medical Investigator has nourished anthropology as an integral part of the operation. The Office not only has made possible training opportunities for fledgling forensic anthropologists but also has encouraged the collection of materials for a forensic collection and a documented skeletal collection as well. Building plans call for the addition of a forensic anthropology lab as part of the facilities.

Table 3-I portrays the cases in which forensic anthropology has played a major role since the inception of the Medical Investigator's Office in New Mexico. The table illustrates a number of phenomena. First, there has been a tendency for an increase in the number of cases handled each year. Apparently as anthropology demonstrates its value, more opportunities are recognized and the case load increases. For the fiscal year 1973–74, the Office of the Medical Investigator in New Mexico reported 2,448 deaths, while for 1979–80, the total was 3,938, an increase of 60.8 percent. In the same period, autopsies increased by 55.8 percent (Office of the Medical Investigator, 1980). The figures from Table 3-I show that between 1974 and 1980, anthropology cases increased by 533 percent. That would mean that there has been an 866 percent increase between 1974 and 1981. This is not a fair comparison, however, since all reports of death must by law emanate from the Medical Investigator. Thus, the reported death figures represent the total number of deaths in New Mexico for those years and are related to the increase in population of the state. On the other hand, cases referred for anthropological analysis depend upon the perspicacity of the investigators and pathologists in recognizing those situations in which anthropology can contribute useful information. A better sense of the increase in anthropology case load in New Mexico can be derived from a "normalization" of figures by comparing the three early years 1974–76 to the three last years, 1979–81. By this method, the increase in anthropology case load amounts to 277.5 percent. Given the sharp upward trend in the last three years, this figure may be on the conservative side.

However one wishes to juggle figures, it is patent that the work of anthropology in New Mexico has increased at a rapid rate, much faster than the rate of increase in death or in autopsies. One might thus conclude that the efficacy of anthropology may be measured by the "excess case load increase" (277% − 60% = 217%). This measure of efficacy would suggest that anthropology has proven its merit in New Mexico. Clearly, however, this rate of increase cannot be sustained. Limitations in time, personnel, and potential case load would set an upper limit well before a projected 240 anthropology cases would be reached by 1990, were future increases to continue at past rates. The figures driving an increase in rates of death are those for increase in state population, while the figures for increase in case

TABLE 3-I
FORENSIC ANTHROPOLOGY CASES IN NEW MEXICO

Material Recovered	1974	1975	1976	1977	1978	1979	1980	1981	Totals	Av/Yr
Fresh Bodies	—	—	—	—	—	—	—	7	7	0.8
"Complete" Skeleton*	1	6	4	1	6	4	1	6	29	3.6
Skeletal Portions	3	2	3	3	—	3	6	1	21	2.6
Skull Only	1	4	—	2	2	3	3	2	17	2.1
Decomposed Body	—	1	5	4	6	4	4	11	35	4.4
Mummified Remains	—	1	—	1	1	5	1	2	11	1.4
Incinerated	—	1	—	1	—	1	9	20	32	4.0
Prehistoric	1	1	2	8	4	5	4	2	27	3.4
Nonhuman	—	3	1	3	1	2	4	1	15	1.8
yearly totals	6	19	15	23	20	27	32	52	194	22.7

*Skeletons in which essentially all portions of the body are represented.

load are driven by the pathologist's perceptions of the worth of anthropological consultations.

The increase is not an isolated circumstance. Data on case loads were also gathered from Walter Birkby at the Arizona State Museum. Adjusted for direct comparison to Table 3-I, these figures show the increase in Arizona to be 297 percent. However, Birkby handles a different mix of cases. He is the forensic anthropologist for a state in which there is no statewide medicolegal system as there is in New Mexico. Many decomposed and "fresh" cases are referred to him by county medical examiners that would be routinely handled by the forensic pathologists in New Mexico. In addition, he consults on types of work not done in New Mexico. This is not uncommon, as many forensic anthropologists have developed specialties for which they are often consulted by agencies outside of the states in which they are located. As a consequence, the actual increase in case load in Arizona forensic anthropology cases is 323 percent (Table 3-II).

Though at least some other forensic anthropologists may be expected to handle a similar total number for a given year, it is unlikely that the same mix of cases would prevail nationwide. A comprehensive case load survey should provide interesting nationwide comparisons. Worthy of contemplation, however, is the sudden increase in forensic cases in both New Mexico and Arizona. The reasons for this increase deserve reflection. Over the years, as Birkby has observed (personal communication) there has been an increase in publicity. The value of forensic anthropology has been successfully conveyed to law enforcement officials and forensic pathologists. This has been enhanced by anthropological participation in the annual Medicolegal Investigation of Death seminar each August in Albuquerque and by similar short courses offered at intervals in both New Mexico and in Arizona. Similar offerings in other states have not always presented anthropology's role as an

TABLE 3-II
FORENSIC ANTHROPOLOGY CASES IN ARIZONA

Material Recovered	1974	1975	1976	1977	1978	1979	1980	1981	Totals	Av/Yr
Fresh	—	1	1	1	4	1	13	15	36	4.5
"Complete" Skeleton*	—	1	3	1	2	5	2	6	20	2.5
Skeletal Portions	1	4	5	7	5	2	5	8	37	4.6
Skull Only	2	3	5	3	3	2	1	6	25	3.1
Decomposed Body	1	4	9	2	12	15	17	15	75	9.4
Mummified	1	—	—	1	2	3	1	3	11	1.4
Incinerated	1	—	—	2	9	13	10	9	44	5.5
Prehistoric	—	—	—	—	—	1	1	—	2	0.25
Nonhuman	—	—	—	—	—	—	—	—	—	—
Photo or x-ray	1	2	1	2	—	1	1	—	8	1.0
Hair Analysis (only)	1	1	3	3	5	3	2	4	22	2.75
yearly totals	8	16	27	22	42	46	53	66	280	35.0

important or an integral one in medicolegal investigations. As noted earlier, though forensic anthropologists have been in short supply, there has been a recent burgeoning in the number of forensic anthropologists. Accompanying this increase in the number of practitioners, one would expect, would be an increase in the total nationwide anthropological case load. As we become more visible, we also become more consulted.

Second, as the tables illustrate, there is a volatility in the relative frequency of the various types of cases dictated by the fortunes of discovery. Judging from this fractiousness, one cannot predict either the case load or the mix of cases from year to year. The discovery of a light plane crash, or the hunter's fortuitous find, cannot be anticipated, and thus, the particular combination of cases varies greatly from year to year. For example, the great leap in the number of incinerated remains in 1980 in New Mexico (Table 1-I) is partly explained by the penitentiary riot, which accounted for 5 cases. The other incineration cases resulted from a car-truck crash and a murder-suicide, a striking example of the shifting fortunes of occurrence. Incidentally, the even more startling leap in 1981 rates may be due, at least in part, to the demonstrated value of anthropological consultation.

Figures from Arizona (see Table 3-II) show the same sort of fluctuation in frequency of cases as noted here for New Mexico, including a similar overall low percentage of mummification cases. One might anticipate that mummification would be more common in the aridity of New Mexico and Arizona, but mummification is a process requiring a rather narrow range of climatological and other conditions (Wells, 1964). The first three categories of skeletonized material vary in a totally unpredictable pattern; however, one might expect that the number of decomposed bodies and incinerated remains would show a tendency to increase, since it is in these areas particularly that anthropology can demonstrate merit unanticipated by law enforcement personnel and pathologists. The figures for New Mexico demonstrate this tendency, but not as clearly as the Arizona data. There, once again, referrals from outside the local area, having produced satisfactory results, are likely to continue to increase as a result of anthropology having provided a useful service.

Third, the arid climate of New Mexico and many other states west of the 20″ isohyet provides unexcelled opportunities for long-term preservation of skeletal remains. But since New Mexico encompasses four physiographic regions, elevations from around 3,000 to over 10,000 above sea level, annual temperature ranges from below − 20°F to well over 100°F, vegetation ranging from coniferous forest to desert grass (Hunt, 1967), annual precipitation ranging from 8″ to 40″ per year, with snow accumulations varying from 2″ to 300″ (Beck & Haase, 1979), local conditions vary greatly. In some areas of the state, preservation of even desiccated soft tissue may extend over many centuries, while in others, less than a decade of exposure will seriously degrade even the skeleton. Hence, conclusions about time since death must be judiciously leavened with information about the source of the remains. Estimates of time since death without accompanying environmental data are thus to be regarded more in the realm of legerdemain than science. Eleven papers presented at the 1978 meeting of the American Academy of Forensic Sciences clearly illustrate the unpredictability of skeletonization rates and point up the need for detailed information about the recovery area (AAFS, 1978). Bass (Chapters 11 & 13) and Sundick (Chapter 29) also document problems of this sort.

Fourth, insofar as even seasoned practitioners of medicine are generally not well equipped to distinguish unerringly between human and nonhuman remains, much nonhuman skeletal material is sent to Albuquerque for identification. We thus tabulate both nonhuman material and human skeletons that, by their antiquity, are beyond the jurisdiction of the Medical Investigator. Strangely, even those who count cattle and sheep as their constant companions are sometimes unable to distinguish between the skeletons of those quadrupedal friends and their bipedal ones. This is particularly the case when fragmentary remains are discovered or when the skull is absent.

INITIATING AN ANTHROPOLOGICAL CONSULTATION

What conditions determine whether a forensic anthropologist should be summoned to examine a given set of remains? It would appear that some jurisdictions, without regular access to a forensic anthropologist, are unaware of the utility of anthropological consultation. Others, though making occasional use of a forensic anthropologist, have not had an opportunity to experience the full range of medicolegal problems that can be addressed in an anthropological context. Medical examiners have been known to proclaim publicly, "I have no need of anthropology," or, "If anthropology is required, I can do it myself." Anthropologists feel keenly that both of these viewpoints bespeak an impoverishment of attitude. Anthropologists feel that their hard-won insights into human skeletal variability are a prized possession, and not one simply to be turned over to anyone with a mere medical school understanding of skeletal biology.

Perhaps one reason for this independent streak on the part of many medical investigators is that many of the basic references in forensic science fail to provide examples of the use of anthropologists. In a survey of some of the basic texts, eight by pathologists include no anthropology at all (e.g. Watanabe, 1968; Curran, 1970), while five contain some anthropology written with the help of an anthropologist or dentist. Of the edited volumes, three contain no anthropology (e.g. Bear, 1973), two include anthropology by a pathologist (e.g. Spitz & Fisher, 1973) one has an anthropology section written by a dentist (Curran et al., 1980), and only three contain anthropology sections written by anthropologists (e.g. Camps, 1968; Tedeschi, Eckert & Tedeschi, 1977). It is a sad commentary on the effectiveness of forensic anthropology that nineteen of twenty-two authors or editors were apparently unable to locate a forensic anthropologist to write an accurate and relevant section.

Perhaps the reluctance to consult a forensic anthropologist lies in our cultural matrix. We are, after all, a nation of dabblers; we are committed do-it-yourselfers. Many pathologists and dentists seem to feel that with a copy of Krogman (1962) and limitless self-confidence, an anthropologist is born. Indeed every large meeting of a group of forensic experts reveals some instance of an expert in another field cheerfully galumphing into anthropological analysis. Not only do they commit significant errors, they seldom know enough to realize it.

There is an allied problem with the legal profession. Most lawyers are in no position to challenge the osteological opinions of the physician-expert impersonating a forensic anthropologist. They, too, are unaware of the value and merits of forensic anthropology as practiced by the informed and experienced osteological anthropologist. In many instances, consultation with a forensic anthropologist would enable a competent attorney to make such a witness decidedly uncomfortable at having overstepped the bounds of his or her expertise. The issue is not really one of comfort or discomfort of the nonanthropologist dealing in anthropology, nor is it one of giving anthropology its "due." The issue is more fundamental than that: that justice truly be served. We increase the probability of correct conclusions being drawn and thus justice being done when we apply the best informed talent to the analysis (Kerley, 1972). Why should we expect physicians or even superbly trained and experienced forensic pathologists and talented dentists to jeopardize their good names and perhaps the future of a defendant as well by testifying to matters with which they are not intimately familiar? This is, of course, a rhetorical flourish . . . we should not. We should not encourage, nor should we condone, this sort of behavior, as it clearly goes against the medicolegal watchword: to venture beyond one's own area of expertise is an action fraught with peril to all concerned and sets a trap that we should all be scrupulously careful to avoid. The reverse also quite clearly applies to anthropologists.

When, then, should a forensic anthropologist be consulted? In those cases where the soft tissue that the forensic pathologist is trained to evaluate is degraded to the point that structures are not clearly recognizable, or where they are missing, there is a clear need for anthropology. The anthropological focus on the skeletal apparatus makes the anthropologist the obvious choice for assessment of those tissues. In the case of mummification or incineration, the soft tissues in most cases will yield insufficient information upon which to draw more than a gossamer conclusion and little upon which to base an identification.

The evaluation of scattered bones or bone fragments is another type of case that cries out for anthropological analysis. Many physicians, having had but a brief encounter with bones early in medical school, are often unable to extract much information from them. Perhaps a classic example is an incident fondly remembered by one of the older faculty members at the University of New Mexico, a cultural anthropologist, who in those long-ago days of General Anthropology also functioned as the department bone man. On that occasion, he was visited by a physician who discovered a "human skeleton" while digging in his backyard. The professor summoned all his considerable dignity to break the news gently that the physician's "human" remains consisted of the south end of a northbound turkey. Often, therefore, the anthropologist may be called upon to answer the most basic of questions: Are these bones human? By replying in the negative, he or she can save a great deal of investigative time as well as remove the potential for future embarrassment (Angel, 1974). Hoffman, in Chapter 7, offers another example of anthropological analysis of nonhuman bone in a forensic setting.

In the case of incinerated remains, the anthropologist, still working in the familiar medium of bones, may be able to restore structures shattered by heat and thus demonstrate features that may lead to the establishment of identity. Bass (Chapters 11 & 13 this volume) and several presentations at the 1982 AAFS meetings document the success of anthropological involvement in such circumstances. Further analysis may also provide data on features that are consistent with ante- or postmortem trauma (Rhine, London and Condon, 1981). Our experience with incinerated remains suggests that Civil Defense agencies and disaster teams should ensure that forensic anthropologists be included in both the recovery phase and in the analysis of remains (Rhine, 1982). This, in turn, requires that anthropologists also be incorporated into the planning for disaster handling to assure that recovery is properly done. Careful and exacting recovery is the key to sophisticated and detailed analysis and identification. The ever-present potential for sudden disaster, such as Colorado's Big Thompson flood (Charney, 1978; Chapter 8) or the prison riots in New Mexico, demonstrates the utility of the inclusion of anthropology in disaster analysis and in instances of multiple deaths.

ANTHROPOLOGICAL ANALYSES

What can the anthropologist do with bones? Besides the determination of sex, age, race, and stature that should be derivable from any reasonably complete specimen (Krogman, 1962; Olivier, 1969; Bass, 1971; Stewart, 1979), the anthropologist may be able to add a host of idiosyncratic details: occupational markings, bone pathologies, malformations, healed fractures, perimortem injuries, cause of death, and many others (see, for example, Brothwell, 1981; Steinbock, 1976). All leave their marks on bone and are lying there waiting to be discovered by the perceptive observer. Numerous examples are included in this volume.

In cases where identity has been tentatively established on the basis of pocket contents or circumstantial evidence, the case for identity may be strengthened by isomorphism between age, sex, stature, and other osteological characteristics derived from skeletal analysis. Forensic odontology also plays a large part in this process, as the peculiarities of dental restorations provide an independent assessment and, in many cases, can be the sole and very powerful basis for establishing a positive ID (Gustafson, 1966; Harvey, 1976).

It has been our experience that a combination of dental and anthropological investigations can be extremely valuable in establishing identity, and the two, working in concert, provide the medical examiner with a degree of certainty that is difficult to match in any other way. In those cases where there is no dental work, or important teeth have been lost (an unfortunately common phenomenon in dried bone cases), an anthropological analysis may be the only way of deriving information about the deceased from the remains.

THE ANTHROPOLOGIST AT THE CRIME SCENE

Ideally, the forensic anthropologist should be called to the scene of discovery of skeletonized, partly skeletonized, or incinerated remains. Police officers, though trained in the recovery of artifacts ("evidence" in the medicolegal context), are not usually experienced in recovery by scientific excavation. As a consequence, even skilled investigators fail to apply the same careful techniques out in the south 40 as they do, say, in the bedroom. Osteological anthropologists have usually had training in the recovery as well as the interpretation of human remains. A prudent policy would be to include an anthropologist wherever there is likelihood of complications in the recovery. Unfortunately, potential complications cannot invariably be anticipated from merely inspecting the area where the body is located.

Practical considerations, such as teaching obligations, may preclude the routine participation of the forensic anthropologist in the recovery of remains. Nonetheless, if sufficient advance notice is provided, most forensic anthropologists can escape the halls of ivy for the necessary time or arrange for a trusted advanced student to participate.

Though Morse and others (Morse et al., 1976; Morse & Daily, 1982) have done excellent work in instructing law enforcement officials in the techniques of skeletal recovery, few officers possess such an advantage. Sophisticated as they are in the recovery and processing of physical evidence, they are quite inexperienced at excavation. It is true that such recovery represents only a small fraction of casework, but it is unfortunate that most of the standard texts do not even allude to the topic. Especially frustrating to the forensic anthropologist is the receipt of a jumbled box of bones curiously lacking in components ("Why is only the 11th thoracic vertebra missing?") and lacking critical information about the context. Exactly where were the remains recovered? What was with them? How were they found? Often these and other critical points of information are missing.

The general feeling seems to be that "bones aren't worth much" and since one cannot get much information from them ("Dead men's bones tell no tales"), it isn't worth spending a lot of time on them. The recovery of a decomposed body can be even more trying. No one, understandably, is anxious to become particularly chummy with a bloated, oozing, and odiferous body. The recovery of incinerated remains is also unpleasant. The complete recovery of any remains, however, and the little osseous scraps surrounding a charred body can yield a boney bonanza to the dedicated forensic anthropologist.

Though such work is, on the surface, a good deal less exciting than gathering up a homicide scene, the ultimate production of data from such cases depends greatly on the recovery having been done thoroughly and correctly. To treat such cases casually is to run the risk of neglecting an important scrap of bone or bit of evidence upon which a case might turn. Many forensic anthropologists have dealt with cases in which a tiny piece of bone, maybe less than 2 inches long, has made the difference between success and failure. For example, in one case, a scrap of anterior tibia showing a healing callus was evidence of a recent fracture. Medical records showed that one of the victims of this airplane crash had fractured his tibia some months before.

LABORATORY ANALYSIS

The standard anthropological analysis may be said to consist of an assessment of bones that are present and an evaluation of those bones in terms of age, sex, race, stature, and idiosyncratic features such as pathologies and anomalies. The ultimate goal is the identification of the remains (Warren, 1978). Individual anthropologists will often indulge their own research interests and specialties in working up a specimen and may even be sent materials from some distance for treatment because of their analytical specialties. Among such special interests are dental aging by tooth sectioning (Maples & Rice, 1979), footprints (Robbins, 1978), aging by counting of osteons in bone thin sections (Kerley, 1965), hair analysis (Birkby, n.d.; see also Bisbing, 1982), and the reproduction of faces on skulls (Snow, Gatliff, & McWilliams, 1970). All of these and many others represent departures from the familiar anthropometric-anthroposcopic skeletal analysis that has been a constant feature of physical anthropology for more than a century. Indeed, with the increase in numbers of physical anthropologists working in forensic anthropology today, there has been a proliferation of research specialties, ranging from reinvestigation of traditional topics to research in topics well beyond the traditional boundaries. Kerley has observed that there are perhaps "a few more research areas than areas of practical expertise" (1978).

CONCLUSIONS

Forensic anthropologists clearly have something to offer in cases where unknown or human or potentially human remains are decomposed, mummified, partly or completely skeletonized, incinerated, or scattered and commingled. The greatest successes for forensic anthropology are in those regions in which there is a specific, regularized means for incorporation of anthropology into the investigative machinery. There are presently no means for objective assessment of anthropological worth, other than citation of specific cases in which anthropology has been of value, or comparison of rates of exploitation of anthropology. The literature abounds with examples of the former, and the earlier part of this chapter presents some data on the latter. Though figures for forensic anthropologists are not available nationwide at this writing, it may be assumed that the case load is tending to increase in those areas in which the utility of forensic anthropology has been demonstrated and a mechanism for their incorporation exists.

REFERENCES

AAFS (1978). Program and Abstracts Book, 30th Annual Meeting, American Academy of Forensic Sciences, Rockville, Maryland.

AAFS (1980) Membership Directory, American Academy of Forensic Sciences, Colorado Springs, Colorado.

Angel, J. Lawrence (1974). *Bones Can Fool People*. FBI Law Enforcement Bulletin, pp. 16–30.

Bass, William (1971). *Human Osteology*, 2nd ed. Missouri Archaeological Society, Columbia.

Bear, Larry Alan (Ed.) (1973). *Law, Medicine, Science and Justice*. Charles C Thomas, Springfield, Illinois.

Beck, Warren A. and Ynez A. Haase (1979). *Historical Atlas of New Mexico*. University of Oklahoma Press, Norman, Oklahoma.

Birkby, W. H. (n.d.) Unpublished case reports.

Bisbing, Richard E. (1982). The forensic identification and association of human hair. In *Forensic Sciences Handbook*, Richard Saferstein (Ed.). Prentice-Hall, Englewood Cliffs, N.J.

Brothwell, Don R. (1981). *Digging Up Bones*, 3rd ed. British Museum (Natural History) London.

Camps, Francis E. (1968). *Gradwohl's Legal Medicine*. John Wright & Sons, Bristol, England.

Charney, Michael (1978). The temporary morgue and the identification of bodies. *The Police Chief*, October, pp. 285–288.

Cleveland, Alan P., Ronald E. Cook, Raymond W. Taylor, Paula R. MacDonald, and Daniel J. Scanlon (1978). *Death Investigation: An Analysis of Laws and Policies of the United States, each State and Jurisdiction*. Department of Health, Education and Welfare (PHS), Publication # (HSA) 78-5252.

Curran, William J. (1970). *Law, Medicine and Forensic Science*, 2nd ed. Little, Brown, Boston.

Curran, William J., A. Louis McGarry, and Charles S. Petty (1980). *Modern Legal Medicine, Psychiatry and Forensic Science*. F. A. Davis Company, Philadelphia.

Eckert, William G. (1974). The forensic sciences—anthropology's role. *INFORM*, Vol. 6, #1, Jan., pp. 3–7.

FSF (1979). *Forensic Sciences Certification Program*. Forensic Sciences Foundation, Inc., Rockville, Maryland.

Gustafson, G. (1966). *Forensic Odontology*. American Elsevier Publishing Company, N.Y.

Harvey, Warren (1976). *Dental Identification for Odontologists*. Henry Kimpton Publishers, London.

Heglar, R. (1978). Presentation at Physical Anthropology Section Meeting, American Academy of Forensic Sciences, St. Louis.

Hunt, Charles B. (1967). *Physiography of the United States*. W. H. Freeman and Company, San Francisco.

Kerley, Ellis R. (1965). The microscopic determination of age in human bone. *American Journal of Physical Anthropology*, Vol. 23, pp. 149–163.

————— (1972). Special observations in skeletal identification. *Journal of Forensic Sciences*, Vol. 17, pp. 349–357.

————— (1978). Recent developments in forensic anthropology. *Yearbook of Physical Anthropology*, Vol. 21, American Association of Physical Anthropology, Washington, D.C.

Krogman, Wilton M. (1962). *The Human Skeleton in Forensic Medicine*. Charles C Thomas, Springfield, Illinois.

Maples, William R. and P. M. Rice (1979). Some difficulties in the Gustafson dental age estimations. *Journal of Forensic Sciences*, Vol. 24 #1, pp. 168–172.

Morse, Dan, James Stoutamire, and Jack Duncan (1976). A unique course in anthropology. *American Journal of Physical Anthropology*, Vol. 45 #3, pp. 743–747.

Morse, Dan and R. C. Dailey (1982) A Florida Story. Paper presented at Annual Meeting of American Academy of Forensic Sciences, Orlando.

Olivier, Georges (1969). *Practical Anthropology*. Translated from the French by M. A. MacConaill. Charles C Thomas, Springfield, Illinois.

Office of the Medical Investigator (1980). Administrative Audit, Sept. 1980. Unpublished Ms. School of Medicine, University of New Mexico, Albuquerque.

Rhine, J. Stanley (1979). Bones in the backyard: Physical anthropology and medicolegal investigation. *Pathologist*, Vol. 33 #6: pp. 300–306.

————— (1982). The Physical Anthropology of Arson and Fire. Paper presented at the Plenary Session, Annual Meeting of American Academy of Forensic Sciences, Orlando.

Rhine, J. Stanley, Marilyn R. London, and Paul Condon (1981). Forensic Anthropology and the New Mexico Penitentiary Riot of 1980. Paper presented at Annual Meeting of American Academy of Forensic Sciences, Los Angeles.

Robbins, Louise M. (1978) The individuality of human footprints. *Journal of Forensic Sciences*, Vol. 23 #4, pp. 778–785.

Snow, Clyde C., Betty Pat Gatliff, and K. R. McWilliams (1970) Reconstruction of facial features from the skull: An evaluation of its usefulness in forensic anthropology. *American Journal of Physical Anthropology*, Vol. 33, pp. 221–227.

Spitz, Werner U. and Russell S. Fisher (1973). *Medicolegal Investigation of Death*. Charles C Thomas, Springfield, Illinois.

Steinbock, R. Ted (1976). *Paleopathological Diagnosis and Interpretation*. Charles C Thomas, Springfield, Illinois.

Stewart, T. Dale (1979). *Essentials of Forensic Anthropology*. Charles C Thomas, Springfield, Illinois.

Tedeschi, C. G., William Eckert, and Luke G. Tedeschi (1977). *Forensic Medicine*, Vol. 11. W. B. Saunders Company, Philadelphia.

Warren, C. P. (1978). Personal identification of human remains: An overview. *Journal of Forensic Sciences*, Vol. 23 #2, pp. 388–395.

Watanabe, Tomio (1968). *Atlas of Legal Medicine*. J. B. Lippincott Company, Philadelphia, Toronto.

Wells, Calvin (1964). *Bones, Bodies and Disease*. Frederick A. Praeger Publishers, New York.

Section II
CIRCUMSTANCES OF DEATH

The case studies in this section illustrate the range of contributions made by forensic physical anthropologists in attempting to establish the circumstances of death. Although the various phases of analysis are frequently interrelated, these presentations provide concrete examples of applications of particular physical anthropological expertise to forensic situations. Establishing the circumstances of death is usually a cooperative task conducted under the direction of a legal or law enforcement agency, and the anthropologist functions as a consultant in the process. As these case studies exemplify, the specific activities required will depend upon the unique aspects of each forensic situation. Forensic physical anthropological expertise that may be relevant to establishing the circumstances of death includes determining if bone is human or not, systematic recovery of all materials during exhumation with archaeological techniques, and estimating time since death for extensively decomposed remains. Dismembered and fragmented human remains from mass disasters and fires can be identified through anthropological analysis, and commingled remains of more than one individual may be segregated by various anthropological methods. Careful examination of the physical evidence may also allow the anthropologist to suggest avenues of investigation to establish cause of death.

Since success of analysis and identification of human remains are often directly proportional to the amount of the skeleton recovered, it is important that a forensic physical anthropologist with archaeological expertise become involved in a case as early as possible. Most physical anthropologists have had training in archaeology as well, and the techniques of this specialty should be a boon to any crime scene investigator in the collection of physical evidence. The investigator and the bio-archaeologist share a common aim. Both attempt systematically to collect and correctly interpret the indicators of past human behavior through physical, circumstantial, and inferred evidence.

In this section, Morse et al. illustrate the basic techniques of archaeology applied to a forensic context. These workers have developed courses and workshops in forensic archaeology for law enforcement personnel. Brooks (1975) and Bass and Birkby (1978) have also published materials on the training process and the importance of careful exhumation. Training manuals for law enforcement, reference books for medicolegal staff, and textbooks for criminal justice classes infrequently, if ever, mention the resources available from archaeologists and physical anthropologists. Levine and co-workers document an unusual application of archaeological and physical anthropological techniques. In both surface and buried contexts, the association of body parts and other materials at the site of discovery may be critical for correct identification and interpretation of the circumstances leading to the deposition of the remains.

Although exhumation is a critical process when criminal activity is suspected, the legal ramifications associated with human remains may also occur when cemeteries are to be disturbed by contemporary construction. In the case presented by Brooks and Brooks, the range of information gleaned from historical and forensic techniques is impressive. Not only are known historical cemeteries subject to purposes of the law, but prehistoric remains must also be identified and processed in a legal context in many states. Rosen (1980) examined some of the legal and ethical problems for this type of exhumation.

Although the services of an archaeologist or an archaeologically trained physical anthropologist are invaluable when buried remains are indicated, they may also provide service when human remains are found on the surface. Snow and Luke, in a later section, illustrate the expertise of the physical anthropologist when the site of discovery is examined. On-site identification of skeletal or body elements, although tentative, may indicate further search to ensure that all parts present are identified and collected before the area is further disturbed by investigative activity. Animal activity, as well as natural forces, can scatter remains over a wide area. In some instances, it might be possible to document the subsequent disturbance of the remains after initial deposition. Careful mapping and photography are essential whenever human remains are encountered.

Hoffman provides an unusual example of the problems of distinguishing human from nonhuman bone. Since few laymen or investigators have detailed anatomical knowledge, determining if a bone is human is frequently requested. In most instances, if the bones are not human, then investigative interest wanes. There are instances, however, where animal bones have been planted to simulate human remains to cover criminal activity. Gross examination of key areas of the skeleton such as skull, teeth, pelvis, limbs, and joints will indicate humanness if the bones are intact. When bones are fragmented, however, identification is more difficult. Cases presented by Kerley, Heglar, and Finnegan provide additional examples of this problem. Radiographic and microscopic examination of specimens may be necessary to evaluate the probability of human status. Serological and protein comparisons might also be valuable if the highly fragmented material retains these structures. Hoffman's bibliography includes the standard references for skeletal comparisons with common species of animals in North America. Direct comparison of the unidentified specimen with a documented animal skeletal collection can also lead to identification. Many universities and museums have zoologists who will cooperate in identification of the specific species. In addition, many forensic anthropologists have developed reference collections in their own physical anthropology laboratories.

Mass disasters with multiple deaths pose significant problems for law enforcement, civil defense, and the military. Charney and Wilber document the contributions made by forensic physical anthropologists in a civilian disaster. Organization and logistics, as well as identification skills, were extremely important. State and national agencies concerned with civil defense and disaster management thus benefit from consultation with forensic physical anthropologists in contingency planning. Identification of multiple individuals in a crisis situation, especially when the remains are fragmented or highly decomposed, necessitates cooperative work from a number of professionals, especially pathologists, odontologists, and anthropologists. Some anthropologists have worked with the Federal Aviation Administration and other mass transportation agencies when disasters have occurred. Commingling of disarticulated parts in such situations is a special problem. Warren and Buikstra and co-workers in this volume discuss procedures and approaches with commingled remains.

Physical anthropology has had a long-standing relationship with the military. Many significant advances in anthropological methodology resulted from efforts to identify casualties from World War II and the Korean conflict. Snow (1982), Stewart (1979), Kerley (1978), Thompson (1982) and Snow (1948) discussed many of the relevant findings. Of special importance was the opportunity to verify and revise earlier standards that were developed from prehistoric and historic materials or dissecting room specimens. Estimation of adult stature (Trotter and Gleser, 1952, 1958) and documentation of age changes (McKern and Stewart, 1957) for modern, well-nourished young Americans were especially significant. Several senior contributors to this volume participated in the military efforts to identify casualties.

Warren provides a first-hand account of the field and laboratory problems encountered in identification during the recent conflict in Southeast Asia. Again, organization and planning before a crisis situation appear as significant elements in successful identification of multiple individuals. Warren shows that the chain of possession, as well as maintaining associated materials for identification, is an important consideration in any identification attempt. Warren and also Rhine indicate the need to convince investigation agencies, both military and civilian, of the importance of systematic evaluation of *all* materials. Commingling and even circumstantial means of identification through clothing or identity cards is easier to unravel if all materials are kept together with the skeleton. Cooperation and overt statements of the needs of all personnel involved should be worked out in the planning stage and not situationally determined.

Disasters are not the only instance when commingling of body parts of more than one individual is a problem in the identification process. Criminal dismemberment of body parts may also be a problem requiring anthropological analysis. Although a number of methods have been applied to problems of commingling and are reviewed by Stewart (1979), matching body parts to establish individual integrity is probably the most widely used method. As Buikstra et al. indicate, evaluating anatomical congruity may be a matter of judgement and experience of the scientist. This case, which incorporates both historical and contemporary perspectives, illustrates the importance of continued refinement of methods and expanded data bases to improve the degree of certainty for conclusions. Their work serves as another example of a particular forensic problem stimulating further scientific research that may have wider applications. Metric and statistical analyses developed in this case promise to advance anthropological efforts in this area.

Changes in soft tissue and body organs after death are frequently used by pathologists and other medicolegal investigators to determine time since death. Natural decomposition rates, however, vary considerably with local environmental circumstances. Most forensic pathology and forensic medicine texts review the major changes used in evaluation; see for example Snyder (1977), Gresham (1975), Camps (1968), and Spitz and Fisher (1980). Anthropologists are often asked to estimate time since death when decomposition is advanced or the remains are skeletonized. Important considerations are odor, feel, degree of ligament and tissue decomposition, presence of adipocere, insects, and other postmortem alterations. The case presented by Bass with the combination of historical and contemporary factors illustrates the importance of approaching each situation with no prior assumptions and considering all possibilities. In addition, this unusual case illustrates that initial conclusions may be revised as more information becomes available and the investigator has had a chance to reflect upon the findings. Although there are regularities in analysis, each case is unique and we, as scientists, must base our probabilistic conclusions on documented data bases.

Since local conditions vary so widely, uniform rates of decomposition are extremely difficult to establish. Morse et al. (1983) have attempted to document alterations of various materials in a range of contexts, and Warren (1980) examined the role of plant activity in the decomposition process. Many logistical problems must be faced in the systematic collection of decomposition data with human remains. Not only are legal aspects involved, but individual sensibilities may be also. Bass indicates the relative paucity of data on verifiable indicators of intervals between death and discovery. Initial steps have been taken under Bass's direction to provide such a base through systematic observation of the decay process and the activity of carrion insects (Rodriquez, 1982; Rodriquez and Bass, 1983). This is another instance when analytical problems in a forensic situation led to further scientific research and academic findings.

Alteration of human remains by fire can be extreme. Not only are soft parts transformed and frequently unidentifiable, but the heat may shrink, distort, fragment, and disassociate the bones as well. Forensic physical anthropologists can contribute to identification of victims of accidental burning, criminal activity, and in some instances even commercial cremations. The second case presented by Bass and the one by Heglar illustrate the importance of systematic collection of all materials at the scene of the fire and the applicability of archaeological techniques. The evaluation of circumstantial materials at the fire scene and the associations or absence of physical evidence need to be evaluated. Bass also provides references for empirical research with bone burned in a number of contexts. Both cases illustrate the importance of cooperative analysis among the forensic specialists. Anthropologists' expertise with bone, especially fragments, was critical in leading to the successful solution of the case. Commingling and individual identification are special problems when bones are fragmented in fires. Heglar nicely illustrates the importance of multicomponent investigation and the range of anthropological techniques that can be applied in a particular situation. The innovative use of radiology in his case is particularly illustrative. Suchey (in Chapter 20) documents other techniques for establishing age at death that may be used with burned remains.

The role of the forensic physical anthropologist in helping to establish manner and cause of death is usually subsidiary to the medical experts. In most jurisdictions, a physician must sign the death certificate and attest to the medical cause of death. Coroners, in some areas, are charged with establishing the manner, mode, and cause of death in any unattended death. They usually rely on the services of a physician, but in some cases a coroner's jury may be asked to determine if criminal activity is probable and should be investigated further. Sauer, besides illustrating skeletal evidence for blunt and sharp instrument wounds, argues that manner and cause of death should be distinguished. In most instances, the anthropologist can suggest lines of investigation to a pathologist or a physician for the final determination of cause of death. Establishment of the manner of death may eventually have to be determined by a coroner's or court trial. Again, the anthropologist may suggest probable events using physical evidence from the remains.

The case presented by Angel and Caldwell is an excellent example of the importance of extensive experience with human remains to be able to determine probable causes of death. Angel's wide experience and examination of thousands of skeletons served well to establish his competence as an expert witness on cause of death, even after initial objections by an attorney that only a physician may be qualified to determine cause of death. The ability to distinguish between fractures around the time of death from those with dried bone some time after death is an important aspect. Angel's final admonition, however, should be remembered: We must stay within our own areas of expertise. This is an important point to maintain credibility. Direct experience and detailed knowledge of anatomy with fractures were keys in the successful presentation of findings in court. As more anthropologists are qualified as expert witnesses, the hesitancy of accepting this sort of scientific testimony should diminish. Care must be taken, however, to distinguish among opinion, scientifically verified data, and circumstantial or inferred probabilities.

Many events can lead to a person's death, and the cause of death may not be readily apparent if the remains are decomposed or if the lethal event did not affect the skeleton. Trauma, either criminal or accidental in origin, can, however, be indicated by careful examination of the skeleton. Care must be taken to evaluate breaks and other alterations that could have occurred after death. Postmortem breaks of bones, especially if they have been exposed to the elements and animal activity, can be extensive, but they are relatively easy to distinguish from perimortem changes. Examination of coloration and the nature of the break or lesion may indicate when the trauma occurred.

Sauer includes a list of protocol that should be followed when suspected lesions are discovered. Coordination of the examination with a pathologist, especially one trained in the forensic aspects, is recommended. Differential diagnosis of potentially lethal lesions from animal toothmarks and other postmortem alteration of the skeletal remains is essential. The anthropologist's attempt to document criminal activity through reconstruction of probable lethal events affecting the skeleton should be integrated with efforts of others in the investigative context. Careful presentations of findings through both the written report and oral court testimony will enhance the acceptance of the conclusions.

Snyder et al. document the importance of a coordinated effort in unraveling the course of events to determine manner as well as cause of death. Few forensic anthropologists have the experience and expertise for this sort of analysis. Snyder, with training in physical anthropology as well as experience in aviation, was especially qualified to document the events described and to coordinate the analysis. This case also illustrates the importance of proper photography and documentation of the entire area with related materials. Associations of physical and circumstantial evidence were critical to the successful reconstruction of the results of this accident. This case illuminates the potential role of anthropological expertise in analysis of situations beyond skeletal identification. Forensic implications involved with product liability and civil litigation, as well as criminal litigation, benefit from coordinated multidisciplinary efforts. The application of anatomical knowledge to particular events in wider contexts appears to be an area for forensic anthropological expansion.

As the following case studies illustrate, the activities of physical anthropologists vary widely with individual forensic situations and significantly contribute to establishing the circumstances of death. A number of osteological methods developed through academic research and experience have direct application in the legal setting. Even though many of these standard methods are creatively applied to particular cases, specific problems in forensic analysis have spurred expanded research and refinement of technique. As more of our colleagues in the other forensic sciences and law enforcement have the opportunity to collaborate successfully with anthropologists, recognition of the relevancy of our expertise increases. The following examples reflect the importance of our specialized analytical skills and experience in integrated investigations concerning the circumstances of death.

REFERENCES

Bass, W. M. and Birkby, W. H. (1978). Exhumation: the method could make the difference. *FBI Law Enforcement Bulletin,* 47:6–11.

Brooks, S. T. (1975). Human or not? A problem in skeletal identification. *Journal of Forensic Sciences,* 20(1):149–153.

Camps, F. E. (Ed.) (1968). *Gradwohl's Legal Medicine.* Bristol: Wright.

Gresham, G. A. (1975). *Color Atlas of Forensic Pathology.* Chicago: Year Book Medical Publishers, Inc.

Kerley, E. R. (1978). Recent developments in forensic anthropology. *Yearbook of Physical Anthropology,* 21:160–173.

McKern, T. W. and Stewart, T. D. (1957). Skeletal Age Changes in Young American Males. Tech. Rep. EP-45. Natick, Mass: Environ. Port. Div., US Army Quartermaster Res. Dev. Ctr.

Morse, D., Duncan, J. and Stoutamire, J. (Eds.) (1983). *Handbook of Forensic Archaeology and Anthropology.* Published by the editors, distributed by Bills' Book Store, Tallahassee, Florida.

Rodriquez, W. C. (1982) "Insect Activity and Its Relationship to Decay Rates of Human

Cadavers in East Tennessee." Master's thesis, University of Tennessee: Knoxville.

Rodriquez, W. C. and Bass, W. M. (1983). Determination of time of Death by Means of Carrion Insects. Paper presented at 35th Annual Meeting of the American Academy of Forensic Sciences, Cincinnati. Typescript on file at Department of Anthropology, University of Tennessee, Knoxville.

Rosen, L. (1980). The Excavation of American Indian burial sites: a problem in law and professional responsibility. *American Anthropologist, 82(1):5–27.*

Snow, C. C. (1982). Forensic anthropology. *Annual Review of Anthropology, 11:97–131.*

Snow, C. E. (1948). The identification of the unknown war dead. *American Journal of Physical Anthropology,* 6:323–328.

Snyder, L. (1977). *Homicide Investigation,* 3rd ed. Springfield: Thomas.

Spitz, W. U. and Fisher, R. S. (Eds.) (1980). *Medicolegal Investigation of Death.* Springfield: Thomas.

Stewart, T. D. (1979) *Essentials of Forensic Anthropology.* Springfield: Thomas.

Thompson, D. D. (1982) Forensic Anthropology. In F. Spencer (Ed): *A History of American Physical Anthropology.* New York: Academic Press, pp. 357–369.

Trotter, M. and Gleser, G. C. (1952). Estimation of stature of American whites and Negroes. *American Journal of Physical Anthropology,* 10:463–514.

_____ (1958). A re-evaluation of estimation of stature based on measurements of stature taken during life and of long bones after death. *American Journal of Physical Anthropology, 16:79–123.*

Warren, C. P. (1980). Plants and Related Decomposition Vectors of Human Skeletal Remains. Abstract, Program American Academy of Forensic Sciences, 32nd Annual Meeting, New Orleans.

Chapter 4

FORENSIC ARCHAEOLOGY

DAN MORSE, R. C. DAILEY, JAMES STOUTAMIRE, AND JACK DUNCAN

Forensic archaeology is simply the application of standard archaeological techniques slightly modified to meet the requirements of crime scene processing where a skeleton(s) or a buried body(ies) is present (Morse et al., 1976). The use of archaeological techniques in processing crime scenes is a rather recent development and has emerged with the realization that, in many instances, significant evidence has been inadvertently overlooked or lost where inaccurate and unsystematic methods of collecting and processing human remains and associated evidence were used. It is still the case that many surface skeletons are collected with a garden rake and buried bodies with a backhoe. The purpose of this chapter is to describe the kinds of modified archaeological techniques that we have used successfully and that we would recommend to be used when a crime scene is processed. If these techniques and procedures described herein are used, the following results can be obtained:

1. greater accuracy in evidence collection
2. increased probability of collecting all physical evidence
3. recovery of the maximum amount of skeletal remains
4. prevention of postmortem damage to the remains

The basic required equipment in a typical tool kit to process a crime scene is similar to that used by archaeologists in small-scale excavations and should include the following:

1. Masons pointed and square trowels — 4.5– or 5-inch size.
2. Pruning shears and saws.
3. Wooden and metal stakes.
4. Small shovels such as entrenching tools. These can be used for collecting dirt after it has been visually searched. They should not be used for digging except for skimming thin slices of dirt to produce a horizontal profile.
5. Visual markers such as thin metal pins for use in photographs and thin wooden sticks with one end painted red to mark positive metal detector readings.

6. Five gallon plastic buckets for the transportation of excavated soil.
7. Plastic (not metal) screens—⅛-inch mesh or smaller.
8. Paint brushes—½– to 4-inch width
9. Wooden digging implements such as shaped bamboo sticks.
10. Containers, including paper with plastic bags, cardboard boxes, and plastic bottles with cotton padding.
11. Mapping equipment, including compass, tape measure (inches or 10ths of feet), line level, transit or farmer's level with stadia rod (if possible), graph paper, and protractor. Feet are used as the measurement system as this remains the simplest system to present in the average courtroom situation.
12. Notebook with pens and pencils.
13. String, twine and/or surveyor's tape.
14. Cameras; 2¼″ format is preferable, but 35mm is acceptable (photographs should be taken in black and white and color if possible), a small slate board with chalk for an inphotograph label, and an arrow with a scale in inches or tenths of feet painted on it. This can be used as a scale and/or a north marker.
15. A metal detector sensitive enough to penetrate several inches of soil.
16. Evidence tape for sealing of evidence containers (Note—this is a special crime scene processing tape.)

Surface bodies

Should a skeleton be located on the surface, the first priority is to establish security. This is done by roping off the area, establishing checkpoints for entrance and exit, and restricting access to authorized persons only. This is the responsibility of the person in charge of the crime scene. The general area should then be photographed prior to searching. Following this, the limits of the crime scene must be determined. This includes locating the original position of the body and all associated evidence by a controlled and patterned visual search. Concentrations of clothing or a number of bones (commonly vertebrae) in or close to their normal anatomical position will help to establish the original location of the body. All bones and evidence should be flagged during the search to prevent them from being stepped on by other searchers. It should be noted that the total crime scene may be larger than the immediate vicinity of the body, making it necessary to avoid concentrating on the body and overlooking other evidence in the search.

The next step is to clear the vegetation from around the remains and any associated evidence to provide working space. Before cutting with shears or saw, get a clear view and be sure no evidence is damaged. Cut all vegetation, except trees, to within ½ inch to ¾ inch of surface, unless it will result in movement of evidence. All vegetation that has been cut should be collected, carefully placed in a suitable receptacle, removed from the cleared area, and examined to determine if the cuttings contain any concealed evidence. The site selected for this should be some distance from the scene and free of any items that might be confused with evidence.

After clearing, it is necessary to set up a grid to include most of the bones and physical evidence. Usually a 10 or 12 feet square unit is sufficient. If scattering is severe, a larger grid or several smaller grids separated from each other may be necessary. The sides of the grid should be oriented as nearly north/south and east/west as practical. A wood or metal stake should be placed at each corner and connected by twine or ribbon (colored ribbon will show up best in photographs). To get a perfect square or rectangle the formula $X = \sqrt{A^2 + B^2}$ is used, where A and B are the sides of the grid and X is the diagonal (in a 10×10 foot grid, $X = 14'\ 1\ \frac{3}{4}''$ and in a 12×12 foot $X = 16'\ 11\ \frac{3}{4}''$).

A *datum point* (permanent mark to which all measurements are tied) should be established so that one can relocate the grid should reinvestigation be necessary. This may be done by measuring distances and angles, relative to magnetic north, to a permanent mark, such as the corner of a building, from two corners of the grid. A second method is to measure distances and angles from a permanent mark to two corners of the grid. A third method is to permanently mark the grid using a $\frac{3}{4}$-inch galvanized water pipe driven 18 inches into the ground at the corners. Later the pipe can be relocated by bearings from a permanent structure and then precisely located with a metal detector. If one has exactly located the grid relative to magnetic north (example: the grid is 5° 15′ east of north on the axis) and recorded that information, then the grid's permanent location may be recorded using one corner only, as the others may be reset by triangulation.

Upon completion of these operations, use a metal detector freely within and outside the grid. All positive recordings should be marked with a wooden stick. If metal corner stakes or other markers are used, the preliminary metal detector survey should be done prior to their placement. Then photograph the entire cleared area using a scale, arrow pointing north, and providing a caption on the slate. Use a ladder or scaffolding if possible. To provide a map, take grid coordinates (measurements from the sides of the grid) of all exposed objects, recording and describing them in detail (example: shotgun casing, red color with brass head, 12-gauge—located 2′4″ north and 5′ east of southwest corner) and locating them on a rough scale map.

Before removing any piece of physical evidence, a close-up photograph should be made, including caption, scale, and north arrow. After the photography is completed, all remains and physical evidence must be removed. During removal of the skeleton, the bones recovered should be checked off on a list of skeletal elements and bagged in units such as left hand and left ribs. Each item should be bagged and the bag labeled as to its evidence number, contents, location, initials of collector, and date of collection. A trained and experienced crime scene investigator should supervise the removal, packaging, sealing, and transportation of all physical evidence to the laboratory. Positive metal detector readings should be excavated using tools and methods discussed below.

Any physical evidence or skeletal remains lying outside the grid should be photographed separately and indicated on the final sketch by triangulation or by recording the direction in degrees and the distance in feet from any of the four corner stakes.

After all evidence is removed, the surface dirt within the grid should be screened, using water pressure and plastic screen. Also, dirt at a depth of 4 to 6 inches under the original position of the body should be passed through a screen.

Buried Remains

In the event that a body is buried, the grave can be located by the use of standard search techniques such as visual observation and the cautious use of a steel probe. The probe is used only to determine the difference in the softness of the soil and to outline the boundaries of the grave, starting from the outside. Never use the probe to locate the body, since the probe can produce postmortem bone damage. The limits of the crime scene are then determined, and the area is treated as noted above, including the following:

1. Photograph the scene.
2. Clear the scene of vegetation.
3. Grid the area and establish datum point.
4. Locate and map all surface evidence and the grave boundaries.
5. Recover and photograph all surface evidence.
6. Search the grave area with a metal detector.

The datum point established in this situation must also include some method of measuring elevation, as the vertical position of the evidence in the grave is important to interpretation. If a transit or farmer's level and stadia rod are available, they should be used to measure depth, and a permanent mark should be made at the level of the instrument plane on the item used to locate the grid (nail in a telephone pole or tree or mark on a building corner). If these instruments are not available, the depth below ground surface can be measured using string and a line level or a board and a carpenter's level.

The grave is then excavated using trowels, paint brushes, pointed sticks, the hands, etc., in 2 to 4 inch levels. The exact levels depend on the strength of the available metal detector. All dirt removed is screened using water pressure and plastic screens as a backup, since it is desirable to locate and leave all physical evidence in place. A metal detector is passed over the grave before each new level is started, and all positive readings are marked. Areas with a positive reading should be screened separately. Use only wooden tools in the area of metal readings to avoid damage to such things as rifling marks on bullets.

When any part of the remains is exposed, digging should be done with soft tools only. If the grave is deeper than about 8 inches, one wall may be sacrificed so that the excavators will be able to work in a more comfortable position. It is unnecessary to screen the dirt removed from the wall. All bits of evidence should be recorded, located on the grid, mapped, and photographed before being moved. Where soft tissues adhere to the remains, they should be removed as intact as possible by undercutting and placing a board or blanket underneath. The body should then be examined by a forensic pathologist.

The excavator should have some knowledge of osteology so that an inventory of the bones may be kept while the skeleton is being removed. The bones of each hand and foot should be packaged separately and labeled. The ribs should be marked with a soft pencil while being removed: 1, 2, 3, 4, etc. As far as possible, elements of the right side of the body should be packaged separately from those from the left and labeled.

After all remains are removed, a soil sample should be taken. Finally, dirt from the bottom of the grave should be removed to a depth of 4 to 6 inches and screened after survey with a metal detector.

It should be remembered that death investigation is a matter of teamwork. The crime scene investigator is trained in methods of collecting, packaging, and transporting various kinds of evidence, including the body. The forensic pathologist has the obligation to determine the cause and manner of death. The forensic anthropologist has the responsibility to reconstruct the individual from the skeleton. These experts and others should work together as a team and should be aware of the capabilities of other members of the team.

CASE NUMBER ONE

Early in 1977 an informant directed investigators to some skeletal remains adjacent to a wayside station near a main highway in northern Florida. The area was secured, and a team of crime investigators and anthropologists, under the direction of the Florida Department of Law Enforcement, processed the death scene (Fig. 4-1).

Investigation revealed that, according to a witness, the victim was shot in the lower chest from above while on his knees and that the event occurred

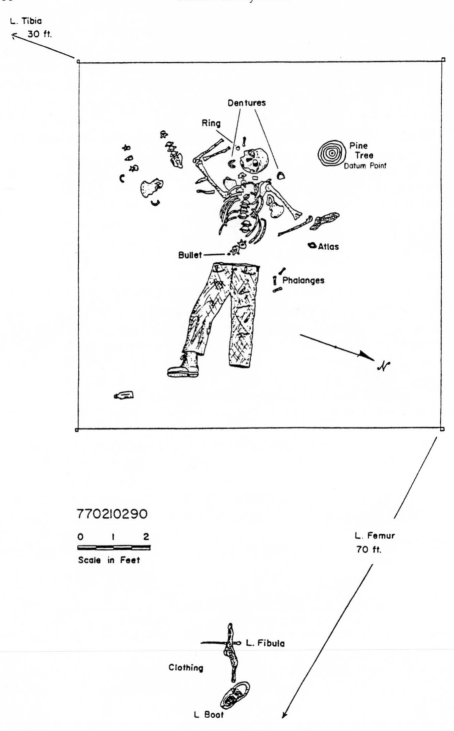

770210290

Scale in Feet

Figure 4-1.

about seven months prior to discovery of the remains.

Most of the skeleton was covered with vegetation, debris, and sand as a result of repeated rainfall. The area was cleared, mapped, and photographed, and a 10-foot-square grid was established. All physical evidence, consisting of a .38 calibre fired bullet, clothing, shoes, dentures, and a ring, was removed to the Florida Department of Law Enforcement Regional Crime Laboratory in Tallahassee; the skeleton was sent to the Department of Anthropology at Florida State University for examination.

All bones were recovered except the lower jaw, the hyoid, and some carpals and hand phalanges. All foot bones were recovered because they were still inside the socks. Most of the bones showed evidence of being gnawed by animals.

Examination

General:	All bones were of good density, indicating probable good health at the time of death.
Sex:	*Male*
Age:	36 to 39 years of age
Race:	Caucasoid
Stature:	5' 8½"
Pathology:	1. Healed overriding fracture of right humerous
	2. Nondeforming healed fracture of right clavicle
	3. Antemortem loss of all maxillary teeth. Since both upper and lower dentures were recovered, the diagnosis of acquired edentia was made.
	4. Slight lipping of lumbar vertebrae, indicative of mild osteoarthritis.

Significant Anomalies

1. The seventh cervical vertebra has a rudimentary rib on the right.
2. The right mastoid process is double the size of the left.
3. There is a double bilateral supra-orbital foramen.
4. There are multiple wormian bones along the lambdoidal suture.

Victim Identification

The suspected victim was a thirty-eight-year-old male, Caucasoid, 5 feet 8 inches in height, with a full set of dentures. Several months before his disappearance, a small chip broke off the upper denture, which his wife saved. There was a perfect fracture match of the broken piece with the broken upper denture recovered at the death scene.

The suspected victim had been in an auto accident several years previously. Though the x-rays of the injury had been discarded, his medical record described a severe fracture of the right upper arm. Chest and abdominal x-rays had also been taken one year before the suspected victim disappeared. These revealed a rudimentary cervical rib on the right and lipping of the lumbar vertebrae, which matched the postmortem films of the skeleton. The recovered U.S. Army ring was identified as belonging to the suspected victim. When he acquired the ring it was too large, so a fit was achieved by pounding it with a hammer.

Based on these data, the identity of the skeleton was considered to be that of the suspected victim.

Cause of Death

A fired bullet was located with the metal detector and recovered 3 inches below the surface of the ground where the upper abdominal region would have been. This confirmed the testimony of the witness, who stated that the victim was shot in the chest from above while kneeling.

Disposition

Suspects were charged, convicted, and sentenced.

CASE NUMBER TWO

Circumstances of the find

Investigation by the sheriff's department of a northeastern county in Florida revealed that a young woman gave birth to a baby in her parents' home. An eyewitness saw her bury the infant in a shallow grave and later rebury it nearby. No physician was in attendance at the time of the delivery.

At the request of the sheriff, a team of anthropologists and crime scene specialists from the Tallahassee Regional Crime Laboratory of the Florida Department of Law Enforcement and Florida State University processed the scene (Fig 4-2).

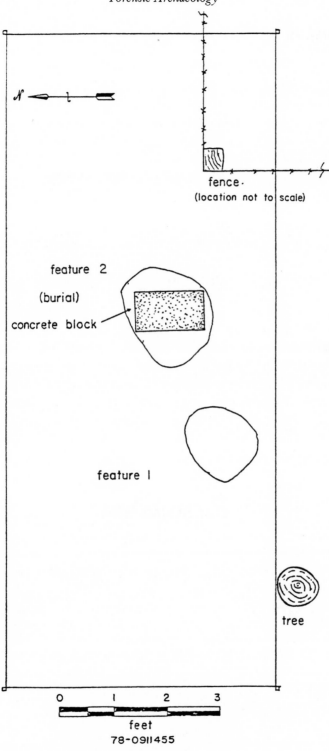

feature 2

(burial)

concrete block

feature 1

tree

fence.
(location not to scale)

feet

78-0911455

Figure 4-2.

Description of the scene

Prior to the start of processing, an area in the yard had been roped off for security purposes. A portion of the ground that seemed relatively free from leaf cover, giving an appearance of possible recent disturbance, was observed near the southwest corner of the roped area. A 12- by 15-foot grid was set up using stakes and string. This included all of the disturbed ground. A depressed area measuring 1 foot in diameter and 4 inches deep and surrounded by loose fill dirt was located 4 feet east and 1 foot north of the southwest stake. This was classified as Feature 1. It was later determined to be an empty grave.

Procedure

The entire area was scanned initially with a metal detector. Repeated scans during the excavation produced no significant results. After removal of surface debris and loose fill, a well-defined circular area of disturbance became apparent (Feature 2). This was characterized by light brown mixed fill surrounded by undisturbed light gray soil. The location was 6 feet 9 inches east and 2 feet 11 inches north from the southwest corner.

Feature 2 proved to be the grave and was excavated first. A concrete block oriented north/south was encountered. At its north end it was 2 inches below surface and its south end was 3 inches below the original surface. The block was removed and found to measure 16 by 8 by 4 inches. Beneath the block was a pink blanket, which filled the remainder of the pit. This was removed and was partially unwrapped. It contained a black-haired infant in a stage of partial decomposition. The boundaries of the pit were determined by careful excavation. It was found to be 18 inches in the north/south direction, 12 inches in the east/west direction, and 16 inches deep. All four walls gave the impression that the grave was dug with a square-bladed shovel with slightly rounded ends. Several clumps of dirt were encountered, which were actually partial "shovel molds." Their shape also indicated a nearly flat-bladed shovel with rounded edges.

Feature 1 was excavated next. The measurements were 19 inches square and 10 inches deep. It was empty.

All dirt removed from the surface and from the two features was water screened through a 3/16 inch mesh plastic screen. Nothing was recovered except a few small pieces of glass and broken china.

The concrete block was taken by the sheriff for evidence. The infant, still wrapped in the blanket, was sent to the Medical Examiner. A shovel, which was found in the home of the parents, was confiscated and retained by the sheriff. It was flat-bladed with curved edges.

Disposition

The results of the investigation were submitted to the sheriff for his attention.

DISCUSSION

It cannot be too strongly emphasized that death investigations are a matter of teamwork. The crime scene investigator is trained in the methods of collecting, packaging, and transporting various kinds of evidence, including human remains, so as not to break the chain of possession. It is the crime scene investigator who is solely responsible for the conduct of the investigation. He should make the decisions as to what is done, how it is to be done, and when. In many states, the matter of jurisdiction in crime scene investigation is not clear, with the result that untrained people often interfere with the orderly process of the investigation.

Once the remains are found and systematically removed along with associated evidence, it is the task of the medical examiner or coroner to determine the cause and manner of death. Usually what the investigator finds at the scene will materially assist in this determination. The forensic anthropologist, when called upon, can greatly assist the other experts in reconstructing the individual with respect to such vital information as age, sex, stature, weight, and anomalies. Together these several specialities, with their knowledge of one another's areas of expertise, can develop significant information with respect to the identification of a crime and its perpetrator(s).

CONCLUSION

In this chapter we have outlined the essential techniques and procedures, including the minimum equipment necessary, to remove and recover human remains and associated evidence systematically in crime scene investigations. Two cases were cited demonstrating the need for teamwork and the methods and kinds of results that can be anticipated.

REFERENCES

Morse, D., D. Crusoe, and H. G. Smith (1976). Forensic archaeology. *Journal of Forensic Sciences,* *21*:323–332.

Morse, D., Jack Duncan and J. Stoutamire (Eds.) (1983). *Handbook of Forensic Archaeology and Anthropology.* Published by the editors, distributed by Bills' Book Store, Tallahassee, Florida.

Morse, D., J. Stoutamire, and Jack Duncan (1976). A unique course in anthropology. *American Journal of Physical Anthropology, 45*:743–747.

Chapter 5

PROBLEMS OF BURIAL EXHUMATION, HISTORICAL AND FORENSIC ASPECTS

SHEILAGH T. BROOKS AND RICHARD H. BROOKS

INTRODUCTION

The exhumation of human remains in various areas of the world is usually conducted by archaeologists concerned with the reconstruction of past cultures, either historic or prehistoric. A higher frequency of burial exhumation is associated with prehistoric archaeological excavations, although recently there are increasing numbers of research projects relating to historic cemeteries (Sublett 1965, 1966, 1969). In Nevada the common pattern for family plots or private cemeteries to be associated with individual historic ranches dating to the 19th century has created some problems during urban expansion and construction. As the large historic ranches are broken up and later sold by present owners, these private historic burial plots must—by law—be excavated and the burials exhumed and reinterred in local cemeteries, unless the family specifies otherwise.

This relocation of private historic burial plots has occurred twice in the past several years in southern Nevada. Each case presented a different set of problems, but they were similar in that the original ranch family had sold their land. In the Stewart Ranch case there was a contractual obligation for exhumation of the private historic cemetery and reinterment of the burials. In the Kiel* Ranch case there was only the assumption that the burials would be protected somehow prior to construction on the land.

Given the legal/forensic importance of these cases, an archaeologist, R. H. Brooks, and a physical anthropologist, S. T. Brooks, from the University of Nevada, Las Vegas, were requested to conduct the exhumation and subsequent identification of the historic burials in both cases. Location of the graves and identification of the deceased were necessary in these instances, since the grave markers had either been destroyed or lost, and in the Kiel Ranch case the land had changed hands several times in the interval since

---

*The spelling of the name has since been changed to Kyle, but the original spelling has been retained in this chapter.

the presumed most recent burials were interred in AD 1900. The overall problems of burial exhumation that relate to archaeological or forensic excavation will be reviewed first. Then specific difficulties experienced during the excavation involved in these two cases will be discussed.

TECHNIQUES OF EXHUMATION

"One can never dig in the ground and put the dirt back exactly as nature had put it there originally" (Bass and Birkby 1978:7) — the digging of a grave leaves clues visible in the soil disturbance. Effectively, the archaeologist destroys the site during exposure of the remains either historic or pre-historic. In consequence, archaeological techniques of excavation have been developed to retain as much of the contextual information or evidence as possible. Through systematic recordations,* mapping of the burial locale, photography, and precise excavation controls, the interrelationships and associational provenience of all materials encountered are maintained. "Excavation cannot be conducted in a haphazard manner, or valuable information will be lost. The association of objects and the sequence of strata and intrusive elements with all their implications must be interpreted with three dimensional principles" (Joukowsky 1980:139). The horizontal (length and width) dimension is represented by the grid system, the vertical (depth) dimension by specifically measured depth levels (10 centimeters usually), beginning at zero or the ground surface. An alternate method of vertical control is through observed stratigraphic changes in the exposed side walls as the excavation proceeds.

"The excavation grid divides the area to be excavated into exact squares which are parallel to the site baseline" (Joukowsky 1980:139), generally related to a north-south axis. A specific stake on the baseline is frequently designated as the site datum point to which all measurements are correlated. Where possible a bench marker is used to assist in relocation of the site at a later time, subsequent to the excavation and the back-filling of the exposed trenches. The grid first is measured and marked on the ground using stakes and string to delineate the squares, which are usually 1 meter in size. The metric system is used in both archaeological and physical anthropological mensuration, but when necessary can easily be converted to the English system for law enforcement agencies or to clarify information for those not accustomed to its use. These meter squares are then mapped, numbered in

---

*Recordation is the maintenance of detailed written records, accompanied by photography (when possible), line drawings of burial position, and associated artifacts or other objects. The recordation of data commences with the beginning of the excavation, through to the removal of the skeleton, ending with line drawings of the stratigraphic profiles of the side walls. In addition, there should be an overall map of the cemetery site showing the burial relationships.

one direction as length, and lettered in the other direction as width, giving each 1 meter square or excavation unit a designation of a letter and number on the gridded site map. Both on the surface and at depth, designating each excavation unit through a number and a letter preserves through a permanent record the interrelationships and associational provenience of artifacts, skeletal remains, and other relevant materials encountered during the excavation. Excavation of each unit then proceeds by the measured level—usually 10 centimeters—and the removed earth or midden in an archaeological site is screened through a 3/16-inch mesh screen. This facilitates the recovery of any objects encountered that have been overlooked during the excavation removal procedure. If a significant object is found during the excavation of a level, its location is recorded in all three dimensions, photographed *in situ* prior to removal, and placed in an appropriately labeled bag. All materials recovered through screening are recorded as to excavation unit and level and also placed in a labeled bag, but separate from specifically recorded items. Simplistically these are the basic outlines of archaeological recovery during historic or prehistoric site excavation, which may be modified as specific circumstances dictate.

Exhumation of historic or recent forensically related burials requires special excavation strategies. Historically in the United States cemetery burial implies a normal interment depth of approximately 6 feet (c. 2 meters) below the ground surface. In these circumstances, where known, 10 centimeter vertical control during depth excavation will not be necessary, and 30 centimeter levels should be adequate. In forensically related exhumations where the grave may be shallow it is advisable to rely on the smaller vertical levels. For both types of exhumation the grid system for horizontal control should be followed to insure the contextual association of interrelated materials encountered during the excavation. "It is a wise practice to photograph the excavation at various stages and include identification and direction markers" (Bass and Birkby 1978:7). As soon as the grid is laid out, a photograph should be taken of the presumed burial locus within the grid system, which is designed to extend outside the perimeters of the actual grave locale. The original excavation for the grave may be immediately visible on the surface of the ground, or will become apparent usually a few centimeters subsurface, below the organically stained soil. The disturbance of the soil composition by the original interment of the body will clearly outline the perimeters of this first excavation of the grave, and the soil itself will be softer in this area (Fig. 5-1).

Depending on the presumed depth of the burial, various implements can be used for exhumation, ranging from shovels for deeply buried cemetery graves to trowels, dental picks, and toothbrushes if the body is close to the ground surface.

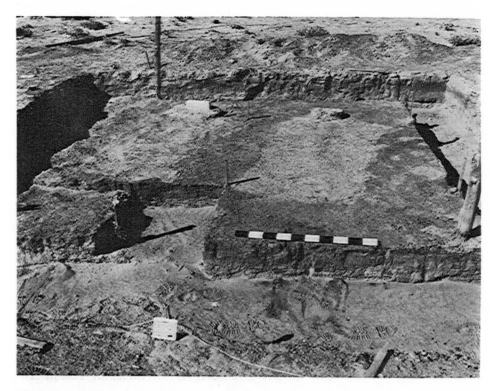

Figure 5-1. Evidence of the soil change clearly delineates the perimeters of these two Kiel family graves. The soil change was caused by the original excavation for the burial and the disturbance created by this activity.

> As soon as a burial is discovered, the excavator must try to determine its position. Since the skull is usually highest, it will most often be discovered first in stripping operations, but several points on the skeleton must be found and identified in order to pinpoint its exact location and position. This should be done before further exposure is attempted, and should itself expose as little of the skeleton as possible in order to protect it from rough handling.... One of the most satisfactory methods of exposing a burial is by blocking it out as soon as the position and extent are determined; that is, by leaving the burial embedded in its matrix on a pedestal while the surrounding dirt is cleared away and a level floor established. (Hester, Heizer, and Graham 1975:172)

Then the bones should be exposed gently, not cutting into the area of the burial from the upper surface, but removing the dirt carefully from the sides as well as the top with brushes and dental picks. The skeleton and all associated artifacts are left *in situ* (in position) and "under no condition should any bone or artifact be removed until the entire grave is exposed" (Bass and Birkby 1978:8). It is during the first contact with the burial and the subsequent cleaning of the bones that photographs should be taken to record this exposure.

Individual line drawings should be made in addition to the photographs for each burial indicating its exact position and any associated artifacts such as rings, coins, pocket knives, the coffin, or related teeth and bones. The position of the arms, legs, head, and directional orientation of the whole body are noted in this line drawing. Certain patterns of burial position characterize particular prehistoric and historic cultures, and information on burial position can be significant for identification. If a coffin is present, size measurements should be taken and dirt in the interior of the coffin screened and examined to insure that no artifactual items, other bones, or teeth have been included. The size of screen mesh is the same as used previously during the excavation, although a smaller mesh size can be used if necessary. Any materials recovered during this screening are placed in a labeled bag indicating the burial with which they were associated.

Once this recordation has been completed, each bone should be carefully brushed, removed, and wrapped in a soft tissue such as toilet paper. Paper bags of appropriate size can be used as bone containers to be placed in cardboard or wooden boxes for transit. Skeletal elements can be grouped for placing in bags labeled by excavation unit, grave, depth, and bones. If in the field anatomical units of the skeleton are bagged together and each bag labeled with site name as well as anatomical information, laboratory identification is facilitated. The following groups are recommended: the skull with mandible and isolated teeth; the ribs and sternum; all vertebrae except the sacrum; each arm with the hand bones separate and labeled; each leg with the foot bones separate and labeled; the scapulae and clavicles; and the pelvis with the sacrum. These labeled bags can then be placed within either larger doubled grocery bags or cartons, which also have to be labeled, preferably with a black marking pen (non-water-soluble ink).

From the bones of the skeleton, information can be obtained on age at death, sex, ethnic group, stature, possible length of inhumation, as well as individual skeletal or dental anomalies or pathologies that will assist in positive identification. Unexpected premortem bone breakage or shattering should be noted, since these features may reflect cause of death. It is preferable to conduct this skeletal analysis in the laboratory, but should the situation not permit laboratory examination, this can be done in the field. Field analysis, however, severely limits the resultant quantity and quality of forensic information. The location of associated cultural materials should be fully recorded in relation to specific bones and should be included with the skeleton if the items are allowed to be removed to a laboratory for thorough examination.

THE STEWART FAMILY CASE

The Stewart family, a pioneer Las Vegas family, had sold the land containing their family's historic cemetery to an adjacent mortuary for conversion into a parking lot. A limiting condition was that all the known burials were to be exhumed and reburied in an appropriate location. The mortuary had removed all grave markers and already stripped the surface of the land in their attempt to relocate the graves when the family stopped the bulldozers and asked the help of the archaeologist, R. H. Brooks, and physical anthropologist, S. T. Brooks. Two problems were involved: (1) the location of the graves now that the surface of the ground was completely disturbed and (2) the identification of the individuals buried, since family records were unclear and all the grave markers removed. Neither the family members nor the mortuary staff were certain where the actual graves were located, although they knew that there were five adult graves, one possible newborn infant's grave, and the probability of stillborn twins interred within one of the adult coffins in this section of the historic family cemetery. Two other burials were presumed to be located in a "crypt" cut into a caliche clifflike outcropping to the west of the bulldozed area. This upper crypt had a drainage pipe that had been installed to remove water from usually subsurface spring waters that ran through this entire portion of the old Stewart Ranch. These two graves were not involved in this first request for professional assistance by the Stewart family, but were exhumed several months later by R. H. Brooks, assisted by his field crew.

The mortuary, under pressure from the Stewart family, hired a backhoe to assist in locating the graves. The family members and morticians were all certain the graves were to be found sequentially in a particular area. With the aid of a *skillful* backhoe operator, a trench was cut and gradually deepened and extended with no evidence of soil change that could indicate burial deposition. After a cut of about a 10 meter long trench, interspersed with occasional short cross trenches, extending to a depth of 3 to 4 meters, the family's and mortician's guess of the graves' locale was abandoned. R. H. Brooks and the backhoe operator cooperated to strip off the bulldozed dirt at shallow intervals in the area opposite the section previously trenched and found the edge of the soil color change indicative of the earth's being disturbed during the original excavation of the graves in the cemetery. Then R. H. Brooks, with the backhoe operator and assisted by anthropology student volunteers working with trowels, cleared the area where the color change occurred to the level of the top of the first wooden coffin. The graves had all been placed in the same plane with approximately 1 meter separating each burial. Four of the adults had been interred in wooden coffins, and the fifth had been placed in a copper coffin, with a glass face plate, which had been ensconsed with a cement covering. This burial was of an uncle of the present Stewarts who had died and been embalmed in Los Angeles in 1902 and then sent to Las Vegas for burial in the family cemetery. The wooden coffins apparently had been made locally, so there were no coffin handles. According to historic accounts, the coffin of Archibald Stewart, Sr. was made from the wooden door on which his body had been placed when he was brought by his widow to the Stewart Ranch for burial.

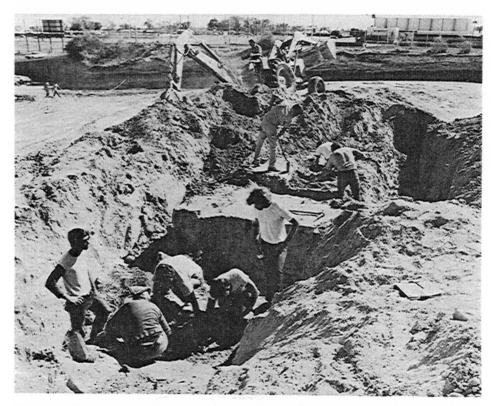

Figure 5-2. The Stewart family cemetery photographed while the backhoe is completing the exposure of the series of five graves. Exhumation has begun on one of the graves, while the others are still in process of removal of the overburden (approximately 6 feet deep).

According to the family there were supposedly at least two Stewarts known to be buried in the cemetery in addition to the embalmed uncle: young Archie Stewart, who had been killed when thrown from a horse, and his father (Archibald Stewart, Sr.), the great-grandfather of the present Stewarts, who had been killed in a gunfight on the Kiel Ranch. Historically the question had never been solved as to whether the great-grandfather had been shot in a fair fight or from ambush by a Kiel ranch hand. Two nonfamily individuals were also presumably interred in the cemetery: an Indian or Mexican girl and an elderly Scotsman, the first schoolteacher in Clark County, Nevada.

To obtain as much information as possible in the short time period allowed for the exhumation and identification—about six days—all five adult burials were exposed through to the upper portion of the grave by the backhoe. (A night watchman was hired by the mortuary under family pressure for protection of the opened grave sites.) This was followed by conventional controlled archaeological excavation, according to the techniques previously described for burial exhumation. Each skeleton (with the exception of the embalmed body) was pedestaled and cleaned with brushes.

S. T. Brooks with physical anthropological student volunteers conducted an *in situ* determination of age at death, sex, pathologies, skeletal injuries, and measurement of long bones for stature estimation. At all times members of the family and frequently the mortuary staff were present, which effectively curtailed photography, mapping, and removal of bones to the osteology laboratory. A complete examination was limited by the family's desire to reinter the remains quickly.

Working closely with several historians, records were obtained as to the age at which the great-grandfather had been killed and the age at death of the schoolteacher. Great-grandfather Stewart had been killed when he was approximately forty-nine years of age, and the schoolteacher was over sixty, perhaps sixty-nine years old at the time of his death. Both men were estimated to have had a stature of 5 feet 10 inches to 5 feet 11 inches during life. The historical records indicated that the schoolteacher had a "dislocated shoulder," which proved to be a broken clavicle that had healed badly from apparently never having been set (Fig. 5-3). This injury had affected his first rib and adjacent vertebrae.

Great-grandfather Stewart's right malar was broken away, and the entire back of the cranium was missing. Although the backhoe in the initial sweep clearing the earth above and lateral to the graves had partially exposed the cranial portion of this burial, the missing parts of the occipital area of the skull were delineated by old breaks, not fresh ones. Had these been recent breaks caused during the excavation of the burial, the color of the broken bone would have been much lighter and the edges of the break sharp rather than rounded. The assumption was made on these bases, without substantiation allowable through x-ray or laboratory examination, that the man had been killed by a shot into his right cheek, which had exited through the back of the skull. No bullet was found during the screening of the dirt in and around his coffin.

Young Stewart and the young Indian or Mexican girl showed no indication of cause of death, although she was supposed to have died as a result of

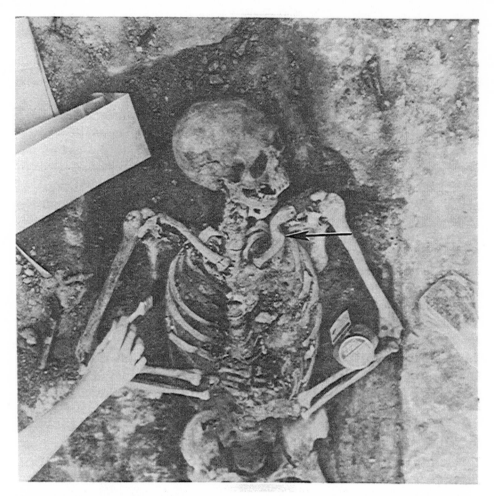

Figure 5-3. This view of the skeleton of the schoolteacher shows the broken and badly healed left clavicle. The arrow indicates the area of the rehealed break.

swallowing a pin and he from being thrown from a horse. The earth from the area around and within her coffin was carefully screened, and no evidence of a pin was found. The adolescent boy's bones were the most poorly preserved of all the skeletonized burials, and little could be determined from the field examination, other than age at death and sex, both of which conformed to the historical records.

The cement covering containing the copper coffin and the embalmed body of the uncle was opened to release the water that had accumulated from the nearby springs, after which a section of the copper cover was cut to expose the lower portion of the embalmed body. This was done at the family's request to determine if the stillborn twins had been placed here, since none of the family knew where they had been buried. The twins were positioned at the level of the lower legs, wrapped in material, but not embalmed. This discovery solved the problem of the burial locus. The newborn infant, who was also supposed to have been buried in the family cemetery in a small box, was not found and was presumed to have been destroyed in the initial bulldozing of the cemetery area.

As soon as all the burials had been identified to the family's satisfaction, by their request the mortuary provided new coffins for all except the embalmed uncle and stillborn twins in the copper coffin, which was removed opened but intact by the morticians. The family further required that each skeleton be placed in anatomical articulated position on the satin linings and pillows — more expensive ones for the family and less expensive for the young girl and the schoolteacher — an unusual experience for the volunteer staff and crew. These coffins were then closed, and the mortuary carried them off for eventual reburial.

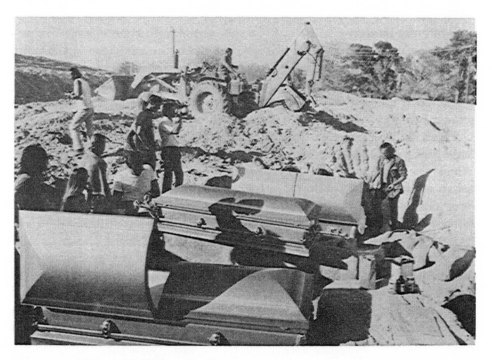

Figure 5-4. The archaelogical crew is placing the exhumed skeletons of the burials in coffins, after which they will be taken by the mortuary to a cemetery area for reburial.

It must be emphasized that ideal exhumation procedures recommended in the techniques section had to be modified under the circumstances that prevailed in this case. The entire exhumation procedure, identification, and placement of the skeletons in the new coffins was completed from one Saturday to the next, with volunteer students or staff participating whenever they had free time. As a joint volunteer project, it successfully combined data from three fields: history, archaeology, and physical anthropology. It also illustrates the solution of problems of locating unmarked graves under a disturbed surface and individual identification within a historical cemetery.

THE KIEL RANCH CASE

The historic family cemetery located on the Kiel Ranch involved some comparable problems, as well as a set of new challenges. There was no apparent concern over the disposition of the land in which the family graves were located during the several times that the ranch changed hands in the interim from the last known interments, AD 1900, to spring, 1975. At this time the City of North Las Vegas had acquired that part of the Kiel Ranch where the ranch buildings are situated. In 1975 City officials decided to renovate the buildings as part of their Bicentennial project. Since the private owner planned to sell the corner plot where the cemetery was located, city officials determined the burials should be exhumed and eventually reinterred on the city-owned land. R. H. Brooks and S. T. Brooks were contacted by the City of North Las Vegas and asked if they would assist in the removal project with their student volunteers.

Elizabeth Warren, then Historian and District Interpreter for Nevada State Parks, was already cognizant of some of the history of the Kiel family. When she was contacted about the proposed exhumation, Mrs. Warren began research on the problem of finding any living relatives of the Kiels so their desires could be expressed in this matter. At the same time she informed the Brookses that although the cemetery locale was identifiable, and two graves (those of a Mrs. Latimer and Conrad Kiel) were known to have had gravestones present earlier in the history of the town, no estimates of total cemetery size had been determined. Conrad Kiel's two sons, who had been killed in a murder/suicide instigated by the elder brother, were reputed to be buried in the cemetery, and there was also the possibility of Indian burials, since a number of local Paiutes worked as ranch hands on the Kiel Ranch.

Process

Initial research on the ranch was begun in part by an archaeological survey of the terrain to ensure that there were no other apparent grave sites on the property now belonging to the City of North Las Vegas. Simultaneously, some of the students under the supervision of R. H. Brooks began gridding the area of the two known grave sites and clearing the surface of debris. As they began the procedure for excavation, the outline of two graves became apparent just below the surface of the ground (Fig. 5-5). At this time a further problem arose in that excavation could not proceed normally using archaeological techniques as had been planned, since there was no way in which the City of North Las Vegas could protect the excavation from vandalism. In fact, the grave of Mrs. Latimer had twice been partially excavated by vandals who were frightened off by a police vehicle driving through the neighborhood. There was a local rumor that she had been buried with a diamond ring. It was then that the tombstone on Mrs. Latimer's grave had disappeared as well as the rail fence surrounding the two graves. In view of the inability to protect the excavation, R. H. Brooks decided to use a backhoe to remove the earth down to the expected level of the burials so that the exposure of the graves and removal of the burials could be accomplished in one day. On the basis of the previous experience in exhuming the Stewart family burials, it was anticipated that use of the backhoe would prove feasible and also that the burials would be situated at an approximate depth of 6 feet, or 2 meters.

Mrs. Warren had contacted members of the Kiel family, one of whom was living in Los Angeles and gave permission for the exhumation. She also allowed the burials to be removed to the physical anthropological laboratory at the University of Nevada, Las Vegas, for examination and analysis. She agreed to be present at the exhumation along with Mrs. Warren and other interested historians.

A backhoe was provided by the City of North Las Vegas, and the operator, working skillfully in coordination with R. H. Brooks, was able to skim off the earth over the two known graves at carefully controlled intervals. After the first indication that Mrs. Latimer's coffin top had been reached, the volunteer crew, following the usual archaeological techniques, began pedestaling and cleaning the burial for complete exposure. The same procedure was used for Conrad Kiel's burial, which was about 50 centimeters north of Mrs. Latimer's and in the same plane (Figure 5-6). An infant burial was located just south of Mrs. Latimer's grave and about 50 centimeters higher. As these three burials were being carefully exposed, the backhoe operator in conjunction with R. H. Brooks continued stripping the area to the north, following the edge of the soil disturbance caused by the original grave excavation for these first two burials. About a meter north of Conrad Kiel's grave, another adult-sized grave outline became visible, and beyond this a fourth adult-sized grave outline. Volunteers began exposing these two additional burials, pedestaling and cleaning them for recordation. The dirt in and around all burials was screened

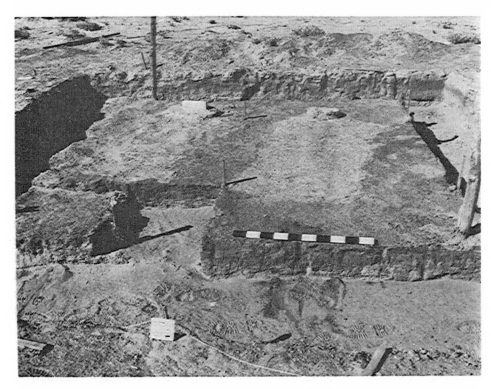

Figure 5-5. Evidence of the soil change clearly delineates the perimeters of these two Kiel family graves. The soil change was caused by the original excavation for the burial and the disturbance created by this activity.

during the procedure to recover small inclusions such as teeth or artifacts.

All four adults had been buried in wooden coffins and the infant apparently in a small box (Fig. 5-7). As with the Stewart burials, the adults were lying face up, with legs fully extended and their hands placed across their bodies. The single exception was the fourth adult burial, which had the shattered left arm extended. All five of the burials exhumed in the Stewart cemetery, and the two Stewarts exposed at a later date in the upper crypt, and three of the adult burials in the Kiel Ranch cemetery were lying with their heads to the west. The skeleton of the third of the Kiel burials was positioned similarly but with his head to the east. According to information obtained from local ministers, historic Christian burials are placed face up with heads to the west so that on "Judgment Day" all the "good" will be able to sit up and face east appropriately. A person who had committed murder and suicide would not be judged "good," so it might be assumed that this third burial was the accused murderer/suicide. Alternatively, the persons burying a closed coffin may not have paid attention to position orientation.

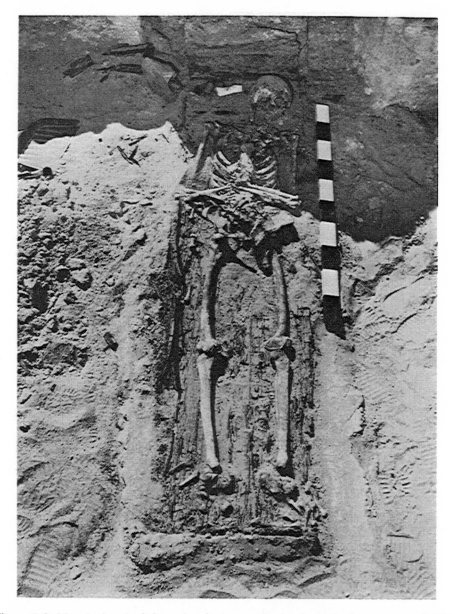

Figure 5-6. Mrs. Latimer's skeleton has been completely cleaned prior to removal. This photograph shows the position in which she had been placed, and the wooden remains of the coffin.

As the exposure of the five burials proceeded, the excavation area became surrounded not only with historians, the officials from the North Las Vegas City who initiated this project, the press, and members of the Kiel family,

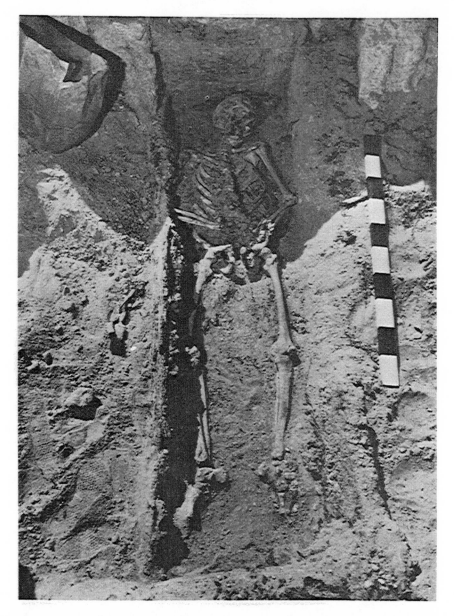

Figure 5-7. Conrad Kiel is lying in the same position as Mrs. Latimer, only his arms and hands are placed further down on his pelvis. The wooden sides of his coffin are still intact.

but also with innumerable other curious bystanders. The backhoe operator assisted by clearing an area adjacent to the large trench, which was now opened to a depth of over 2 meters, so that no one would accidentally be precipitated on top of the volunteer workers and staff.

The first adult burial was identified as Mrs. Latimer, a woman well past her fifties, who had been buried in 1891. The second burial, that of Conrad Kiel, buried in 1893, was in an excellent state of preservation and was identified as a male over sixty at the time of his death. The two Kiel brothers were known to be fifty-three and fifty-one years of age at the time of their deaths in 1900. On the basis of the premortem breaks in the facial portion of Burial #3 (Fig. 5-8) and the cranium and face of Burial #4 (Fig. 5-9), these were identified as the Kiel brothers. Burial #4, subsequently identified as William Kiel, had a shattered left radius and ulna (Fig. 5-10) in addition to the breakage of the craniofacial region. Specific identification was based on comparison of the crania in the laboratory analysis with a photograph of the Kiel brothers, taken in their youth, that was obtained from the University of Nevada, Las Vegas Library, Special Collections historical photographs.

Edwin Kiel had been accused of killing his brother William Kiel with a shotgun and then committing suicide with a handgun. The bodies had been

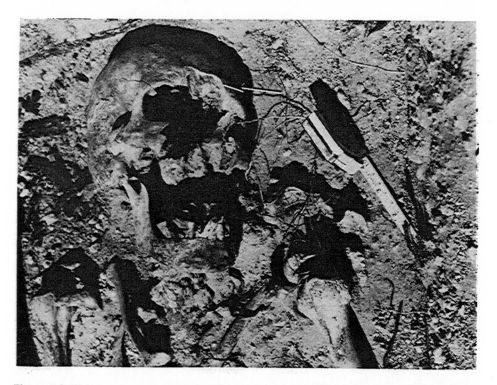

Figure 5-8. This is a close-up of Edwin Kiel, Burial #3, showing his shattered frontal (arrow), broken left malar, and missing nasal bones, resulting from the exit wound of the bullet that killed him.

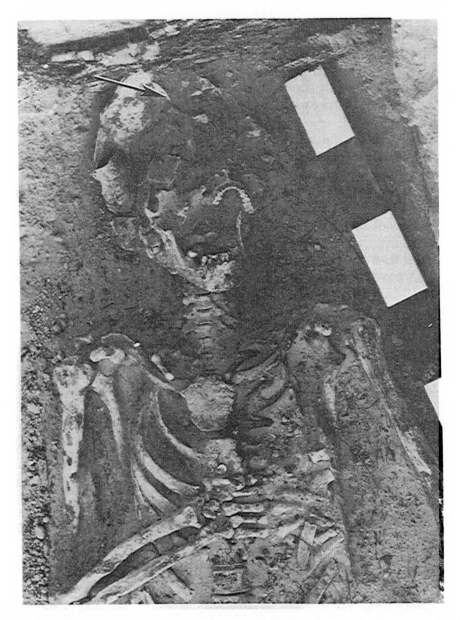

Figure 5-9. This is a close-up of William Kiel, Burial #4, showing the shattered craniofacial region (arrow), the result of apparently two shotgun blasts.

found by members of the Stewart family. One was another Stewart uncle, who on his death had been interred in the upper crypt. The other man was the second husband (also named Stewart but unrelated) of the widow whose first husband, great-grandfather Stewart, had been killed earlier at the Kiel

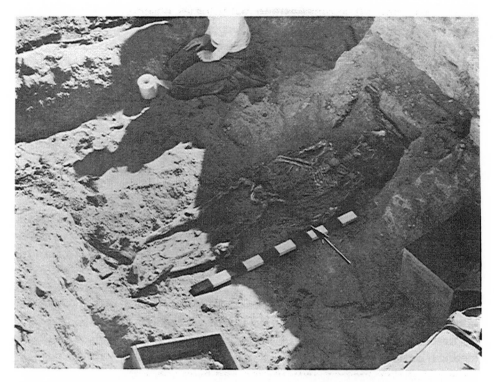

Figure 5-10. It is presumed that William Kiel's left ulna and radius were shattered during one of the shotgun blasts, and the breaks are visible (arrow). The left arm is lying in a fully extended position, which differs from the arm position of any of the other burials.

Ranch. After the discovery of the bodies a Coroner's jury determined at the inquest that the interpretation of the brothers' deaths was murder followed by suicide.

All four adult skeletons were removed according to the usual procedures followed in archaeological methodology. The infant skeleton was taken out as a block, retaining the dirt matrix for protection. With the permission of a Kiel family member all the burials were returned to the laboratory that night. The following day R. H. Brooks and the backhoe operator carefully stripped a number of trenches out from the area where the five burials had been removed, extending these trenches for several meters in each of the cardinal directions, with some cross-trenching. No further historical or skeletal materials were encountered.

Findings

In the laboratory the four adult burials were thoroughly analyzed anthropometrically; discrete morphological traits were recorded, age and sex determined, and all anomalies and pathologies observed. The work was done by volunteer students under the supervision of S. T. Brooks. During this examination two of the students discovered what appeared to be a bullet entrance wound just to the left of center in the occipital of Burial #3. Dr. Sheldon Green, Clark County Assistant Coroner, later confirmed that this could be the correct size for a .44 or .45 bullet entrance hole, with the shattered anterior frontal, left malar, and both nasal bones showing the characteristics of an exit wound. The entire cranium and upper facial area of Burial #4, William Kiel, was indicative of a shotgun blast, although the palate and mandible were intact.

The crania of both these burials were taken to the 1976 American Academy of Forensic Sciences meetings, and colleagues were able to confirm Dr. Green's explanation of the entrance and exit wounds in Edwin Kiel's cranium, as well as suggest that the breakage pattern of William Kiel's cranium was characteristic of shotgun blasts. Another suggestion was to x-ray both crania to determine whether there was any evidence of metal from the bullet or shotgun pellets remaining in the crania that might give further clues as to the direction of the shots. One colleague also theorized that in 1900 the interpretation of the exit wound through the face of Edwin Kiel could easily be mistaken for an entrance wound unless there had been a thorough medical examination. From the historical documentation of the case, it appeared that no medical examination had been conducted.

Both crania, as well as the earth block containing the infant burial, were x-rayed by Dr. Raymond Rawson, D.A.B.F.O. Evidence of metal traces in the frontal bone of Edwin Kiel and in opposite sides of the cranial vault of William Kiel seem to substantiate the proposal that the former had been shot from the rear and the latter shot at least twice by a shotgun. The conclusion reached by S. T. Brooks and Rawson was that this had been a double murder; Edwin Kiel was probably ambushed as he walked out of the ranch house and shot with either a .44 or .45 revolver, and William Kiel was shot twice with a shotgun as he came towards the murderer. The one shot had shattered his left radius and ulna, perhaps as he threw up his arm to protect his face. A second shotgun blast apparently struck his head from a different angle, further indicating that this also was murder and not a suicide.

Dr. Rawson's x-ray of the infant showed a metallic chain, small cross, and two safety pins. In addition, his x-ray analysis of the teeth indicated that the infant had passed through birth trauma and apparently died shortly afterwards. As yet Mrs. Warren in her researches has found no historical documentation of identity of the infant or its parentage.

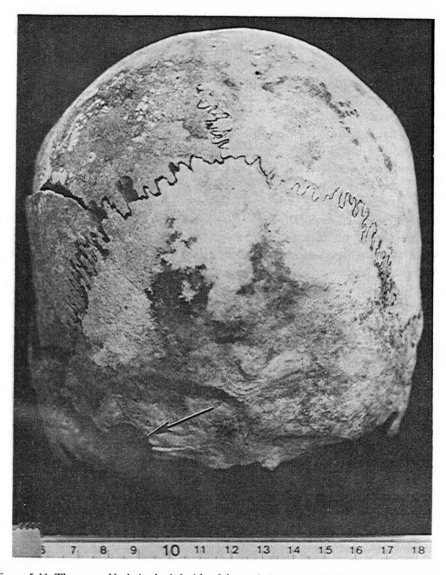

Figure 5-11. The curved hole in the left side of the occipital (arrow) is the result of the entrance wound left by the bullet that killed Edwin Kiel. The bullet exited through the face, as is shown in Figure 5-8.

DISCUSSION AND CONCLUSIONS

In reviewing these two cases some emphasis must be placed on the depth to which the graves in both cemeteries had been excavated by the original grave diggers, probably ranch hands, family members, or neighbors. All of the adult burials in both cemeteries were at a depth of at least 2 meters, a confirmation of the historically known burial pattern of Western culture. Considering the extreme difficulty of digging through the local caliche soils and hard pans in this desert area, using only the physical strength of the grave diggers and hand tools, it is an interesting reflection on the significance of known burial practices (burial at a depth of 6 feet or 2 meters) for the participants in that culture.

During the exhumation the marked soil change at the perimeters of the graves and the softer fill of the graves were the evidence used by R. H. Brooks to determine the location of the nine adult burials and the infant's burial. The coordinated use of the backhoe was important in locating the Stewart burials because of the surface destruction of the grave sites. In the Kiel case, the backhoe enabled completion of the exhumation in one day's time. Excavation problems were solved through the skill of the backhoe operator working in coordination with the archaeologist, so each burial was contacted and blocked out by the backhoe with no damage to the skeleton itself or the coffin. By leaving the matrix around the burials intact, the volunteer crew members were then able to employ archaeological techniques of exhumation to pedestal, clean, and fully expose the burials. Screening of the dirt in and around the coffins was done for all burials to determine if there were associated artifacts, loose teeth, bullets, or other relevant items.

Although the Stewart family expected to find rings or other individual keepsakes with their family burials, none were found, not even with the two burials in the upper crypt (which were removed at a later date by R. H. Brooks). A quarter was found within the coffin of the schoolteacher in a position that suggested it had been in a trouser pocket. The young Indian or Mexican girl had in association with her burial several metal rings, numerous beads of small colored glass types (perhaps for a necklace or pendant), a necklace of perforated dimes, and a Mexican quarter. With the exception of the stillborn twins, the only other associated objects in the coffins encountered at the Stewart Cemetery were fragments of buttons.

Despite the rumors that Mrs. Latimer had been buried with a diamond ring, only buttons from her dress were recovered during the screening of the dirt in her coffin. Parts of shoes were still preserved adjacent to the foot bones of both Edwin and William Kiel. No other cultural items were encountered during this excavation except the chain and cross fragments and safety pins observed in the x-ray photography by Dr. Rawson. Dr. Rawson also examined the fillings in Edwin Kiel's teeth and from the technique of manufacture estimated they had been made by a midwestern dentist prior to Edwin Kiel's move out to join his father, Conrad Kiel, on the ranch. These fillings are slightly visible in the photograph from the

Library's Special Collections, which may confirm this estimation, as the historians have presumed the picture was taken at the Kiel farm in the Midwest.

Both of these cases were conducted under time constraints, that of the Stewarts to have the burials identified and reinterred as soon as possible, so that the work had to be completed *in situ*. It was assumed from the pattern of facial bone breakage and the evidence of an apparent preinterment loss of the back of the cranium of great-grandfather Stewart that these were evidence of a facial entrance wound and an occipital exit wound. No confirmation of the direction of the bullet could be made through a laboratory examination or the use of x-ray to find possible indications of metal from the bullet, either in the facial bones or around the broken area of the back of the skull. Lack of a full laboratory examination and analysis, as well as the curtailment of photography and sketching, limited the physical anthropological investigation of the Stewart burials.

Despite the pressure to complete the Kiel family exhumation in one day, the controlled use of the backhoe, the volunteer efforts of staff and students, and the preliminary archaeological examination conducted by R. H. Brooks before the excavation began enabled the removal of the burials to be completed. It was through the permission to analyze and examine the Kiel burials in detail in the physical anthropological laboratory and x-ray them that the positive identification was accomplished. This further allowed forensic analysis to be developed through the substantiating evidence indicative of a double murder of the Kiel brothers ("by person or persons unknown").

These cases involved the field cooperation of members from three disciplines: archaeology, physical anthropology (including forensic physical anthropology and odontology for the Kiel case), and history. The historians are still researching the identity of the infant buried in the Kiel Ranch cemetery. Speculation is of course continuous as to the interrelationship of the three murders, especially as great-grandfather Stewart was killed on the Kiel Ranch, but no historically valid conclusions have yet been reached.

REFERENCES

Bass, William M. and Walter H. Birkby (1978). Exhumation: The method could make the difference. *FBI Law Enforcement Bulletin, 47*:6–11.

Hester, Thomas R., Robert F. Heizer, and John A. Graham (1975). *Field Methods in Archaeology*, 6th ed. Mayfield Publishing Company, Palo Alto, California.

Joukowsky, Martha (1980). *A Complete Manual of Field Archaeology, Tools and Techniques of Field Work for Archaeologists*. Prentice-Hall, Englewood Cliffs, New Jersey.

Sublett, Audrey J. (1965). The Cornplanter cemetery: Skeletal analysis. *Pennsylvania Archaeologist, XXXV*:74–92.

_____ (1966). Seneca Physical Type and Changes Through Time. Unpublished Ph.D. Dissertation. S.U.N.Y. at Buffalo, New York.

_____ (1969). To conduct *in situ* analysis of Mohawk Indian burials. *Year Book of the American Philosophical Society, 1969*:333–334.

Chapter 6

PERPENDICULAR FORENSIC ARCHAEOLOGY

Lowell J. Levine, Homer R. Campbell, Jr., and J. Stanley Rhine

THE PROBLEM

We were requested by the District Attorney of one of the Lake States to recover a body that, according to an informant, had been cast into a well about ten years earlier. The well was located on an abandoned dairy farm. The only building remaining was the old, dilapidated farmhouse, which was frequented by hunters in season. We were brought to the scene in an unmarked police car. The farmhouse was a beehive of police activity, swarming with unmarked police cars and police officers in mufti.

Ordinarily, this region would have been swathed in snow in late November, but the weather had been so unusually mild as to be the subject of much baffled conversation. In lieu of snow, however, Mother Nature provided us with a steady drizzle. The ground had been transformed into a damp sponge, and the entire hillside rising away from the house and nearby well oozed with the product of many days of determined sogginess.

The well was unimpressive at first sight: a clay pipe, some 78 cm in diameter, standing about 30 cm above ground level. Just beneath the surface of the water could be seen a mass of beer cans, rusty food cans, and assorted trash, which would prove to be part of a solid fill to the bottom of the well. It had previously been decided that the best method for attacking the problem would be to dig down adjacent to the well casing, simultaneously draining the water off the well and exposing the casing to view. Then we could smash the casing and remove the fill.

THE FIRST DAY

Following traditional archaeological practice, we established a master datum point on the lip of the well (Fig. 6-1). Such a datum point is "a permanent measuring point for future reference" (Meighan, 1966). This enables reconstruction of the site, as all features and items of importance are located in reference to the datum. The backhoe operator went to work and soon exposed a sizable section of casing. He also dug a ditch to carry off the water.

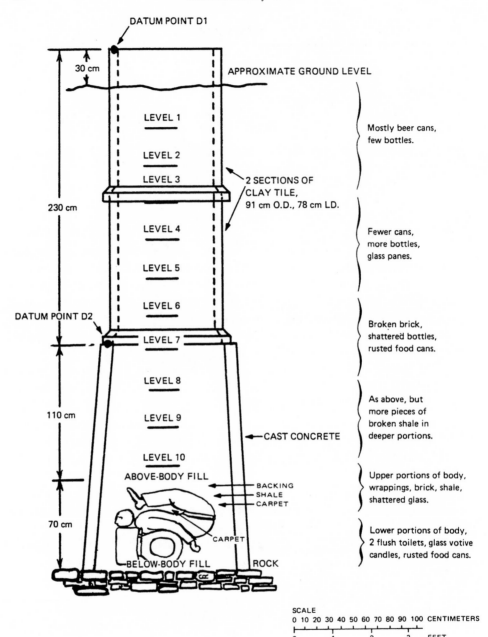

DATUM POINT D1

30 cm

APPROXIMATE GROUND LEVEL

LEVEL 1

Mostly beer cans, few bottles.

LEVEL 2

LEVEL 3

2 SECTIONS OF CLAY TILE, 91 cm O.D., 78 cm I.D.

230 cm

LEVEL 4

Fewer cans, more bottles, glass panes.

LEVEL 5

LEVEL 6

DATUM POINT D2

LEVEL 7

Broken brick, shattered bottles, rusted food cans.

LEVEL 8

As above, but more pieces of broken shale in deeper portions.

110 cm

LEVEL 9

CAST CONCRETE

LEVEL 10

ABOVE-BODY FILL

BACKING
SHALE
CARPET

Upper portions of body, wrappings, brick, shale, shattered glass.

CARPET

70 cm

Lower portions of body, 2 flush toilets, glass votive candles, rusted food cans.

BELOW-BODY FILL   ROCK

SCALE
0 10 20 30 40 50 60 70 80 90 100 CENTIMETERS
0   1   2   3   FEET

Figure 6-1.

Following the archaeologists' "golden rule," to "excavate one layer at a time—and nothing in that layer should escape his or her detection" (Joukowsky, 1980), we worked up one layer at a time. We chose an arbitrary 30 cm layer as the prevailing unit of excavation until we should discover a body. The well proved to be brimming with cultural fill, which, as used here, is defined as Canadian beer bottles and domestic bottles and cans.

To excavate, one of us would slide down into the saturated hole and, perching on the edge of the backhoe scoop, pick and shovel the fill into the scoop. Each handful or shovelful was cursorily inspected in the pit. Then the scoop was raised to the surface, where we washed the dirt through a 1/4 inch screen and sorted and evaluated the fill. A random sample was set aside, bagged, and tagged. This deliberate progress made for slow work, but we wished to work carefully, assessing each layer to gauge its contents. We were ever mindful of Kenyon's constraining, "all excavation is destruction" (1957). We wanted to be sure of finding material of potential importance, and the discovery of a .22 caliber casing in one of the upper layers is evidence of our success. This casing, however, had no direct connection with what was found in the lower levels. Thus, each layer was removed as a unit, evaluated as a unit, and sampled as a unit. Then we would return to the well to break out the next section of clay pipe and recover the next 30 cm of fill.

Anyone who has ever watched an archaeological excavation knows that it is an exacting and slow process (see Hole and Heizer, 1977), and at times the watching throng of newspersons and police became decidedly impatient with our testudinarious pace. However, even the most alacritous archaeologist would have been slowed down by the problems inherent in the excavation of a vertical cylindrical site, some 2 feet in diameter and sheathed in a resistant tube.

Our first day's work (see Fig. 6-1) carried us down to 230 cm of fill (about 7'6"), and at dusk we retired to the farmhouse to review the day's work and to anticipate problems of the morrow.

THE NEWS MEDIA

The news media provide an incessant counterpoint to many forensic investigations. They were fascinated by this spectacle for several reasons. First, the District Attorney (DA) had called in expert help (an expert being defined here as someone from more than 100 miles away). Second, the peculiar mix of two dentists and one anthropologist apparently intrigued and mystified them. Third, perpendicular forensic archaeology is seldom undertaken in such a grand manner, and fourth, the prospect of a body in the well sent them into transports of expectation. The scene had been closed to the public, and armed State Policemen stood guard around the perimeter. The DA, however, took pains to keep the media informed, providing them with background information, progress reports, and numerous statements.

Our work was encapsuled in banner headlines, ran as the top item on the late TV news, and seemed to be second only to the unusually clement weather in the general conversation list of the region. The afternoon of the second day, having been deprived briefly of direct access to the scene, the more enterprising reporters chartered helicopters, which would suddenly loom flup-flupping out of the drizzle, and carefully skirted the periphery with their long lenses focused on the site. They acted as though they felt some danger of being shot down should they venture too close. This brought considerable amusement to the mud-encrusted laborers below.

Curiously, despite all of the media attention, there was never any attempt to interview us beyond our brief introduction to the press by the DA and a couple of subsequent short statements. We were grateful and quite pleased to have been left alone to contemplate late evening repasts after having chipped and rinsed the mud away. We were thus able to review, to plan, and to conduct the work unmolested by the constant attentions of the media. Perhaps this is a regional peculiarity, a willingness not to pry, or perhaps they did not know where we were and had been discouraged by the DA and by those two patrolmen who were always with us.

In this particular instance, the handling of the news media by the District Attorney was exemplary. Given the curiosity of the public and their right to know the nature of the investigations being undertaken, it is entirely appropriate to deal with the media representatives in an open, frank, and forthright manner, providing them with all possible information about what is being done; how, why, by whom, and why it is important that it be done this way. That does not mean that one should call a press conference if he or she feels that a particular forensic investigation has been neglected. Rather, investigations such as these, in the public's behalf, should be characterized by the presence of an informed spokesperson. That individual may be the forensic specialist, or it may be someone else, but the identity of the media contact should be agreed upon in advance, and all communications should be channeled through that person.

Clearly, anticipating the findings of a forensic investigation is hazardous, and such prognostication should be shunned. The media will best be served and the public's interest fulfilled if the media representative states clearly and concisely the goal of the investigation and how that goal is being met. Tidbits of information about the forensic investigators, why they have been called, what they do, and how they do it should round out the information needed for an accurate, informative piece. Genuine concern for helping the media and for assuring their comprehension will repay the investigators many times over in getting the true story out and garnering good will for the forensic profession as a whole.

THE SECOND DAY

Water was constantly being replenished by springs and seeps gurgling down into the great cavity that had grown adjacent to the well and by repeated drizzles through the night. About dawn, the pumps that were manned by police support people shuddered to a stop. Our arrival was greeted by the sight of a brimming lake, which required a couple of hours of hard pumping to reduce to a working level again. In the meantime, we salved our disappointment with a fresh supply of coffee and doughnuts. The proximity of such inexhaustible sustenance made an otherwise grim job much easier to take. As the water level fell, the hole was enlarged further, and equipped with rubber boots, we resumed our progress into the lithosphere.

Having reached the depth at which the clay pipe gave way to a tapering concrete section, we measured in a second datum point, D2. The first datum point, D1, on the lip of the well was to be sacrificed. The shattered segments of pipe teetered precariously above us, and they had to be removed for reasons of safety. Typically a master datum point is sacrosanct and remains inviolate throughout the course of the excavation. Uncommon circumstances call for uncommon solutions, however, hence the establishment of a second datum point 230 cm below and rotated 90° from the first.

About noon, one of the patrolmen spotted the foot and then the left lower leg of a fully clad human body. Long-term submersion in the cold water of the well had formed adipocere (a waxy substance formed when soft tissue decomposes under moist conditions) on the leg. The tibia, uppermost in the well (see Fig. 6-1) was 110 cm below our second datum point D2, or about 11 feet below ground surface. The yawning cavity next to the well was opened up still further, and the backhoe bucket swung to break out a larger area of the well casing, which had changed from a clay tile to poured concrete at datum point D2. The body was protected by a covering while this work was going on. With the discovery of the body, we abandoned our arbitrary level procedure and systematically removed the remainder in two large levels: (1) vicinity of body, and (2) beneath the body.

After the discovery of the body, the area was fully sealed off and not reopened until the body was being removed. At that time, a press conference was convened by the DA on the brink of the abyss. The DA then provided the group of newspersons with an excellent view of the process replete with coroners, pathologists, lawmen, dentists, and anthropologist scurrying around in the waning afternoon light.

Portable lights were set up around the excavation after removal of the body to the morgue. In their yellow glow, we cleared the remaining material from the bottom of the well: two porcelain toilets, a large number of glass votive candle holders, and other miscellany. The final 20 cm of water was being replenished as rapidly as it could be sucked out. Thus the last half hour was spent probing barehanded through the murky and very cold water at the bottom of an immense dank hole, filtering slimy strings of decomposing flesh, a few hand bones, rusted cans and broken glass carefully through our fingers. Night having fallen, and there being some indication that the backhoe was in some danger of following its example, a conference with the patrol chief and the DA unanimously declared the recovery phase to be complete.

CONTENTS OF THE WELL

What follows is a brief summary of the well contents. As noted above, samples were extracted from each level and preserved in numbered plastic bags. In general, the bulk of the fill consisted of beer cans and bottles, broken panes of glass, bits of wood, broken bricks, pieces of shale, and a number of wrappings around the body. Beneath the body were the two toilets, more cans (mostly food cans), and the votive candle holders.

The upper levels contained mostly cans. For example, Level 1 contained a total of 60 cans, 5 bottles, 8 pieces of wood, several pieces of what appeared to be melted glass, and a considerable volume of trash, consisting mostly of glass fragments. By Level 5, there were many more bottles than cans, and much broken glass, but in Level 6 broken bricks began to appear in large numbers. Glass panes, both single and double strength, which began in Level 3, disappeared in Level 6 and were replaced by the first traces of shale. Changes that could be seen in can morphology and certain isolated items gave a hazy picture of the passage of time, though a dating would be less precise than an archaeologist might wish (Watson, 1972). The body itself would furnish little due to the length of immersion. Clothing would be of some value, as pointed out in the now-famous case of the burial of Colonel Shy (Bass, 1978, see Chapter 11), where clothing confirmed the Civil War era.

Directly over the body was a large piece (c. 2 sq. meters) of carpet padding. Around and immediately on top of the body was a plastic wrapping, a number of very large pieces of shale, and a sprinkling of broken brick and shattered glass. The body was resting on its chest with the legs doubled over its back, directly on top of one of the toilets. There was no evidence of any sort of bindings around the body, nor did there appear to have been a binding holding the body to the toilet, but it is difficult to imagine how even a determined group of assassins could have managed to stuff the toilet and body at the same time into the narrow top of the well.

From the juxtaposition of these elements it seems possible to suggest that the body had been tucked into the well and came to rest on the toilet, and then a considerable quantity of shale and brick had been added to keep the body down. Then, for good measure, a carpet pad (perhaps used to transport the body) had been inserted, and additional brick and shale used to secure it. In the intervening ten years or so, the well slowly filled with the accumulated discards of hunters visiting there.

THE AUTOPSY

On Monday, we joined a host of patrolmen and officials to witness the autopsy. The body had been fully extended and radiographs taken. Most of the soft tissue had turned to adipocere. Organs below the diaphragm were recognizable. The x-rays showed the presence of small radiopaque objects in the right upper chest, and dissection revealed defects that were consistent with the entry of a projectile from the rear, between the sixth and seventh ribs, with fracture of the third rib anteriorly in such a way as to suggest bullet exit. Holes in the shirt corresponded with these observations.

We began our detailed dental and anthropological examinations at conclusion of the formal autopsy. We performed the usual analyses, determining age, sex, race, and stature from the bones, a description of the shape of the skull and face, observations of osteoarthritis, skeletal damage (healed nasal bones), and other relevant features useful in establishing the identity of the person. Numerous observations and measurements of the skull and long bones provided the bases for a description as follows: The individual was a male Caucasoid of middle European antecedents, around thirty-five years of age at death, and with a stature of about 5 feet 9 inches. He had a broad head, surmounted by a broad forehead, a face tending toward narrowness, a small chin, and a medium-wide nose.

The teeth were charted. There were no pocket contents, nor were the hands complete enough for fingerprints to be taken. Identity was thereby established on the basis of the agreement of dental and anthropological findings with antemortem records.

On the grounds thus provided by the identification of this murder victim, the credibility of the State's witness was authenticated, and the accuracy of his testimony was verified.

CONCLUSIONS

The involvement of the forensic specialties of odontology and anthropology in a case of this nature is quite unusual and provides a good example of the recovery of a body guided by anthropological practice (Hume, 1969) under rather difficult circumstances (see also Ward and O'Leary, 1959). There is no doubt that the body could have been recovered by the State Police. As in every case where experts are called in, it certainly was a cooperative venture. Without their equipment, a superb backhoe operator, and the able assistance of some of the patrolmen, we might still be digging there. However, we did add important elements to the task.

What did we do that the State Police might not have done? Our presence provided them with three disinterested investigators, unbiased by prior publicity, who had only a scientific interest in either recovering a body or in conclusively demonstrating that no body was present. The employment of outside investigators removed the state agencies dealing with the case from charges of conflict of interest. In approaching the problem as we did (that is, in a painstaking and deliberate fashion), we were able to reconstruct the context later in the same way that an archaeologist reconstructs a site from field notes. As Hume says, "Excavation, no matter how skillfully conducted, is sheer wasted effort unless the results are properly recorded and passed on" (1969). Law enforcement people, rarely trained in archaeology, generally do not think in these terms. However, they can readily appreciate the need for precise control in an excavation as well as in the recovery of evidence from a room (Bass & Birkby, 1978). The complicating factor here is the existence of a third dimension, depth.

In searching carefully through each layer, we were in a position to recover ancillary evidence that might prove important in later analysis. As it happened, the layers above the body could be regarded as "sterile" in the context of the body. Of course, one does not know this before one does the excavation, so, as in archaeology, one has to approach a perpendicular site (or scene) with an open mind and a willingness to interpret continually and to alter methods when confronted with new circumstances.

In the final analysis, the local authorities had the means for excavation of the well and might have accomplished it in much the same manner, that is, by clearing dirt away from the well and breaking the casing down little by little. Under the circumstances prevailing at this scene, the results may have been exactly the same. Nonetheless, if circumstances had been different — an alteration in the nature of the fill, more than one body, the body positioned higher up in the well, etc. — the outcome might have been drastically different.

Thus, in the present case, with the use of a modified archaeological technique and with anthropologists and odontologists working at the scene, the officials had taken all of the right steps to maximize return of information. A forensic excavation is like an archaeological one in that once it has been done, it can never be redone. As Piggott notes, "The excavator bears a very heavy burden of responsibility: as he excavates, he does in fact destroy the site he is excavating" (Piggott, 1959).

REFERENCES

Bass, William (1978). Skeletonization Rates in the Southeast United States. Paper presented at meetings of American Academy of Forensic Sciences.

Bass, William M. and Walter H. Birkby (1978). Exhumation: The method could make the difference. *FBI Law Enforcement Bulletin*, Vol 47, No 7, July, 1978.

Hole, Frank and Roger F. Heizer (1977). *Prehistoric Archaeology*. New York: Holt, Rinehart & Winston.

Hume, Ivor Noel (1969). *Historical Archaeology*. New York: Alfred A. Knopf.

Joukowsky, Martha (1980). *A Complete Manual of Field Archaeology*. Englewood Cliffs: Prentice-Hall, Inc.

Kenyon, Kathleen M. (1957). *Beginning in Archaeology*. New York: Frederick A. Praeger.

Meighan, Clement W. (1966). *Archaeology: An Introduction*. San Francisco: Chandler Publishing Co.

Piggott, Stuart (1959). *Approach to Archaeology*. New York: McGraw-Hill Book Company.

Ward, Charles W. and Timothy J. O'Leary (1959). "A Preliminary Investigation of an Early Man Site in the Delaware River Valley." In *Readings in Anthropology*, Vol. 1. Morton H. Fried, Ed. New York: Thomas Y. Crowell Co.

Watson, P. J. (1972). "Explanations and Models: The Prehistorian as Philosopher of Science and the Prehistorian as Excavator of the Past." In *The Explanation of Culture Change*. C. Renfrew, Ed. London: Duckworth.

Chapter 7

IDENTIFICATION OF NONSKELETONIZED BEAR PAWS AND HUMAN FEET

J. MICHAEL HOFFMAN

The initial question facing the forensic investigator, whether an anthropologist or not, is "Are the remains human?" The forensic physical anthropological literature is filled with studies (e.g. Angel 1974; Stewart 1959, 1979) documenting the skeletal differences of humans and a wide variety of animals—pig, primate, sheep, horse, dog, etc. One of the more difficult problems of skeletal differentiation and identification involves human hands and feet and those of bears, usually the common North American species *Ursus americana*, or black bear.

The literature of the skeletal differences between human and bear hands and feet is rather complete and indicates little diagnostic problem for the trained osteologist (Angel, 1974; Gilbert, 1973; Olsen, 1973; Schmid, 1972; Stewart, 1959, 1979). A bit more difficult, however, might be the identification of fully or nearly fully fleshed appendages of these two mammals, wherein the specific osseous criteria for identification are hidden from direct view. The following case involves such a find.

CASE PRESENTATION

One fall afternoon a resident of Colorado Springs noted the family dog had brought a "meaty-looking" object onto the family's back patio. Since the dog had not recently been given any leftovers, and in the face of a spate of recent neighborhood pet poisonings through tainted meat tossed into backyards, the woman became concerned and investigated closer. The object appeared to her to be a "foot," whereupon she immediately called the Colorado Springs Police Department.

A preliminary search of the neighborhood environs turned up no additional material. The "foot" was brought to a local hospital for examination and identification by a forensic pathologist. Gross anatomical and radiographic examination by the pathologist and a radiologist could not positively rule out the possibility that the specimen was human. The police were concerned

96

because if the specimen was human, this would necessitate an immediate, full-scale search of the neighborhood. The search would have been quite difficult because by that time it was very late at night. I was then contacted and arrived at the hospital shortly before midnight.

The gross specimen was, indeed, a foot that had been sawed and broken off from the lower leg several centimeters above the tibiotalar articulation. Compared to a human adult of "normal" size, the foot appeared rather short (c. 15 cm in length), had little or no discernible arch, and lacked the middle and distal phalanges on all digits. Notable gross anatomical features included—

1. relatively large muscle mass in the immediate region of the tibiotalar articulation;
2. a large plantar pad of fat or adipose tissue;
3. rather deep central grooving of the distal ends of the exposed phalanges; and
4. a "reversed" curvature of the distal row of phalanges, i.e. with fragments of tibia and fibula present the foot was identified as being a left, yet the longest metatarsal and associated digit was on the fibular or lateral side of the foot.

Radiographic examination (anteroposterior and lateral views) supported several features noted grossly and revealed several new things. These included—

1. a very "flat" foot with virtually no longitudinal arch present;
2. an adult (i.e. no epiphyses unfused) foot of very short dimensions;
3. a relatively long (compared to overall foot length), laterally compressed calcaneus of short height;
4. a short anterior projection of the talus, which did not project beyond the anterior surface of the calcaneus;
5. a very short (i.e. total and relative anteroposterior length) distal tarsal region;
6. five rather equally proportioned metatarsals, even though differing in overall length;
7. a well-defined central ridge on the distal ends of each complete metatarsal.

The *combination* of the above anatomical and radiographic features led to the following conclusions the night of the initial examination: (1) The "foot" was not human but (2) was probably the left hind paw of a bear. Definitive identification as bear remains was made the following morning when additional comparative references and materials were available. The police were notified and the case was closed. A request by this author to retain the specimen for inclusion in a comparative collection was granted.

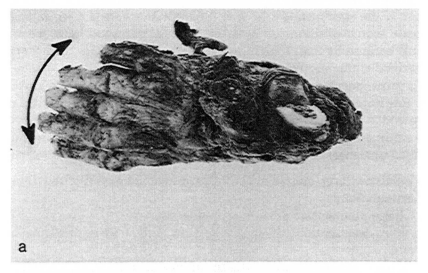

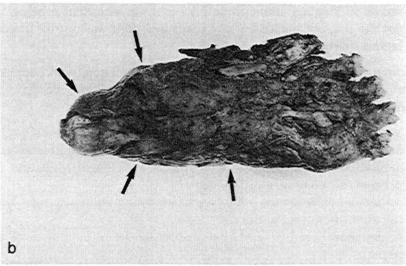

FIGURE 7-1. a. *Left* hindpaw of black bear, *Ursus americana*, superior view. The curve formed by the ends of phalanges makes this appear to be a normal *right* human foot. The lateral surface is at the bottom of the figure, identified by exposure of the sawed and broken surface of the medially located tibia. b. Left hindpaw of bear, plantar surface. Note the large expanse of fat covering the surface and extending onto the sides of the paw.

ANATOMY OF HUMAN AND BEAR FEET

As most of the previously cited authors have noted, many of the distinguishing features of human and bear feet relate to the quite different locomotor patterns exhibited, the former being habitually bipedal while the latter

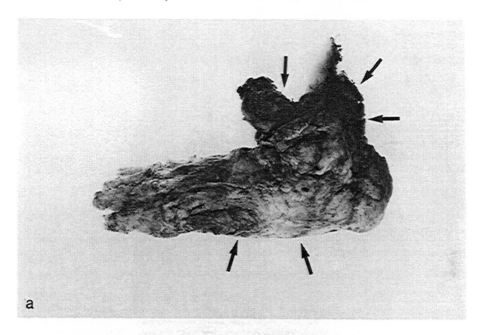

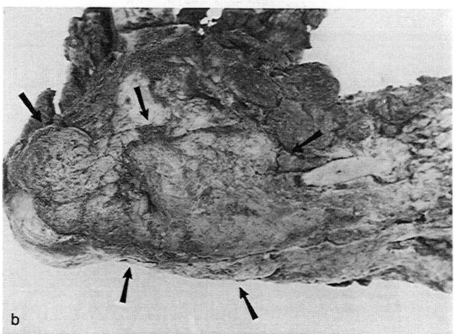

FIGURE 7-2. a. Left hindpaw of bear, lateral surface. Note the large amount of soft tissue in the tibiotalar ("ankle") region and the bulging caused by the plantar fat pad which gives a very "flatfoot" appearance. b. Close-up view of the medioinferior surface of the bear paw to illustrate the continuous extension of fat tissue from plantar to medial (as well as lateral) surfaces, typical of clawed quadrupeds with a large central pad.

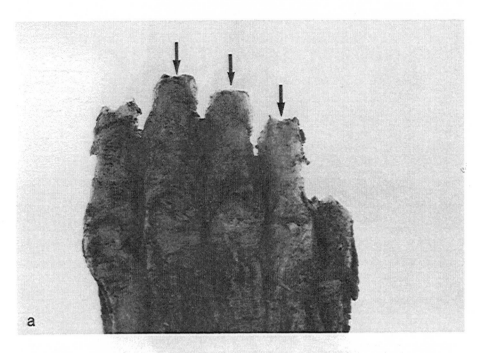

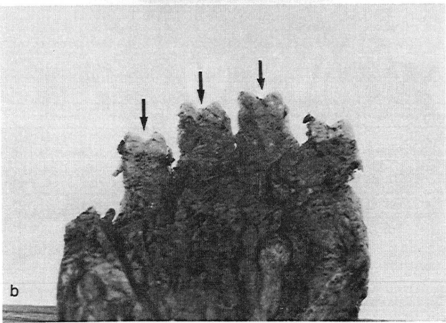

FIGURE 7-3. a. Superior view of the proximal phalangeal row. b. Inferior view of the proximal phalangeal row. Note how much more apparent is the deep central grooving of the exposed phalangeal ends in this view versus that in a.

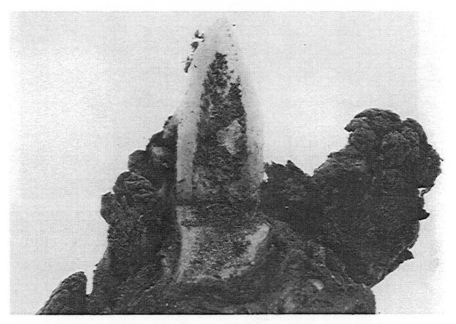

FIGURE 7-4. Close-up view of the sawed and broken tibia, medial view. Again, note the heavy musculature in the surrounding region, which in humans would be mostly tendinous and ligamentous structures.

walks plantigrade with an occasional bipedal stance. The human foot, therefore, is structurally modified to meet the demands of the peculiar striding nature of human bipedality plus weight bearing for the whole organism. These differences are seen in the much greater size and robusticity of the bones of the human foot, especially given the small relative body weight compared with that of the black bear. The larger articular surfaces plus the presence of arches in the human foot also belie the additional flexibility necessary for human bipedal striding. Further details about the evolutionary aspects of human bipedality and structural-functional relations in the human foot appear in Napier (1967), Warwick and Williams (1973), and Wells and Luttgens (1976); bear locomotion is briefly discussed by Vaughan (1972).

Although the definitive identification of this specimen rested with the osseous evidence, there were several major gross anatomical features that ruled out the possibility of human origin, particularly when these features were seen in combination. Among the most important was the presence of the large plantar fat pad covering nearly two-thirds of the central portion of the sole and extending beyond the medial and lateral borders of the foot proper. Humans have some plantar adipose tissue, but it is not nearly as extensive, well demarcated, and thick as in this specimen. The appearance here was the typical one expected in a carnivore having a large central and several distal foot pads.

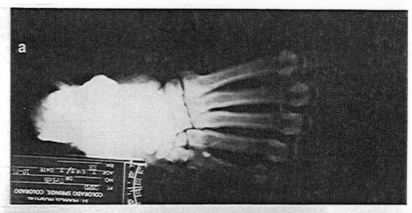

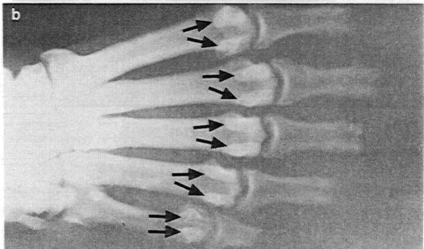

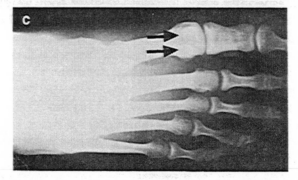

FIGURE 7-5. a. Superior X-ray of the bear paw. b. Close-up of X-ray of the metatarsal and phalangeal region of the bear paw. Note the presence of two sesamoid bones at the distal end of each metatarsal. In comparison, humans consistently have sesamoids only at the distal end of the first metatarsal. c. X-ray of human metatarsal and phalangeal region. Note: (1) lack of sesamoids except at first metatarsal and (2) the shallow grooving of distal surfaces of proximal phalanges in contrast to deep *V*-shaped grooves in the bear, faintly visible in b.

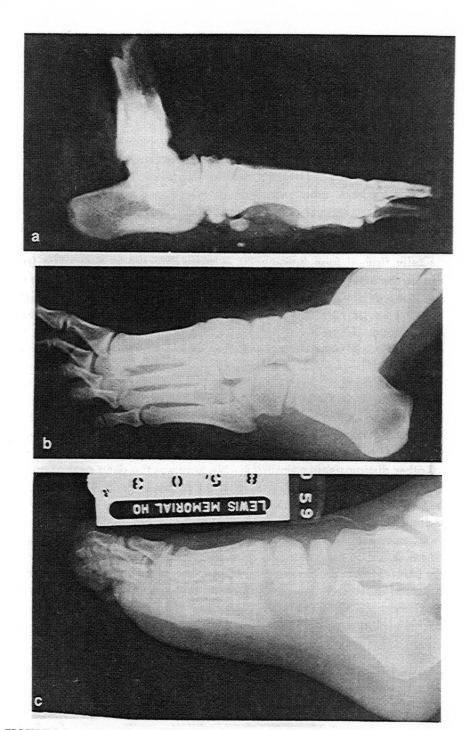

FIGURE 7-6. a. Lateral X-ray of bear paw. Note: (1) foreshortened anterior tarsal region; (2) long, narrow calcaneus; and (3) overall "flatness" of bony structure. b. Lateral x-ray of adult human foot. Note contrasts with structures in a. c. Lateral X-ray of subadult human foot. Note contrasts with structures in a.

The other major gross anatomical feature distinguishing this foot from a typical human was its reversed (left to right) or mirror image appearance. Angel has noted, "The fact that bear toes look like a mirror reversal of human ones is our immediate give away" (Angel, 1964:18). In the human, the first or second toe projects most anteriorly with digits III–IV–V projecting less anteriorly in succession, so that the fifth toe projects the least anteriorly of all the toes. For the most part this is a reflection of the length of the metatarsals in humans, where the second (II) is the longest. The longest metatarsal in the bear is the fourth (IV), a reflection of the bear's walking on the outer edge of its foot to some degree; thus the shortest and least anteriorly projecting digit in the bear is the first (I). We thus understand the basis for Angel's statement regarding the reversed mirror appearance. With a skinned, nearly fully fleshed foot, however, it is more difficult to determine from which side the foot is. Only when we can correctly side the foot can we tell whether the toes' projections are normal or reversed as in the bear. With this specimen, it was an easy task given the presence of the distal ends of both tibia and fibula. Given their normal medial and lateral positions in the lower leg, we could immediately tell that this specimen was from the left side. This made the toes appear reversed and, therefore, like the pattern seen in bears. If the tibia and fibula were not present, we could still correctly side the foot radiographically because of the medial position of the navicular and other anterior tarsal bones. Also, the talus overhangs the medial edge of the foot and is in line with digits I and II in both species, and both have a prominent sustentaculum tali.

The other distinguishing feature visible here was the deep central groove present on the exposed distal ends of the proximal phalanges. This is in marked contrast to the human situation where a groove is present but instead is much shallower and broader.

It was noted that the definitive differential diagnosis lies with the finer structural detail of the individual's bones. Many of these details can be readily identified on a radiograph of suspect specimens. The details of these finer skeletal differences have been well described and illustrated by Angel (1974), Gilbert (1973), Schmid (1972), and Stewart (1959, 1979) and are summarized in outline form in Table 7-I.

SUMMARY AND CONCLUSION

Nonskeletonized bear and human feet can readily be distinguished by any one or a combination of gross anatomical features. Presence of a large, well-demarcated plantar fat pad, heavy musculature in the immediate tibiotalar joint region, reversed or mirror image of curvature of toes or metatarsals,

TABLE 7-I

INDIVIDUAL BONE DIFFERENCES IN HUMAN AND BEAR FEET*

Region	Bone	Differences
Lower Leg	Tibia	Very pronounced medial malleolus in *Homo*; larger circumference (distally) relative to overall size of foot in *Homo*
Tarsus	Talus	Neck of talus is long in *Homo*, short in *Ursus*; lateral tubercle (= posterior talar process) typically present in *Homo*, absent in *Ursus*; posterior calcaneal articular surface mediolaterally oriented in *Homo*, antero-posteriorly oriented in *Ursus*
	Calcaneus	Much narrower (side to side) in *Ursus*; posterior projection beyond talus — relatively shorter and higher in *Homo*, longer and lower in *Ursus*

Remaining tarsal bones have much the same position and relative size to one another in both *Homo* and *Ursus*, but compared with *Ursus* those in *Homo* are relatively larger to the foot as a whole.

Region	Bone	Differences
Metatarsus	MTI	Much thicker and rugged compared to metatarsals II-V in *Homo*; same overall size and proportions relative to others in *Ursus*
	MTII	Longest foot bone in *Homo*
	MTIV	Longest foot bone in *Ursus*
	All	Distal ends more "sculptured" in *Ursus*, more smoothly rounded in *Homo*; usually a pair of sesamoids at each distal, plantar surface in *Ursus*, fewer and less consistent in *Homo*
Digits	Proximal Phalanges	Notched proximal-plantar edge in *Ursus*; distal ends more deeply grooved in *Ursus*, groove broader and shallower in *Homo*
	Middle Phalanges	Proximal-plantar edge notched in *Ursus* as above; concave flexor surface in *Homo*, concave extensor surface in *Ursus*
	Distal Phalanges	Flattened with "tufted" distal ends in *Homo*; rarely present in skinned bear specimens, remain attached to claws in skin

*Summarized from Angel (1974), Gilbert (1973), Schmid (1972), and Stewart (1959, 1979).

and distinctive distal ends of both metatarsals and phalanges all serve to distinguish bear hind paws from human feet. Definitive diagnosis is made with analysis of fine skeletal detail seen radiographically or after skeletonization, either partial or complete, of specimens.

Regarding why such remains turn up in the first place, Stewart (1959, 1979) has detailed the process for the interested reader. His remarks are fully supported by my discussions with local hunters.

The final question of why these remains cause such a problem for some investigators is summed up succinctly and directly by Brues:

The medical school curriculum allows very little time for the study of the skeleton, and the medical graduate has only a casual acquaintance with bones. The error most commonly made by the doctor is to identify an animal bone as human, not realizing how similar bones of different species may be in general outline. . . . In all cases correct judgement could be made instantly by a person who was thoroughly familiar with the human skeleton. *Experience is the essence of recognizing bones; it is as easy for the expert as it is impossible for the beginner.* [Emphasis added] (Brues, 1958:554)

REFERENCES

Angel, J. Lawrence (1974). Bones can fool people. *FBI Law Enforcement Bulletin, 43(1)*:16–20, 30.

Brues, Alice M. (1958). Identification of skeletal remains. *Journal of Criminal Law, Criminology and Police Science, 48(5)*:551–563.

Gilbert, B. Miles (1973). *Mammalian Osteo-Archaeology: North America.* Columbia: Missouri Archaeological Society.

Napier, John (1967). The antiquity of human walking. *Scientific American, 216(4)*:56–66.

Olsen, Stanley J. (1973). Mammal Remains from Archaeological Sites. Part I: Southeastern and Southwestern United States. Papers of the Peabody Museum of Archaeology and Ethnology 56(1).

Schmid, E. (1972). *Atlas of Animal Bones.* New York: Elsevier Publishing Co.

Stewart, T. D. (1959). Bear paw remains closely resemble human bones. *FBI Law Enforcement Bulletin, 28(11)*:18–21.

———(1979). *Essentials of Forensic Anthropology.* Springfield: Charles C Thomas.

Vaughan, Terry A. (1972). *Mammology.* Philadelphia: W. B. Saunders Co.

Warwick, Roger and Peter L. Williams (Eds.) (1973). *Gray's Anatomy*, 35th British ed. Philadelphia: W. B. Saunders Co.

Wells, Katharine F. and Kathryn Luttgens (1976). *Kinesiology: Scientific Bases of Human Motion*, 6th ed. Philadelphia: W. B. Saunders Co.

Chapter 8

THE BIG THOMPSON FLOOD*

MICHAEL CHARNEY AND CHARLES G. WILBER

On the weekend beginning 31 July 1976, the centennial celebration in Colorado was in high gear. Numerous persons and groups of tourists were enjoying the natural attractions of the famous Big Thompson Canyon located in the front range of the Rocky Mountains in northern Colorado. The Canyon carries along its bottom the Big Thompson River, originating in Rocky Mountain National Park and flowing down through the canyon for 25 miles until it runs out into the high plains at the town of Loveland.

A severe thunderstorm system, on 30 July, became immobilized over Rocky Mountain National Park and within four hours poured down 14 inches of rain. The average annual rainfall in Colorado is about 10 to 15 inches. Hence, in this four-hour period the equivalent of one year's rainfall descended, causing a water flow, at peak flood through the canyon, of 40,000 cubic feet per second. The average normal flow is 84 cubic feet per second.

At 9:30 PM during the evening of Saturday, 31 July, a wall of water 19 feet high moved down the canyon, causing astonishing destruction. At about 12:30 AM that same night an even higher wave of water surged down the canyon.

Man-made structures were destroyed. Automobiles, trailers, and campers were demolished. Soot, silt, and sand buried debris, automobiles, and victims. The silt reached depths of 5 or 6 feet.

As soon as the floodwaters subsided on 1 August 1976, body recovery began. A total of 139 bodies were finally recovered; half of these were found during the first week after the waters subsided (Wilber, 1979).

Bodies were whole or partly fragmented; mud, soot, and silt camouflaged many of them *in situ*. Most bodies, as recovered, were not recognizable. Sand and silt had to be washed from the surface of each body and even the body cavities before identification could begin.

Refrigerated trucks were used as morgue storage crypts. The Union Pacific Railroad sent four refrigerated boxcars, which were kept on a siding until the situation clarified as to the expected number of victims.

How long did it take to identify the bodies? Thirty percent were identified

*Reprinted/adapted from *American Journal of Forensic Medicine and Pathology*, 1(2):139–144. Courtesy of Masson Publishing USA, Inc., New York, N.Y.

within one day after recovery: 49 percent within two days; 56 percent within three days; 75 percent within seven days.

BODY IDENTIFICATION METHOD

At the outset, Charney said that there would be no mass viewing of the bodies. Quite apart from the severe emotional shock such a procedure would inflict on already grieving relatives of the missing, it was felt that no identifications would ensue. Gas gangrene had already set in, and the bloated faces bore little resemblance to the features of the victims when they were alive. What people recognize are the clothing; however, the bodies were all naked. Allen, a forensic pathologist and co-director of the temporary morgue, concurred with this approach.

The identification procedure used began with the interview of families for pertinent data as to body description down to such minutae as scars, moles, and anomalies. Carefully noted would be the names of the dentist and physician. This task the Larimer County Mental Health Clinic personnel did admirably. They exercised tenderness, solicitude, and a gentle insistence that brought out the myriad of details that made for identification. The overall identification procedure was as follows:

1. Charney and Allen together, or separately if one was away, made the examination of the body while one of the nurses recorded the details.

2. Lt. Col. Morlang, Air Force Dental Officer, and the local dentists on hand did the same for the teeth.

3. Comparison was then made against the data furnished by the families. These data were broken down by separate category for children, for sexes, and for age in decades. The records personnel were instructed to check the body description information in the age set and also in the decade bracket lower and higher to cover the borderline age individuals. The use of the computer in this effort will be discussed later.

4. When a match was made, and similar sex, age, height, weight, and any other pertinent information checked, Charney and Allen took over the search for the trait or traits that individually, personally identified the body.

The identification picture had to be a total one. In other words, the characteristic that made for an identification, such as similar dental restoration, tattoo, and sinus prints, had to belong to a person answering the sex, race, age, height, and weight of the person. No identification trait was permitted to stand alone. As Morlang remarked, identification was a team effort of the forensic pathologist, the forensic odontologist, and the forensic anthropologist. This team effort, initiated at the start, was responsible for the identification of all 139 bodies.

Dental records accounted for 25 percent of the individualizing traits.

Physical traits, scars of previous operations, tattoos, anomolies such as hammertoes, overlapping toes, x-rays revealing old fractures, distinct jewelry, nail polish on hands and feet that matched with details brought in by the family—combinations of all these accounted for some 65 percent of the identifications. Ear comparison with photographs and home movies allowed for two identifications, those of a five-year-old boy and a man of fifty-five years. Sinus prints and similar skull outline with an older x-ray identified a man of eighty-six years who was reduced to bone with the facial skeleton missing. One lad of seventeen years had a beebee embedded in his hand from an accidental discharge of two years previous.

Fingerprints identified three victims of the flood and might have been more effective in the identification process but for the action of the morticians who, in their cleaning of the bodies before forwarding them to the morgue, scrubbed away the friable skin over the fingers. It is strongly recommended that the mortician, if used in a mass disaster morgue operation, be under the strict control of the morgue director and not act independently as was the case at the Big Thompson scene.

Information on fingerprints did help to confirm identification in some 30 percent of the bodies. It should not be assumed that this confirmation is of little value, for the legal aspects of such a disaster continue for many months. Such confirmatory evidence will have a buttressing effect, especially where there are insurance implications.

TYPES OF TRAUMA

Few of the recovered bodies in the Big Thompson disaster exhibited signs of simple drowning. The spectrum of injuries included multiple fractures, bodies ripped apart, extremities torn from torsos, bruises, abrasions, and avulsion injuries. Many massive blunt injuries caused by floating logs, automobiles, and propane gas tanks were observed. Postmortem lacerations were common.

With the passage of weeks, decomposition was rapid, and data as to sex, age, race, height and weight were obtained in many cases from the bones.

SOME METHODOLOGY

The use of a computer for matching the characteristics of the bodies recorded at autopsy with information obtained from family, friends, and dental and medical records could have been critical. Hewlett Packard did send in a table model computer and the personnel to use it. However, the instrument was used in the main for keeping track of the missing persons.

Over 4,500 were so reported. Five up-to-date bulletins were published daily for the first month. This left only six inputs for identification work. Morlang ran the dental effort by visual comparison. Future morgue operations will certainly see the computer used to its full capacity, with one program for the body data and one for the dental. There are at least three such programs for the dental traits now in publication and several for the body. As has been mentioned, the use of mass lineup of bodies for friends and next of kin to pass along and pick out remains that they can identify is barbaric and ineffective. This was proven at the Big Thompson morgue when two people were permitted to view all the bodies. One was a physician who had grown up in Loveland where his father is also a physician and who claimed to "know everyone." The other was the postmistress of Drake, a hamlet at the confluence of the Big Thompson Rivers. After two days of viewing they recognized no one.

Individual viewings of presentable bodies, generally the face only, that had been cleaned up was resorted to in obtaining confirmation of identification. This procedure was not possible after the second week.

WHY THE CENTER WAS ESTABLISHED

The establishment of the Center of Human Identification at Colorado State University is an attempt to bring some order into the chaotic state of body identification. None of our states nor the federal government has any laws or acts relating to human body identification. Who shall do the analysis of human remains and who is responsible for the study are left up in the air. It is commonly assumed that the coroner or medical examiner is the responsible official, but the statutes establishing these two positions make no mention whatsoever of body identification! The coroner and medical examiner shall determine the cause and manner of death in an unattended death, a death under suspicious circumstances, or a homicide. Thus, one must read the various state statutes.

Where law enforcement agencies involved cannot establish the identification of a body by the usual routine methods, they turn for assistance to the scientific community that they know: the coroner, the medical examiner, the dentist. The medical examiners are essentially pathologists. For all their expertise, they are not conversant with all the factors that go into body identification. The coroners, too frequently, are morticians or other nonscientists.

The dental profession renders the greatest service in the body identification process through dental restoration comparison. However, according to statistics from the dental societies, only some 40 percent of the American public sees a dentist. Where does that leave body identification? Where does that leave the law enforcement agency that has the ultimate responsibility?

Too often do we hear that the police have been advised to bury a body when the dental input was of no avail. Remedies to these hard facts were included in a paper delivered at the Pan-American Conference on the Forensic Aspects of Anthropology, Dentistry, Pathology and Paleopathology, Mexico City, in November 1977. Subsequently the presentation was published (Charney, 1978).

Remedies to the existing chaotic situation were offered in a plea for the formation of a central agency where the services of all the forensic scientists (notably the pathologist, odontologist, and anthropologist) would be available to any and all police agencies faced with the identification of a single case or of many as in a mass disaster.

A TEAM EFFORT

The concept of a team approach to body identification, rather than reliance on the wisdom of a single person such as a medical examiner, has been voiced by Reals and Cowan (1979) in their paper on the Teneriffe air crash. In this article they made a plea for the formation of a national response agency for mass disasters and that this response be a team effort.

Since the temporary morgue effort and body identification endeavor of the Big Thompson flood tragedy of the summer of 1976, Charney has been pleading for the formation on a national scale of a center that would make available teams of forensic experts in future mass disasters. Such a team would be used in mass disasters and also in the everyday cases that law enforcement agencies face with unidentified bodies.

MISSING PERSONS

Quite apart from the very vital need for an organized team effort in body identification in mass disasters, another aspect of identification remains a most trying problem to law enforcement agencies at all levels, from the federal to the local. This problem is the identification of individual cases of unknown bodies against the missing persons lists. At present, there is no country-wide organized approach to such identification; the FBI and the NCIC are working on it. However, it appears that they are concerned, in the main, with the type of body data that can be put on computer: morphological description, dental restorations, etc. Many identifications can be made by techniques that do not lend themselves to computerization, at least for the present. Think of morphological comparison of photographs of ears, teeth, x-rays of any part of the body, including sinuses. Such comparisons proved themselves in the identification of some of the bodies of the Big Thompson flood tragedy.

It is proposed that some facility be a repository for photographs, x-rays, home movies, etc. from families who report such missing persons. The facility can then work closely with all law enforcement agencies in an all-out attack on the identification process rather than the piecemeal effort now in force.

Such an all-out effort is not possible today because of the very fragmentation of identification work and the lack of a central agency that can collate all the work done by any local agency and can bring all the identification aids spelled out above.

THE NEED FOR A NATIONAL SYMPOSIUM

From 9 to 11 December 1968, a symposium in Personal Identification in Mass Disasters was held in Washington, D.C., under the auspices of the U.S. Army Support Services and the Smithsonian Institution. This effort resulted in a fine publication by the Smithsonian (Stewart, 1970). It is now time for another such symposium with a large portion of the event devoted to the problems not tackled at the 1968 meeting. These problems are spelled out in this chapter: Who shall do body identification? What should be done about state and federal statutes that do not now exist on this subject? Should the coroner and medical examiner take an active part in body identification? If so, can we tolerate the destructive input of the many morticians who are coroners and deputy coroners? Can a step be taken towards the establishment of a team endeavor of forensic specialists available, upon need, to all levels of legal jurisdiction?

REFERENCES

Charney, M. (1978). The temporary morgue and identification of bodies. *Police Chief 45.* *10*:285–288.

Reals, W. J. and Cowan, W. R. (1979). Forensic pathology and mass casualities. *Human Pathology, 10(2)*:133–136.

Stewart, T. D. (Ed.) (1970). *Personal Identification in Mass Disasters*. National Museum of Natural History, Washington, D.C.

Wilber, C. G. (Ed.) (1979). *1978 Potpourri of Environmental Pathology*. The Forensic Foundation, Rockville, MD., 71 pp. plus 179 2 × 2 slides.

Chapter 9

IDENTIFICATION OF MILITARY REMAINS
Field and Laboratory Problems

CHARLES P. WARREN

INTRODUCTION

During the recent involvement of American armed forces in Southeast Asia, one of the many problems facing the military in its efforts to locate, recover, identify, and repatriate battle casualties was the need to distinguish deceased American personnel from the military and civilian war dead of allied and enemy groups. This task was accomplished routinely in the U.S. Army Central Identification Laboratory, Camp Samae San, Thailand. Warren (1978a, 1978b, 1981) has described in great detail the procedures of the laboratory; in summary, each set of remains that underwent processing in the laboratory required (1) a thorough examination by an identification specialist (a licensed embalmer who had received additional training in military identification) and a forensic anthropologist; (2) a complete set of highly detailed case papers (including photographs and radiographs); (3) a search of the records in the files of the laboratory for possible associations; and (4) a satisfactory resolution of the case (Fig. 9-1). All of the procedures described above were required for each case regardless of the status of the individual being processed—American, Vietnamese or other nationality, friend or foe, military or civilian, battle casualty or former occupant of a mistakenly disturbed cemetery.

In an effort to reduce the number of cases generated by the introduction of unselected remains into the processing mechanisms of the laboratory, several alternatives were tested. First, the military personnel who were engaged in search and recovery activities were given additional training in the techniques of artifact recognition and discrimination. Particular attention was given to appraising and analyzing the artifacts that generally accompanied the remains, since similar uniforms and common field equipment being used by both American and allied troops reduced the discriminating qualities of clothing and equipment.

Second, when a plane crash was located, rather than bring the entire

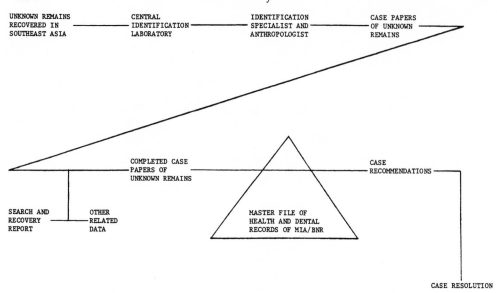

Figure 9-1. Flowchart of the processing of unknown remains recovered in Southeast Asia.

aggregate of recovered anatomical parts to the laboratory in Thailand for segregation and reassembling, a forward operations base was established in the Republic of Viet Nam so as to be closer to the sites of recoveries and to allow for a preliminary processing of the remains. This forward operations base was staffed by trained personnel from the Central Identification Laboratory, Thailand. The laboratory personnel determined what remains (or portions of remains) were to be transshipped to the laboratory in Thailand after a preliminary viewing of the remains. The following report is an account of one such effort.

HISTORY OF THE OPERATION

On 7 June 1974, an American major assigned as an Advisory Desk Officer to Military Region I, Republic of Viet Nam, received information from a group of Vietnamese woodcutters about an aircraft they had discovered in a heavily wooded region on Hai Van Peninsula, north of Da Nang, Republic of Viet Nam. The woodcutters had seen a number of remains that included skulls and limb bones. They had returned with eight tape cassettes and a microphone from the wreckage, which they gave to the major. It was tentatively concluded that the cassettes belonged to an American.

On 12 June, Mr. Tai, Joint Casualty Resolution Center Operations Specialist, briefed the woodcutters on map reading, aircraft identification procedures, precautions concerning the handling of remains, and the possibility that explosives might be associated with the remains (Warren, 1977). Emphasis was placed on the two primary goals, locating the site and identifying the aircraft. After further briefing on the use of the Polaroid® camera, the group of woodcutters departed to charter a boat and head for the site. Sufficient funds ($58.00) were paid to the group for rations and boat rental for three days.

Because of a storm, the anticipated return of the woodcutters was delayed. The party returned on 17 June with an assortment of aircraft parts, personal effects, Polaroid photos, and a map marking the site. An assortment of identification cards with names indicated the presence of at least one American and two Vietnamese victims of the plane crash. Personal papers, a notebook, three handguns, and three hunting knives were also recovered. The Polaroid photographs revealed the aircraft to be a U-17 with the tail number 67-14502. At this time the woodcutters were paid an additional $115.00 to compensate them for five days lost wages and to cover an additional amount that had been demanded by the boat owner for the charter of the boat for two additional days.

The woodcutters were asked how they knew the American authorities might be interested in their discovery of the crash site. Mr. Cu, the leader of the group, indicated that since he was a reserve soldier, he knew that he should report this discovery immediately to someone. Furthermore, he had heard a Joint Casualty Resolution Center radio broadcast asking for information concerning missing human remains. One of the younger helpers said that he knew that the information should be reported because he had seen a TV broadcast requesting casualty resolution information. He gave a detailed and accurate description of both the TV visual and spoken messages.

Further recovery efforts were then coordinated with the Army personnel of the Republic of Viet Nam, and on 26 June 1974 a recovery party consisting of three Vietnamese officers, a squad of enlisted personnel, and two woodcutters departed from Da Nang for the crash site. The party returned on 27 June with the recovery.

As part of the plan to establish a forward operations base, on 11 June the commanding officer of the Central Identification Laboratory, Thailand and one of his noncommissioned officers traveled to the Republic of Viet Nam via Saigon to establish a forward operations base at Nha Trang and to pick up an aggregate of remains that had been recovered from a C-123 crash site in Khanh Hoa Province. In the meantime a crash site of a Navy C-47 had been located in Ninh Thuan Province, and these remains and personal effects were delivered to the commanding officer at Than Rang. The remains from both provinces then were brought to Nha Trang. On 14 June the chief of the laboratory, several search and recovery personnel, and I (the forensic anthropologist) were flown from Thailand to Nha Trang via Saigon with the laboratory equipment and supplies. Processing of the remains in

Nha Trang was initiated at the Central Identification Laboratory forward operations base, and a temporary laboratory was set up in an empty room of the American Consulate building. As the processing of the remains progressed, inquiry revealed that the naval aircraft had crashed on 10 March 1967 with four U.S. Navy crewmembers and twenty-four American and Vietnamese passengers aboard. Search and recovery missions had been conducted on 11 and 22 March 1967, twenty-seven of the twenty-eight casualties had been recovered, and all of the recoveries were subsequently identified. Thus, there was still one individual whose name, nationality, and status were unknown and who presumably was missing. After four and one-half days of examining these remains (17 bags of assorted anatomical parts), it was concluded that the unidentified remains should be sent to the Central Identification Laboratory in Thailand where the identification specialists would have access to the complete records of the incident.

On 26 June I emplaned for Da Nang via Saigon to examine the remains reportedly recovered from the crash site of the U-17 aircraft. I initially examined the remains in Da Nang during the afternoon of the same day at the mortuary of the Army of the Republic of Viet Nam Military Hospital. The remains were packaged in five bags, four plastic and one paper. Upon examination I discovered that each bag contained the commingled portions of several individuals. A preliminary field segregation revealed the presence of three skulls: one with a broken mandible; one minus the occipital bone; and one with shattered facial bones. This information established the presence of at least three individuals. No documents were made available to me at that time, but from the verbal accounts of the aircraft passenger manifest and the personal effects that were reported to have accompanied the remains, it had been presumed by the officials in charge that the three individuals represented by the remains were an American officer and two Republic of Viet Nam officers.

Further examination of the remains and their containers revealed that all of the personal effects that the recovery teams had brought back to Da Nang had been removed from the remains, and the identification cards and other name-bearing belongings of the presumed American casualty then had been forwarded to Nakon Phanom, Thailand, the headquarters of the Joint Casualty Resolution Center. These acts were contrary to good identification procedures.

Under these conditions it was impossible, then, to establish a "BTB" (believed-to-be) identification of any of the remains. Faced with this very serious error—the removal of the objects that provided leads to the names of the individuals—I decided that it was necessary to take all of the remains to the Central Identification Laboratory in Thailand for complete segregation and identification.

In spite of my decision, the Republic of Viet Nam officials in charge requested the Joint Casualty Resolution officials to release the remains of the two Republic of Viet Nam officers to them so that the remains could be returned quickly to the Vietnamese next-of-kin. This required an effort on my part to further separate the commingled parts of the two Vietnamese remains from the remains of the American (assuming that only three individuals were involved) and to identify the two Vietnamese remains by name. To accomplish this I needed the records of the physical characteristics of the individuals listed on the aircraft manifest to verify the reconstruction of the individuals and to establish positive identification. However, the physical records of the Vietnamese servicemen that had been promised by the authorities in Da Nang had not been given to me.

There were other observable major discrepancies. As stated above, the remains were commingled, even though Captain Thinh, one of the recovery officers, said that he had made an attempt to keep the individuals segregated. The skulls had been switched by someone, possibly the woodcutters. There were four pairs of boots and one pair of low-cut shoes (Captain Thinh stated that these possibly had been worn by the pilot). One pair of boots was marked "Hanh." This was the pilot's name as reported by the Vietnamese officials. I also noted that major portions of all of the skeletons were missing, and the eroded condition of the ends of the long bones prevented the reassembling of unique remains by articulation; most rearrangements of skeletal parts possible to make in the field had to depend upon comparisons of relative bone length, not articulation.

Being aware that the releasing of commingled remains without further processing was a poor identification procedure to follow, I convinced the Republic of Viet Nam officials that a more scientific segregation of the remains could be accomplished at the Central Identification Laboratory in Thailand and that positive identification of the remains only could be accomplished in the laboratory, since all items that bore names had been removed from the remains and forwarded to the Joint Casualty Resolution Center headquarters in Thailand. The Republic of Viet Nam officials were reluctant, but they finally agreed to leave all of the remains in the care of the American identification personnel, provided the Vietnamese remains were returned to the Republic of Viet Nam within two weeks.

The political implications of the recovery and identification of the remains became clear during the following days. To honor officially the transferral of the remains of the American officer from the custody of the Republic of Viet Nam government to the government of the United States of America, a formal remains turnover ceremony was conducted at Da Nang Air Base at 1100 hours on 28 June 1974. The ceremony was attended by a number of ranking officers and prominent civilian representatives of the two allied governments involved, as well as by representatives of the local province and city. Newspaper, radio, and TV coverage was provided by members of the local and international newscasting agencies. Proceedings were conducted in an atmosphere of dignity and solemnity that the occasion demanded.

Following the ceremony, the remains, accompanied by the laboratory personnel and the Joint Casualty Resolution Center and Republic of Viet Nam Air Force escorts, were transported via an Air America C-47 to Tan Son Nhut Air Base, Saigon. That evening they were placed aboard a C-130 military aircraft and flown to U-Tapao Royal Thai Air Force Base, Thailand. The remains were then trucked to the Central Identification Laboratory and logged in at 2300 on 28 June. Since other recoveries also had been made during the time that the laboratory team was in Viet Nam, the three sets of remains from the U-17 crash were assigned Evac Numbers THCIL 0058-74 through 0060-74.

In subsequent official reports it was opined that the entire activity was well planned and most effectively implemented. Further, the coordination and cooperation extended by both the military and civilian elements of the governments of the United States of America and the Republic of Viet Nam were truly outstanding. In addition, the major who had supervised the recovery (and who also removed the identification cards) was given high praise and recognition for his consistently superior duty performance. Overall, it was felt that this activity well exemplified the positive casualty resolution results that could be achieved when United States and Vietnamese officials worked harmoniously in an atmosphere of candor and cooperation. No mention was made of (1) the mixing of the anatomical parts upon recovery, (2) the deliberate removal of the personal effects and identification cards from the remains, or (3) the exerting of undue pressures on the identification team by the authorities to make positive identifications of the remains using incomplete data.

Following routine procedures, the remains and the personal effects were simultaneously processed in the Central Identification Laboratory in Thailand. After rectifying the major and minor discrepancies, the following associations were established from records provided by the laboratory and the Republic of Viet Nam officials (see Table 9-I):

    a. 0058-74, BTB Quamo, George,
    b. 0059-74, BTB Nhan, Nguyen Van,
    c. 0060-74, BTB Hanh, Nguyen Ngoc.

The Vietnamese remains, positively identified, were returned to the Republic of Viet Nam within the two-week period as promised. The case papers of the American officer were accepted as an individual identification by the

TABLE 9-I
COMPARISONS BETWEEN LABORATORY FINDINGS (L) AND
RECORDED PHYSICAL CHARACTERISTICS (R) OF THREE RELATED CASES

Characteristic	0058-74 BTB Quamo, George	0059-74 BTB Nhan, Nguyan Van	0060-74 BTB Hanh, Nguyen Ngoc
Sex	(L) Male	(L) Male	(L) Male
	(R) Male	(R) Male	(R) Male
Race	(L) Caucasoid	(L) Mongoloid	(L) Mongoloid
	(R) Caucasoid	(R) Mongoloid	(R) Mongoloid
Dentition	(L) Conclusive	(L) Inconclusive	(L) Inconclusive
	(R) Matching	(R)	(R)
Age	(L) 24–27y	(L) 25–30y	(L) 22–25y
	(R) 27y 9m 24d	(R) 27y 2m 21d	(R) 21y 9m 24d
Stature	(L) 67.4" (FEMUR + TIBIA)	(L) 64.3" (TIBIA)	(L) 65.7" (FEMUR + FIBULA)
	(R) 69"	(R) 63.8"	(R) 65.7"
Hair Color	(L) None Found	(L) None Found	(L) None Found
	(R) Brown	(R) Not Recorded	(R) Not Recorded
Healed Fractures & Bone Malformations	(L) Exostosis on right tibia above tuberosity; possible old injury of left tibia, proximal third	(L) None Found	(L) None Found
	(R) Not Recorded	(R) Not Recorded	(R) Not Recorded
Osteological Evidence of Cause of Death	(L) Severe trauma of right side of mandible, left scapula, and rib cage; portions of upper and lower limbs, shoulder and pelvic girdles, and vertebral column missing	(L) Severe trauma of bones of face and postcranial skeleton; portions of upper limb bones missing	(L) Severe trauma of skull, appendicular long bones, and pelvic girdle; portions of long bones missing

Department of the Army, Washington, D.C., on 15 August 1974 (Helgesen, 1974).

DISCUSSION

After the occurrence of military mass disasters, as exemplified by this case, as well as in civilian mass disasters, there is a serious lack of understanding and awareness of the need for maintaining an unbroken continuum of association of the human remains recovered and the identification documents that are found with them. This lack of understanding and awareness occurs at all levels of the recovery, the transportation, and the laboratory examination of the remains and their accompanying artifacts, but throughout the period reported it was most serious during the intermediate stages of the recovery and handling of the remains prior to their delivery to the Central Identification Laboratory, Thailand.

Some observations that are applicable to the handling of remains and their associated artifacts during times of disaster have been drawn from the reported efforts in the Republic of Viet Nam. First, it is feasible neither to attempt to segregate commingled remains nor to make tentative identifications at a forward operations base, especially in those cases involving a large number of casualties. Imposed staff, space, and time limitations require deviations from acceptable laboratory procedures and protocol, and these shortcuts invite errors and omissions. Second, there is a tendency for personnel who come in contact with remains to remove the personal effects that may lead to identification of the individual. It cannot be stressed too strongly that these items must accompany the remains to the processing laboratory, along with all other applicable documents (Warren, 1978b). Furthermore, unnecessary handling of the remains and attempts to examine and segregate commingled portions by other than laboratory personnel should strongly be discouraged. These field examinations serve no useful purpose, and the possible contamination of the remains and the identification artifacts—or loss of portions thereof—places the laboratory personnel at a disadvantage during subsequent processing of the remains.

In predisaster planning, whether military or civilian, additional instruction should be given to all personnel responsible for recovering remains, stressing the importance of maintaining an unbroken linkage of the personal effects with the remains, from the time of recovery to the receipt of the remains in the processing laboratory. If untrained personnel are enlisted to recover the remains and the accompanying artifacts from the scene of a mass disaster, contamination of the site and the recoverables will inevitably occur. However, after the remains are turned over to the authorities, military or civilian, then all efforts should be expended to maintain the integrity of the recovery from the time of the turnover through the final identification.

REFERENCES

Helgesen, H. T. (1974). Status Summary. Typescript Manuscript, Department of the Army, U.S. Central Identification Laboratory, Sattahip, Thailand, 1 November.

Warren, C. P. (1977). Field forensic anthropology: The excavation of human remains under adverse conditions. *Proceedings of the Indiana Academy of Science for 1976, 86*:104–109.

———— (1978a). Personal identification of human remains: An overview. *Journal of Forensic Sciences, 23*(2):388–395.

———— (1978b). Forensic anthropology—Theory and practice. *Proceedings of the Indiana Academy of Science for 1977, 87*:83–89.

———— (1981). Forensic anthropology in a military setting. *Human Organization, 40*(2):172–180.

Chapter 10

THE CASE OF THE SEVERED SKULL*
Individuation in Forensic Anthropology

JANE E. BUIKSTRA, CLAIRE C. GORDON, AND LUCILE ST. HOYME

INTRODUCTION

Individuation is a problem frequently faced by the forensic anthropologist. Body parts may become dispersed in mass disasters, as a result of fortuitous postmortem events, or by criminal intent. In any of these circumstances, the forensic anthropologist is likely to be called upon to present arguments concerning the minimum number of decedents and the probable association of remains that may represent one individual.

Anthropologists have responded to the challenge of individuation with varied strategies. Krogman's text (1962) contains a chapter on individuation that emphasizes such topics as postmortem alterations because of bone desiccation, age/sex differences in the rib and sternum, and bone density. Stewart (1979) emphasizes the special problems presented by commingled remains and includes a critique of Baker and Newman's (1957) strategy for sorting based upon dry bone weights. Snow and Luke (1970) and Snow and Folk (1970) have published a technique for estimating the probability that only one individual is present when dispersed elements are discovered. Individualized patterns of fluorescence have also been investigated (McKern, 1958; Eyman, 1965), as have direct tests of chemical composition (Weiner, Oakley, and Clark, 1953; Guinn, 1970). However, as noted by Kerley (1962), a most convincing line of evidence, when available, is perhaps the most obvious: the degree of congruence between joint surfaces.

Biomedical scientists have presented the most detailed studies of joint congruence, usually as an aspect of arthritis research and frequently emphasizing joints of the lower limb. Greenwold's extensive investigation of degenerative disease in association with congruence of the hip joint (1974) is a good example of this genre. Though anthropologists have collected reams of data concerning bone length and shape variation in osseous structures, most of these data are presented as averages across populations or population samples, and they seldom approach the topic of joint congruence from the perspective of intraindividual patterning or interindividual variability. Fo-

*Portions reprinted/adapted from *Journal of Forensic Science*, 25(1):246–259. Courtesy of ASTM, 1916 Race Street, Philadelphia, PA.

rensic scientists faced with the need to develop a probability estimate based on such data will not likely find published reports suitable for their particular problem and may therefore be forced to discuss, as did the scholars in the oft-cited Ruxton dismemberment case (Glaister and Brash, 1937), observations of "harmony" between adjacent joint surfaces.

The following illustrates our attempt to develop quantified standards for assessing the degree of congruence between bones of the neck. Choice of study sample and analytical procedures were influenced by the recent forensic example (the Bass case) cited here as well as by the earlier Ruxton case (Glaister and Brash, 1937). The recent forensic case also stimulated investigation of vertebral maturation during late adolescence/young adulthood.

THE BASS CASE

The *Detroit Free Press* (1981, 150:3A, 5A) describes a long-standing controversy between Dr. Werner Spitz, Wayne County (Michigan) medical examiner, and his former assistant, Dr. Millard Bass. The newspaper indicates that relations between the colleagues began to deteriorate in 1975, when Bass alerted county officials to the possibility that Spitz was illegally removing and selling pituitary glands from bodies autopsied at the Wayne County Morgue. In addition, Bass is said to have accused Spitz of using bodies in ballistics experiments without obtaining permission from next of kin. The newspaper reports that—

> Spitz countered with charges that Bass was decapitating bodies, removing flesh from skulls and other bones and storing various body parts in a Greektown warehouse.
>
> In May of 1976, after county investigators eventually found a total of 11 human heads floating in a vat in a "skeletonizing" room used by Bass at the Wayne State University Medical School, Spitz suspended Bass. Bass resigned two days later.
>
> Spitz told reporters at the time that he had seen Bass boiling human body parts in the basement of the morgue and that Bass had "a couple of van loads" of bones and skin tissue stored in the Greektown warehouse.
>
> Bass was charged with illegally decapitating 11 bodies and stripping flesh from 14 others. (*Detroit Free Press*, 1981, 150:3A)

One of the charges faced by Bass was specific: the removal of the head and neck from the cadaver of a 23-year-old black female. This body had been exhumed, and it was found to be missing, skeletally, the cranium and the first three cervical vertebrae. Authorities removed the remaining cervical vertebrae from the body and sought the missing elements. A series of cervical vertebrae (C1–C3) discovered in Bass's office was described by Spitz as fitting the cadaver specimens. It was this question—the degree of "fit" or congruence between the "office" vertebrae, specifically the third cervical (C3), and the cadaver C4—that led to the request by attorneys representing

Bass that anthropologists St. Hoyme and Buikstra view the evidence. Both "experts," after independently observing the two sets of cervical elements, determined that the vertebrae could not represent one individual because (1) the inferior aspect of the office C3 body was simply too large to fit between the superiorly directed "lips" of the cadaver C4 (Fig. 10-1) and (2) the epiphyseal rings of the office vertebrae were not present, indicating that they represented an individual developmentally younger than the 23 year old, whose epiphyseal rings had indeed fused.

Although the noncongruence of the office and cadaver vertebrae appeared obvious to St. Hoyme and Buikstra, whose evidence was important in the eventual dismissal of the case, other physical anthropologists and medical scientists did not concur with their opinion. This lack of consensus stimulated the senior author to initiate the following study, designed to develop additional information concerning cervical congruence (individuation) and epiphyseal ring fusion in a reference sample. The previously collected information from the Bass case was then tested against the individuation model, as were published data from the retrospective Ruxton example (Glaister and Brash, 1937). The Ruxton case was included as a preliminary means of assessing broader applicability of the technique, recognizing the limitations imposed by the nature of the reference sample. Although congruence and development for the total cervical region have been investigated (Buikstra and Gordon, 1980), only those data directly relevant to the Bass and Ruxton cases are presented here.

THE RUXTON CASE

The background of the Ruxton case is presented in copious detail by Glaister and Brash (1937). Important for our purposes is that the individuation problem involved two female bodies that had been dismembered and distributed across the English countryside. These were later determined to represent the remains of Isabella Ruxton, the wife of Dr. Buck Ruxton, a Lancaster physician, and of Mrs. Ruxton's nursemaid, Mary Rogerson.

The forensic challenge in the case involved reconstructing the two women from multiple mutilated body parts. Our data are relevant to the suggested fit between a trunk segment that included the last two cervical vertebrae (C6, C7), most of the thorax, and two lumbar vertebrae; and a unit that contained a head (Head No. 2) and five cervical vertebrae (C1–5). A second head (No. 1) with four cervical vertebrae and fragments of a fifth had also been discovered; however, the fifth cervical unit was sufficiently fragmented to render measurement imprecise. Thus, in this case, we are concerned with congruence between the inferior aspect of C5 and the superior aspect of C6.

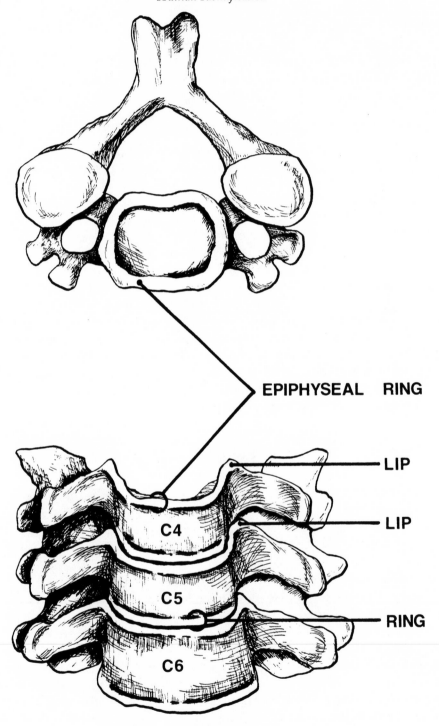

EPIPHYSEAL   RING

LIP

LIP

C4

C5

RING

C6

Figure 10-1.

MATERIALS AND METHODS

The study sample is composed of all the black females between the ages of 16 and 25 from the Terry Collection located in the Smithsonian Institution. There are 33 remains so listed, although on occasion the array of observations is limited by the presence of such conditions as assimilation of the atlas and incomplete neural arches. In no case, however, did the number of observations fall below 32. Two types of data were recorded: measurements and degree of epiphyseal union.

All measurements were taken by the senior author with dial-reading calipers. Taken to the nearest 0.1 mm, each measurement was recorded and later checked. If the second measurement was within ±0.1 mm of the original, then the original observation was retained. Scores of ±0.2 mm were averaged, and broader deviations required a third measurement, which in all cases was within ±0.2 mm of one of the prior observations. In such situations, the two closer measurements were then treated as if they were the first pair.

An initial survey of measurements commonly taken of the region in question disclosed that most had been made in the course of studies of sexual dimorphism (Iordanis, 1961; Van Vark, 1970; Helmuth and Rempe, 1968; Dubreuil-Chambardel, 1907) or as an aspect of population variability (Hasebe, 1913; Anderson, 1883; Martin, 1928; Hrdlicka, 1912; Trotter, 1926, 1929; Cyriax, 1920; Macalister, 1893). The most common measure is that of vertebral body height, which has been most extensively documented in population descriptions and studies of age changes in the lumbar region (Ericksen, 1976, 1978a, 1978b; Allbrook, 1956). Body height measurements have also been taken in studies of changes in the vertebral column during maceration (Todd and Pyle, 1928a), and comparability of radiographic and direct measurement techniques has been investigated (Todd and Pyle, 1928b). Because our investigation was somewhat different from previous work, we decided to generate a new set of measurements, relying whenever possible on previously defined standards. Measurement pairs that would most likely reflect congruence between elements were selected. These are defined in Table 10-I and illustrated in Figures 10-2 and 10-3.

For each paired set of measurements, for example, C3IAP and C4SAP, a new variable (C34AP) was generated by subtracting the measurement for the more caudal (inferior) element from that of the more cranial (superior) unit. In the case of C3IAP and C4SAP, the new variable C34AP would reflect the result if C4SAP were subtracted from C3IAP. To isolate those new variables which denoted close congruence between adjacent elements, measures of dispersion and central tendency were generated for the absolute values of the variables by using the program CONDESCRIPTIVE from the Statistical Package for the Social Sciences (Nie et al., 1975).

TABLE 10-I
DEFINITION OF MEASUREMENTS

Element	Symbol and Definition[a]	Observation Pairing and Variable Definition
1. 3rd cervical vertebra[b]	C3IAP: maximum anterior-posterior distance of the inferior surface of the body, including the epiphyseal ring (when present), sagittal plane	C3IAP − C4SAP = C34AP
2. 3rd cervical vertebra[b]	C3IMLMIN: on the inferior surface, the maximum distance between the inflection points at the lateral aspect of the horizontal surface of the body as this surface meets the articular surface for the lips of the adjacent vertebra, coronal plane	C3IMLMIN − C4SMLMIN = C34MLMIN
3. 3rd cervical vertebra[b]	C3IMLMAX: on the inferior surface, the maximum distance between the most inferior-lateral points of the articular facets for the lips	C3IMLMAX − C4SMLMAX = C34MLMAX
4. 3rd cervical vertebra[b]	C3IZMIN: distance between the most medial points on the postzygapophyses, coronal plane, perhaps corresponding to the measurement described by the researchers in the Ruxton case (Glaister and Brash, 1937, p. 49); Helmuth and Rempe (1968) and Hasebe (1913) also report this measurement	C3IZMIN − C4SZMIN = C34ZMIN
5. 3rd cervical vertebra[b]	C3IZMAX: distance between the most lateral points on the postzygapophyses, coronal plane, perhaps corresponding to the measurement described by the researchers in the Ruxton case (Glaister and Brash, 1937, p. 49)	C3IZMAX − C4SZMAX = C34ZMAX
6. 4th cervical vertebra[c]	C4SAP: maximum anterior-posterior distance of the superior surface of the body, including the epiphyseal ring (when present), sagittal plane	C3IAP − C4SAP = C34AP
7. 4th cervical vertebra[c]	C4SMLMIN: on the superior surface, the maximum distance between the inflection points at the base of the lips as they meet the horizontal surface of the body, coronal plane	C3IMLMIN − C4SMLMIN = C34MLMIN
8. 4th cervical vertebra[c]	C4SMLMAX: on the superior surface, the maximum distance between the most lateral points on the articular surface at the superior aspects of the lips, coronal plane	C3IMLMAX − C4SMLMAX =C34MLMAX
9. 4th cervical vertebra[c]	C4SZMIN: distance between the most medial points on the prezygapophyses, coronal plane	C4IZMIN − C4SZMIN =C34ZMIN
10. 4th cervical vertebra[c]	C4SZMAX: distance between the most lateral points on the prezygapophyses, coronal plane, perhaps corresponding to the measurement described by researchers in the Ruxton case (Glaister and Brash, 1937, p. 49)	C3IZMAX − C4SZMAX = C34ZMAX

[a]All nonpathological extensions of articular facets are included; arthritic structures and ligamentous/tendinous ossifications are not.

[b]These definitions are repeated for the 5th cervical vertebra, used in the Ruxton example.

[c]These definitions are repeated for the 6th cervical vertebra, used in the Ruxton example.

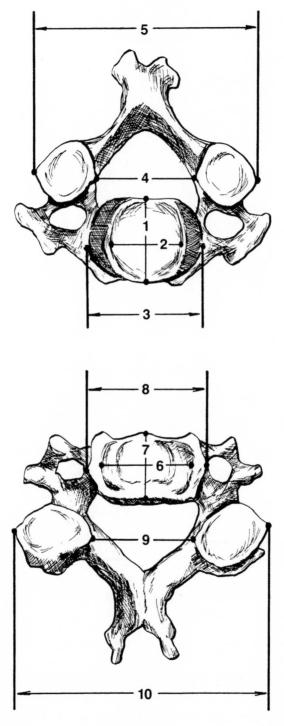

Figure 10-2.

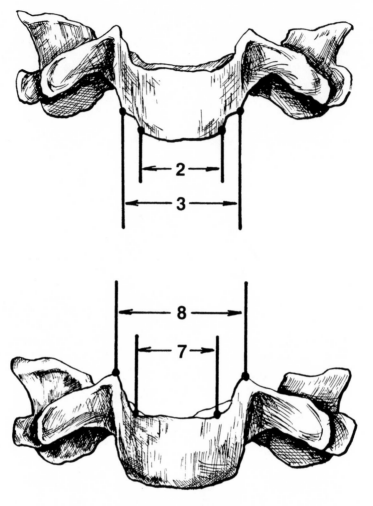

Figure 10-3.

Table 10-II defines and Figure 10-4 illustrates the stages of epiphyseal ring fusion recorded in this study. As indicated by McKern and Stewart (1957), there is little information available concerning the timing of fusion for these secondary ossification centers with the centra. McKern and Stewart (1957) provide ossification data for the thoracic region in a racially mixed sample of males between the ages of 17 and 25. The present study reports ossification patterns for the cervical region in black females of comparable age. Observations were recorded separately for the superior and inferior surfaces of each vertebral unit as well as for the dorsal (posterior) and ventral (anterior) halves of each element. It should be noted that the recorded cause of death for these females frequently included disease states that could have slowed maturation processes, and we therefore believe that our data are best used as a maximum estimate for developmental timing in a population not under similar disease stress. Our results concerning the *pattern* of fusion should, however, be representative. It is important to note that an effort was made to replicate the McKern and Stewart scoring technique. It appears, however, that only the initial two or three stages are comparable (0, 1, 2). For this reason, our data should not be directly compared with data collected through the use of the McKern and Stewart standards. In statistical evaluation of the ossification sequences, program FREQUENCIES (Nie et al., 1975) was used for developing descriptive statistics.

TABLE 10-II
DEFINITION OF STAGES OF EPIPHYSEAL RING FUSION

Stage	Definition
0	unfused, ring absent
1	ring present and partially fused; unfused sections evident
2	ring completely fused; edges of ring clearly defined throughout circumference
3	ring completely fused; edges of ring indistinct, that is, integrated with centrum, in a portion of the circumference
4	ring completely fused; edges of ring integrated with centrum throughout circumference

RESULTS

Table 10-III presents descriptive statistics for the measurements defined in the previous section. We believe that those measurements with the smallest dispersions, that is those with the lowest values for standard deviation and the smallest 0.95 confidence interval, will be those most likely to minimize Type II error, which, in this study, would be the merging of remains from two individuals.

To facilitate identification of those measures with the least dispersion, we have in Table 10-IV grouped confidence interval sizes by 0.05 mm increments, with the values at the higher end of the scale being summarized in larger units. From Table 10-IV it is clear that confidence interval sizes tend to vary by parameter rather than by anatomical location. In other words, AP confidence intervals tend to be smaller than those for MLMAX across all vertebrae. According to Table 10-IV, the measurements of closest congruence are AP, ZMAX, and ZMIN followed by MLMIN. The values of MLMAX are larger than the other cervical parameters. Although it is possible that the variables with relatively large confidence intervals will become useful in certain circumstances, it seems likely that those with least dispersion, such as AP, will be those of greatest utility in forensic science work.

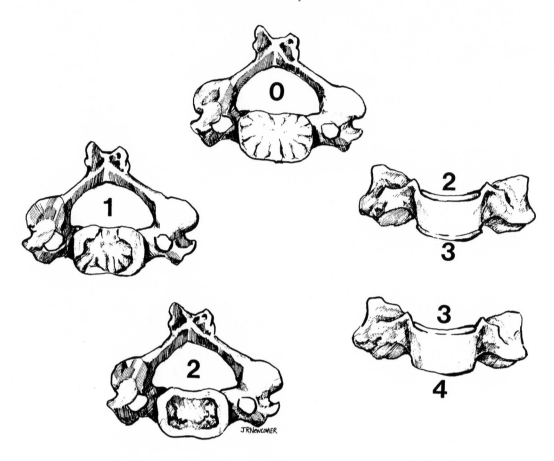

Figure 10-4.

TABLE 10-III
SUMMARY STATISTICS FOR DERIVED VARIABLES (IN mm) n = 33

Variable Name	Mean	Min/Max	Standard Deviation	0.95 Confidence Interval	Confidence Interval Size
C34AP	0.65	0.0/18.0	0.51	0.47 to 0.83	0.36
C56AP	0.59	0.0/12.0	0.41	0.44 to 0.73	0.29
C34MLMIN	0.64	0.0/30.0	0.66	0.40 to 0.87	0.47
C56MLMIN	0.92	1.0/24.0	0.58	0.71 to 1.13	0.42
C34MLMAX	1.73	3.0/44.0	1.04	1.36 to 2.09	0.73
C56MLMAX	2.26	1.0/34.0	0.77	1.98 to 2.53	0.55
C34ZMIN	0.66	1.0/15.0	0.42	0.51 to 0.81	0.30
C56ZMIN	0.76	0.0/29.0	0.63	0.53 to 0.98	0.45
C34ZMAX	0.50	0.0/16.0	0.41	0.35 to 0.65	0.30
C56ZMAX	0.69	1.0/15.0	0.36	0.56 to 0.82	0.26

TABLE 10-IV
SUMMARY TABLE OF 0.95 CONFIDENCE INTERVAL SIZES

Interval Size	Variables
0.20–0.24	.....
0.25–0.29	C56AP, C56ZMAX
0.30–0.34	C34ZMAX, C34ZMIN
0.35–0.39	C34AP
0.40–0.44	C56MLMIN
0.45–0.49	C56ZMIN, C34MLMIN
0.50–0.59	C56MLMAX .....
0.60–0.69	.....
0.70–0.79	C34MLMAX

Table 10-V presents summary data, grouped by age, for epiphyseal ring fusion within the cervical region. In a general sense, it is clear that the anatomy books are correct: by age 25 the epiphyseal rings are fused to the centra. It is also obvious that, at any given age, the more cranially directed cervical vertebrae tend to be at a stage of maturation more advanced than that of the more caudal units. Especially significant for the current study is that by age 23 epiphyseal rings for most upper cervical vertebrae should show at least Stage 3 fusion.

TABLE 10-V
STAGES OF EPIPHYSEAL RING FUSION IN CERVICAL VERTEBRAE
(TERRY COLLECTION BLACK FEMALES, AGES 17 to 25 YEARS)

Vertebral Surface[a]	Stages of Fusion by Age[b]					
	17–19	20–21	22	23	24	25
C2ID	2(2/5)3(3/5)	3(3/4)4(1/4)	2(1/5)3(4/5)	3(5/5)	3(7/7)	3(5/6)4(1/6)
C2IV	3(3/4)4(1/4)	2(1/4)3(3/4)	2(1/4)3(3/4)	3(5/5)	3(6/7)4(1/7)	3(3/6)4(3/6)
C3SD	1(1/5)3(4/5)	3(4/4)	3(5/5)	3(5/5)	3(5/7)4(2/7)	3(6/6)
C3SV	2(2/5)3(2/5)4(1/5)	2(1/4)3(3/4)	3(3/5)4(2/5)	3(5/5)	3(6/7)4(1/7)	3(6/6)
C3ID	1(1/5)2(2/5)3(2/5)	3(4/4)	2(2/5)3(4/5)	2(1/5)3(4/5)	2(1/7)3(5/7)2(1/7)	3(4/6)4(2/6)
C3IV	1(1/5)2(3/5)3(1/5)	2(2/4)3(2/4)	1(1/5)2(1/5)3(3/5)	2(2/5)3(3/5)	3(6/7)4(1/7)	3(6/6)
C4SD	1(1/5)2(1/5)3(3/5)	3(4/4)	1(1/5)3(4/5)	3(5/5)	3(7/7)	3(6/6)
C4SV	1(1/5)2(1/5)3(2/5) 4(1/5)	2(1/4)3(3/4)	2(1/5)3(4/5)	3(5/5)	3(6/7)4(1/7)	3(6/6)

[a]I = inferior surface; S = superior surface; D = dorsal aspect; and V = ventral aspect
[b]Stage (number/total number)

DISCUSSION

The Bass Case

In this example, a determination of probable congruence between a third and a fourth cervical vertebra was required. The third was the last in a series of three units that had been found in the defendant's possession. It was alleged that these, along with the skull, had been removed from the body of the young adult black female. Three of the five measurements reported in the present study, AP, MLMAX, and MLMIN, were recorded by the senior author. Although the evidence was viewed two years prior to the Terry Collection research, data collection techniques should be comparable.

As can be seen in Table 10-VI, values for two of the three variables differ significantly from the Terry Collection means. Of importance is that, as indicated in Tables 10-III and 10-IV, these two parameters are of relatively small dispersion when compared to MLMAX, the variable for which the difference is not significant. Given that two of the three variables show significant differences and that the single parameter that does not had been designated a priori as a poor discriminator, the null hypothesis can be rejected with confidence. Because there is minimal congruence between the third and fourth cervical elements, the remains viewed as evidence are therefore inferred to represent at least two individuals.

TABLE 10-VI
COMPARISON OF FORENSIC SCIENCE DATA WITH TERRY COLLECTION PARAMETERS

Case	Variable	Value	Terry Mean (n)	Terry Standard Deviation	t	P
1	C34AP	3.6	0.65 (33)	0.51	5.699	<0.001
1	C34MLMIN	3.7	0.64 (33)	0.66	4.568	<0.001
1	C34MLMAX	0.8	1.73 (33)	1.04	0.881	>0.2
2	C56ZMAX	0.6	0.69 (32)	0.36	0.246	>0.5

Also important in this case were the observations of epiphyseal ring fusion. Our data indicate that by age 23 there should be obvious fusion of both the superior and inferior rings, as there was in the cadaver. That such fusion had not occurred in the second and third "office" vertebrae lends strong support to the hypothesis that two individuals—not one—are represented.

The Ruxton Case

As noted previously, our concern here is with congruence between C5 and C6. Glaister and Brash (1937) report several observations taken upon the cervical vertebrae of the trunk and head/neck units, including vertical diameter of the bodies, maximum distance between transverse processes, and maximum distances between articular processes. It is assumed here that the last-mentioned measure is comparable to ZMAX, although the textual definition of the measurement is not explicit. Glaister and Brash (1937) also report data for a single control set of vertebrae with age, sex, and population unspecified.

The value for ZMAX in the Ruxton example is compatible with the Terry Collection statistics. In addition, the *t*-test probability estimate of $P > 0.50$ strongly prevents rejection of the null hypothesis that the Ruxton C56ZMAX value is not significantly different from the Terry Collection mean. Although the Ruxton remains are reported to differ from the study sample in both age and racial group, our data clearly do support Glaister and Brash's carefully drawn conclusions of congruence between the cervical vertebrae of the trunk and those associated with Head 2.

Resolution of the Bass Case

Charges against Bass were dropped in 1977 after it was determined in court that the well-publicized maceration was part of Bass's legitimate research efforts. Spitz was not charged, although the *Detroit Free Press* (1981, 150:5A) reports that a Wayne County Organized Crime Task Force discovered Spitz had indeed authorized removal and sale of pituitary glands without permission. Neither had permission from next of kin been obtained for ballistics experiments conducted in 1973 and 1975. A few other irregular procedures are also reported.

In 1981, Federal District Court heard a suit by Bass against Spitz alleging that Spitz "recklessly and wantonly committed perjury at pre-trial hearings in that case" and that Spitz interfered at a national scale with Bass's employment opportunities (*Detroit Free Press*, 1981, 150:5A). Wayne County was also named in the suit. The Federal Court jury awarded Bass, after hearing again the full range of evidence in the case, including the skeletal data described above, significant damages of $150,000 and court costs. An appeal is in process.

Resolution of the Ruxton Case

The trial of Dr. Buck Ruxton for the murder of Isabella Ruxton began in Manchester on March 2, 1936, and ended March 13 of the same year.

Evidence concerning the murder of Mary Rogerson was admitted as evidence, but he was not formally charged with this murder at that time. He was judged guilty of Isabella Ruxton's murder and sentenced to death. The Court of Criminal Appeals dismissed an appeal of the sentence on April 27, 1936. Forensic evidence concerning the identification and individuation of the bodies was judged to be of excellent quality and figured heavily in gaining the conviction (Glaister and Brash, 1937).

REFERENCES

Allbrook, D. B. (1956). Changes in lumbar vertebral body height with age. *Am J Phys Anthropol, 15*:35–39.

Anderson, R. J. (1883). Observations on the diameters of human vertebrae in different regions. *J Anat Physiol, 17*:341–344.

Baker, Paul T. and Russell W. Newman (1968). The use of bone weights for human identification. *Am J Phys Anthropol, 15*:601–618.

Buikstra, J. E. and C. C. Gordon (1980). Individuation in forensic science study: decapitation. *J Forensic Sci, 25(1)*:246–259.

Cyriax, E. F. (1920). On certain absolute and relative measurements of human vertebrae. *J Anat 54*:305–308.

Dubreuil-Chambardel, L. (1907). Variations sexuelles de l'Atlas. *Bulletin et Memoires de la Societie D'Anthropologie de Paris, 8*:399–404.

Ericksen, M. F. (1976). Some aspects of aging in the lumbar spine. *Am J Phys Anthropol, 45*:575–580.

——— (1978a). Aging in the lumbar spine, II, L1 and L2. *Am J Phys Anthropol, 48*:241–246.

——— (1978b). Aging in the lumbar spine, III, L5. *Am J Phys Anthropol, 49*:247–250.

Eyman, C. E. (1965). Ultraviolet fluorescence as a means of skeletal identification. *Am Antiq, 31*:109–112.

Glaister, J. and J. C. Brash (1937). *Medico-legal Aspects of the Ruxton Case.* E. and S. Livingstone, Edinburgh.

Greenwold, A. S. (1974). Joint congruence—a dynamic concept. In *The Hip: Proceedings of the Second Open Scientific Meeting of the Hip Society.* C. V. Mosby Co., St. Louis.

Guinn, V. P. (1970). Forensic neutron activation analysis. In *Personal Identification in Mass Disasters*, T. D. Stewart, Ed. Smithsonian Institution, Washington, D.C.

Hasebe, K. (1913). Die Wirbelsäule der japaner. *Zeitschrift für Morphologie und Anthropologie, 15*:259–420.

Helmuth, H., and U. Rempe (1968). Über den geschlectdimorphismus des epistropheum bein menschen. *Zeitschrift für Morphologie und Anthropologie, 59(3)*:300–321.

Hrdlicka, A. (1912) Examination of the skeletal parts attributed to the tetraprothomo: the Monte Hermoso atlas. *Bulletin 52*, Bureau of American Ethnology 364–369.

——— (1920). *Anthropometry.* The Wistar Institute of Anatomy and Biology, Philadelphia.

Iordanis, P. (1961). Determination du sexe par les os du squelette (atlas, axis, clavicule, omoplate, sternum). *Annales de Médicine Légale, 41*:280–291.

Kerley, Ellis R. (1962). Special observations on skeletal identification. *J Forensic Sci, 17*:349–357.

Krogman, W. M. (1962). *The Human Skeleton in Forensic Medicine.* Charles C Thomas, Springfield, Illinois.

Macalister, A. (1893). Notes on the development and variations of the atlas. *J Anat Physiol, 27*:519–542.

Martin, R. (1928). *Lehrbuch der Anthropologie, Zeiter Band: Kraniologie, Osteologie.* Verlag Gustav Fischer, Jena, Germany.

McKern, T. W. (1958). The Use of Shortwave Ultraviolet Rays for the Segregation of Commingled Skeletal Remains. Environmental Protection Research Division, U.S. Army Quartermaster Research and Development Center, Natick, Massachusetts.

McKern, T. W. and T. D. Stewart (1957). Skeletal Age Changes in Young American Males. Technical Report EP-45. Headquarters, Quartermaster Research and Development Command, Quartermaster Research and Development Center Environmental Protection Research Division, Natick, Massachusetts.

Nie, N. H., C. H. Hull, H. G. Jenkins, K. Steinbrenner, and D. H. Bent (1975). *Statistical Package for the Social Sciences,* 2nd ed. McGraw-Hill, New York.

Snow, C. C. and J. L. Luke (1970). The Oklahoma City child disappearances of 1967: Forensic anthropology in the identification of skeletal remains. *J Forensic Sci,* 15:125–153.

Snow, C. C. and E. D. Folk (1970). Statistical assessment of commingled skeletal remains. *Am J Phys Anthropol,* 32:423–428.

Stewart, T. D. (1979). *Essentials of Forensic Anthropology.* Charles C Thomas, Springfield, Illinois.

Todd, T. W., and S. I. Pyle (1928a). Effects of maceration and drying upon the vertebral column. *Am J Phys Anthropol,* 12:303–319.

———— (1928b). A quantitative study of the vertebral column by direct and roentgenoscopic methods. *Am J Phys Anthropol,* 12:321–337.

Trotter, M. (1926). The movable segments of the vertebral column in Old Egyptians. *Am J Phys Anthropol,* 9:457–466.

———— (1929). The vertebral column in whites and in American negroes. *Am J Phys Anthropol,* 13:95–107.

Van Vark, G. N. (1970). *Some Statistical Procedures for the Investigation of Prehistoric Human Skeletal Material.* Rijksuniversiteit te Groningen, Groningen, The Netherlands.

Weiner, J. S., K. P. Oakley, and W. L. Clark (1953). The solution of the Piltdown problem. *Bulletin of the British Museum* (Natural History) 2(3).

Chapter 11

TIME INTERVAL SINCE DEATH
A Difficult Decision

WILLIAM M. BASS

W hen law enforcement agents ask the help of a forensic anthropologist, one of their first questions is "How old is it?" Actually, two questions relating to age are involved: (1) How old was the individual when he or she died and (2) How long has the individual been dead? The second question is much more complicated and difficult, since few comparative data exist and there are many yet unresolved problems.

This case study, illustrating problems in estimating the time interval since death, has two beginnings—the first on a cold, rainy, and wind-blown day, December 16, 1864, and the second on a cold Friday morning, December 30, 1977.

REMOVAL OF BODY

I will begin with the 1977 day and follow the forensic sequence of events as they actually occurred. Late Thursday afternoon December 29, 1977, I received a call from Detective Captain Jeff Long of the Williamson County Sheriff's Office in Franklin, Tennessee requesting aid in the identification of a recently discovered body in a disturbed grave. Arrangements were made to meet Captain Long on Friday morning, December 30, at 10:30 AM.

That day was cold with a slight mist blowing from low-hanging clouds. On the way to the scene in Franklin, Tennessee, Captain Long explained that a grave in a family cemetery in the backyard of an old home had been disturbed and contained what appeared to be decaying human remains. We proceeded to the location, a large brick mansion that originally had been the Shy home in the middle 1800s. The backyard cemetery contained several marked graves. When I first observed the scene, a large hole was covered by a 4 by 8 foot sheet of plywood over a grave marked:

136

Lt. Col.* W. M. Shy
20th Tenn.
Infantry C.S.A.
Born May 24, 1838
Killed at Battle of
Nashville
Dec. 16, 1864

Beneath the plywood lay a decaying body with no head and various articles of decaying clothing. We used the plywood sheet as a platform on which to lay the bones and began to articulate the skeleton. The smell of decaying flesh was strong, and most of the bystanders stood back as I climbed down into the hole and began removing bits and pieces of clothing, tissue, and bones.

We began to clean out the disturbed soil and expose the body. Decay had advanced to the stage where various parts of the body were no longer in anatomical order, i.e. the legs were separated from the pelvis and the arms were separated from the thoracic cage. Sections of the vertebra were still held together by ligaments, as were the arms at the elbows and the legs at the knees. Neither the skull nor the mandible was present.

My initial impression was that this adult male was originally placed in a squatting position on top of the cast iron coffin after those who dug the hole had broken a 1 by 2 foot hole in the top of the cast iron coffin. As the body decayed, it had fallen into the Civil War coffin. It was difficult to remove this body because of the small dimensions of the grave, the wet conditions of the ground (mud), the partial disarticulation of the decomposed remains, and the smaller hole in the cast iron coffin through which the lumbar and sacral elements of the spinal column as well as parts of the lower legs had descended. Associated with the decaying body were fragments of a tuxedo type of shirt, vest, coat, pants, and a white cloth glove from the right hand.

The skeletal material with associated tissue was arranged in anatomical order. I cut pink flesh from the femur, and the small and large intestines were still morphologically identifiable. I tentatively identified the skeleton at the scene as a male, age 25 to 28, who had possibly been dead from 6 to 12 months. The latter decision was based on the odor and amount of decaying flesh.

At this stage of the investigation, we discussed the possibility that the body was that of Colonel Shy. However, this idea was dismissed because of what I refer to as *mind set*. Mind set refers to preconceived ideas from earlier

---

*Shy was actually a Colonel at the time of his death, apparently having been raised from Lieutenant-Colonel just prior to his death; the family may not have known of his latest promotion (Dowd 1980:61).

experiences that tend to obstruct a clear and analytical analysis.

In the summer of 1973, I had moved a German Lutheran cemetery near Wartburg, Tennessee for the Tennessee Highway Department. This cemetery had been used from 1842 to 1891. All of the skeletal remains of the approximate 17 graves we located and removed could have been held in both hands. My frame of reference (or mind set) was that burials from the Civil War period would be extensively decomposed and certainly would not have pink tissue associated with the bones. Previous excavation of early coffin burials in South Dakota and Tennessee had produced fully skeletonized material of a dark brown color.

ANALYSIS OF MATERIAL

After the bones, tissue, and clothing had been removed from the hole over Colonel Shy's grave late afternoon of December 30, we left the clothing for analysis at the State Crime Laboratory in Donelson, Tennessee. The clothing was too odiferous to be taken inside the laboratory, so it was sorted outside on the driveway—a cold task, as the sun was setting and the temperature was dropping into the low 30s.

On Monday, January 2, 1978, the bones that had been removed to my laboratory in Knoxville were placed in a heated vat to aid in tissue removal. By noon I detected the smell of embalming fluids coming from the vat. I was startled by this and began to rethink the original conclusion that this was not the skeleton of Colonel Shy.

In the meantime, arrangements had been made to extend the excavation and remove Colonel Shy's coffin. After the removal of the bones, tissue, and clothing on Friday and cleaning out the hole above the coffin, I was held by my feet and lowered head first into the opening in the top of the coffin so that I could look toward both the head and foot of Colonel Shy's casket. I was unable to locate a body; however, no attempt was made to inspect the inch or two of debris and decayed matter on the bottom of the coffin. The appearance of this material also tended to reinforce my feeling that the bones in Civil War graves from Tennessee would have disintegrated. Since no skull or mandible was present with the material recovered above the coffin and no skull was seen at the head of Colonel Shy's casket, I believed the burial of Colonel Shy and the body found over his grave were not associated. However, when the coffin was excavated on the following Monday, we discovered that the skull had fractured into 17 pieces from the force of a shot that caused instant death. The tissue over the head did not hold embalming fluids because of two large holes in the skull, and as the tissue decayed the skull fell apart. These pieces were hidden from view in the inch or two of debris and decaying material on the floor of the coffin.

By late afternoon of Monday, January 2, 1978, three separate events had occurred that allowed us to make a correct determination: (A) We had discovered that Colonel Shy's coffin contained a fragmentary skull and mandible. (B) The State Crime Laboratory had found no synthetic fibers, and all of the cloth was cotton. (C) We had noted that the tissue and skeletal material that I had brought back had been embalmed. The original field analysis of a 25 to 28-year-old male who was thought to have been dead from 6 to 12 months was then changed to a 26-year-old male who had been dead 113 years. Though my determination of age at death was entirely accurate, my estimate of length of time since death had been off by 112 years!

COLONEL SHY'S DEATH

An excellent history of the battle of Nashville and the death of Colonel Shy has been written by Dowd (1980:47–72). William Mabry Shy, one of ten children, was born in Bourbon County, Kentucky, on May 24, 1838. His family moved to the home in Williamson County, Tennessee, where the family cemetery was located. He enlisted as a private at the inception of Company H of the 20th Tennessee Infantry. It is reported that he was a man of quiet disposition, a man of deeds rather than words, and he rose through the ranks to Colonel by the time of his death of December 16, 1864.

He was killed in the battle of Compton's Hill at Nashville, Tennessee. The battered Confederates still were in possession of Compton's Hill on the afternoon of the second day. They were surrounded on three sides by thousands of Union soldiers, and the marooned Rebels were receiving fire from all angles; many were shot in the back. Dowd states (1980:59):

> Around 4:00 p.m. it began to rain. The defenders had not slept. They were tired, cold, wet and hungry, but still they fought on. The rain was now coming down in sheets and it was getting much colder. They knew the enemy was massing at the foot of the hill for a full scale attack but could do nothing about it. Suddenly the massive Federal attack that had been building all day began. There were a few minutes of violent fighting and then it was all over. They came so fast with so many that the small force atop the hill was completely overwhelmed. The entire command of defenders was practically annihilated, only 65 individuals escaped (Horn 1968:127). Colonel William M. Shy, and nearly half of his men, were killed while bravely defending this hill (later this hill was to be called Shy's Hill as a tribute for his gallant stand and heroic death).

After the battle, Compton's (Shy's) Hill was covered with the dead and wounded from both sides. Among them was Colonel Shy, dead at the age of 26, with a minnie ball to the brain (Fig. 11-1). Marshall's account of the Battle of Nashville states that he was shot at close range, "his head being powder-burned around the hole made by the shot" (Marshall, 1912:522).

Colonel Shy's death was reported to his family, and Dowd (1980:61) says:

> Being unmarried the unpleasant chore of recovering his body fell to his parents. Colonel Shy's mother and father were divided in their sympathies toward the war; she siding with the South and he with the North. . . .
>
> The area around the Shy farm was still in turmoil due to the recent Battle of Franklin and this confusion was greatly magnified by the retreat and pursuit of the fleeing Confederate army after the Battle of Nashville. For a civilian to obtain permission to travel the busy and cluttered roads into Nashville was near impossible. Fearing to cross through the Union lines the Shy family solicited the help of their close friend, Dr. Daniel B. Cliffe, who held an influential position in the community. . . .
>
> Dr. Cliffe made arrangements for his wife, Mrs. Virginia Cliffe, to go to Nashville to recover Colonel Shy's body. Why he sent his wife instead of going himself is not entirely clear. He might have been unable to leave at this time due to the fact that he was urgently needed to tend the many wounded at Franklin. . . .
>
> Colonel Shy was brought home and laid to rest in the family cemetery at Two Rivers, near Franklin, Tennessee. Since Dr. Cliffe was a good friend of the family and was skilled in the art of embalming, he very likely embalmed the body of Colonel Shy.
>
> The body was placed in a cast iron coffin for burial.

ANALYSIS

What can be learned from this experience? Little appears in the literature concerning the time interval since death. Stewart devotes only seven and a half pages out of 300 to means of determining time since death and states that "there is no escaping the fact that, for most skeletonized remains, estimation of time since death usually is little more than an educated guess" (1979:71). Other texts in forensic anthropology, Krogman (1962) and El-Najjar and McWilliams (1978), devote less space to criteria for determining time since death. The discussions that do exist do not deal with embalmed bodies.

Those of us who have practiced as forensic anthropologists are aware of the pitfalls of making a hasty, tentative identification. It is difficult to refuse to make any decisions when the law enforcement officer brings to your laboratory the bones of an unknown individual and seeks a rapid identification so that his investigation can proceed. However, this case serves as an example of how attempting such an analysis in the field on a cold, rainy day with muddy specimens and incomplete evidence can lead to a marked misinterpretation of the time interval since death. I therefore advise the following.

First, forensic analysis should be based on a careful study of the material with a clear and open mind to all of the possibilities. As stated before, we considered, while in the field, that this could have been Colonel Shy's body, but because of previous experience with Civil War period graves (mind set), I was of the opinion that very little would have remained of the skeleton and thus discarded this possibility. I knew that the bodies from the German

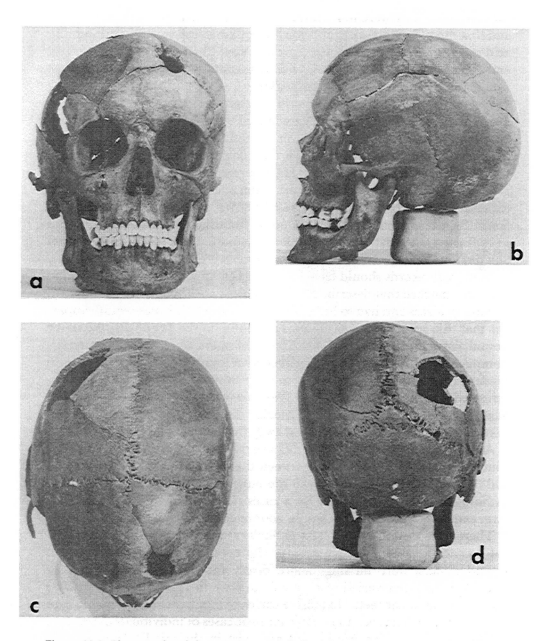

Figure 11-1. Photographs of the reconstructed skull of Col. William M. Shy, a Confederate officer killed in the battle of Nashville, Tennessee, in 1864. a. Norma frontalis. b. Norma lateralis. c. Norma verticalis. d. Norma occipitalis.

Lutheran cemetery were not embalmed and had been buried in pine boxes and that the pH of the soil at the Wartburg Cemetery was 4.8—well into the acid range and a major cause for skeletal decay. I had little experience with embalmed bodies, and this was my first encounter with a well-sealed cast iron coffin that apparently had not leaked.

Second, all of the evidence should be considered before a statement is made. We should have completely excavated the coffin on Friday. We would have then recovered the skull and from at least three pieces of evidence from the cranial bones (the fractured skull, the color of the cranial fragments, and the nature of wound to the skull) made a correct analysis.

The cranial bones were dark brown, almost chocolate in color. Previous experiences with coffin burial (post–Civil War graves from army forts in South Dakota and burials from Tennessee) indicated that skeletonized bones in coffins are often dark brown in color. The postcranial skeleton of Colonel Shy did not show this color because the bones were covered with tissue.

Historical records should have been checked immediately. The wound to the head matched that described for Colonel Shy. Although the skull was in seventeen pieces and had to be restored (see Fig. 11-1), it was readily apparent that this individual had died from trauma to the head with the entry wound above the left eye and the exit wound in the back of the left parietal. Comparison of this wound with published accounts of Colonel Shy's death would have matched. The great force from this shot caused extensive fractures and shattered the entire skull. The force was great enough to split both mastoid processes in an anterior-posterior direction so that the lateral sections of both mastoids were fractured away from the medial halves.

An analysis of the dentition would have provided additional information. The most memorable difference between the forensic cases I had in Kansas and those in Tennessee has been in the larger number of caries and dental pathologies present in the southern cases. Differences in the diet, dental care, and heredity are evident in the poor condition of the teeth.

There were no fillings in Colonel Shy's teeth. Four teeth, the maxillary left second premolar, the mandibular right second, and the left first and second molars, were missing before death and with advanced alveolar resorption. Cavities varied from small to large in most of the remaining premolar and molar teeth. Extensive caries without attempts at dental care are, however, seldom seen in modern forensic cases of individuals of this age. Dental restorations for cavities did not exist in the middle 1800s, so the condition of Colonel Shy's dentition should immediately have been a clue.

Other than an excellent job of embalming and burial in a sealed cast iron coffin, I cannot explain the excellent preservation of the soft tissue. Lack of previous experience with these, the unfavorable field conditions, and pressure for immediate answers all contributed to my making an initial observation that this was a recent death. Three days later, when all of the evidence had been analyzed, our mistake was noted and a correct interpretation made.

TIME SINCE DEATH

As stated earlier, there is little in anthropological literature on the time interval since death. At the Forensic Science meeting in New Orleans in 1980, Morse and Stoutamire (1980:96) reported on the determination of the time since death by the degree of deterioration of associated material (clothing, shoes, leather items, etc.) where the items had been exposed to the elements in Florida. At that same meeting, Charles P. Warren (1980:97) discussed the role that plants and related decomposition vectors played on human skeletal remains from Southeast Asia.

Although not directly related to the determination of time interval since death, Sublett (1966) studied 554 skeletons, the most recent of which died in 1938, from Seneca Indian sites and cemeteries. A paper emphasizing decay rates after death was given by Sublett (1967) at the American Association of Physical Anthropologists meeting in Chapel Hill, North Carolina.

In Ubelaker's analysis of the skeletons (1974b:154) from an ossuary along Nanjemoy Creek in Maryland, he discusses decomposition rates (1974a:66). He also found little data on rate of body tissue decomposition and especially for prehistoric scaffold situations. Ubelaker (1974a:66) states:

> Bodies placed by the mid-Atlantic Indians in death houses or scaffolds may have been protected from many scavengers, but bacteria, maggots, and perhaps birds would insure that decomposition and defleshing would proceed rapidly. Thus, even allowing for deaths during the winter months, it is doubtful that lower-leg bone articulation could have been maintained longer than eight months after death.

During the excavation of many prehistoric American Indian graves from the Northern Plains, we observed fly pupae with some graves and not others. This led us (Gilbert and Bass 1967:534–535) to postulate the possibility of seasonal dating of burials from the presence of fly pupae. Motter (1898:226–229) has the best discussion known to me on insects and flies associated with buried bodies. Motter (1898:227) recognized the problems of insect association when he noted:

> That the presence of certain insects on a cadaver may indicate the exposure of that cadaver to a temperature favorable to the functional activity of these insects, is a conclusion wholly legitimate, and not without entomologic interest. Can it have any Medico-legal weight? To go before a Court of Law and to swear that because a Muscid was found upon a disinterred human cadaver, that cadaver *might* have been interred in June, but *could not* have been interred in January, would be to fly in the face of facts and to assert a proposition controverted by practical experience.

Responding to the article by Gilbert and Bass, Ubelaker and Willey (1978:69–74) suggest that Arikara mortuary practices were more complex and that the presence or absence of fly pupae in a grave does not allow a determination of season of burial in all cases.' T. K. Marshall (1968:80–107) provides a good summary of changes to the body after death.

Most of the literature dealing with decay rates of carcasses appears in the entomological or ecological journals and has to do with insect activity. Readers should check this literature for their particular state, region, or climatic condition, since temperature and seasonal changes are major factors in insect activity. The following references are related to the climate and weather of the Tennessee or mid-south region.

A doctoral dissertation by Reed (1953) on insects that attack decaying dog carcasses in east Tennessee lists 55 references. Of these 55 references, only one (Motter 1898:201–231) specifically deals with human cadavers. Motter observed the disinterment of 150 bodies in Washington, D.C. in the summers of 1896 and 1897. The skeletal material was deposited in the U.S. National Museum. Motter (1898:203) states:

> So varied and so numerous are the modifying conditions and circumstances that it is impossible to say, definitely and absolutely, what is the exact order of disappearance of the several organs and tissues. Looking at the problem from the opposite standpoint, it seems that the bones and the hair are the last to undergo disintegration. I have found the bones, after an interment of seventy-one years, still preserving their general form and appearance, though easily crushed between thumb and fingers; the hair I have seen practically intact after thirty-six years. The brain I have found a still recognizable grayish mass, lying within the skull after all the other soft tissues had disappeared and the skeleton had been completely disarticulated. Indeed, I have found it, after eighteen years and two months (No. 136), lying on the occipital bone after the skull itself had fallen apart. Strange to say, the spinal cord seems to disappear much earlier; I have failed to find any vestige of it—in one case (No. 6)—after three years and five months. The skin and the more superficial connective tissues of the trunk and extremities are converted into a sort of case of adipocere, which preserves the general outline of the cadaver long after the internal organs, and the muscles and tendons even have been completely destroyed and the skeleton within stripped and disarticulated. Under ordinary conditions of interment, some, at least, of this adipocere may persist for ten or twelve years, remaining longest about the pelvis and lower part of the abdomen. I have been able to recognize the skin, fasciae, muscles, tendons, vessels and nerves of the thigh in one cadaver (No. 44) after six years and five months; while, on the other hand, in another case (No. 40) the muscles had entirely disappeared after six years and three months. In most of the cases observed, the thoracic and abdominal organs seem to have disappeared before the muscles. The face, hands and feet seem to be the first parts attacked; I recall at least one instance where the skull was entirely stripped while as yet there seemed to be but little change elsewhere.

Motter, in his studies, found great variation in the rate of decay, and none of his observations appear to have been on an embalmed body buried in a well-sealed cast iron coffin.

Reed's (1953) study of decaying dog carcasses, placed at intervals of about two weeks in hot weather and less frequently in cooler weather, revealed that the total arthropod populations were largest in summer. However, certain species reached their heights of population during the cooler parts of the year. The dog carcasses were placed in pairs in both wooded and nonwooded areas. Insect populations in general were smaller in the nonwooded areas than in the wooded areas, but Reed found (1958:213–245) that decay was more rapid in open areas compared with that in wooded areas (possibly due to increased temperature).

Jerry A. Payne (1965:592–602) conducted a summer carrion study of the baby pig (*Sus scrofa*) in a hardwood-pine community at Clemson, South Carolina. Six stages of decomposition were delimited for carrion exposed to arthropods: flesh, bloated, active decay, advanced decay, dry, and remains. He found that carrion free of insects decomposed and dried slowly.

Payne (1965:592) found: "A definite ecological succession occurred among the fauna of carrion. Each stage of decay was characterized by a particular group of arthropods, each of which occupied a particular niche. Their activities were influenced by physical properties of carrion, rapidity of putrefaction, time of day, and weather." Motter's (1898:228) research on buried bodies from Washington, D.C. led him to state that the modifying conditions were "far too numerous and conflicting" and "the conditions vary far too widely to be thus comprehended in any concise, unqualified manner" (1898:227).

Payne and his associates have published extensively on the insect succession and decomposition of pig carcasses. Payne, Mead, and King (1968:565–567) report on *Hemiptera* associated with pig carrion; Payne, King, and Beinhart (1968:1180–1181) on arthropod succession and decomposition of buried pigs; Payne and King (1970:224–232) on *Coleoptera* associated with pig carrion and (1972:153–162) with insect succession and decomposition of pig carcasses in water; and Payne and Mason (1971:132–141) on *Hymenoptera* associated with pig carrion.

SUMMARY

It should be evident that we have much research yet to conduct to be able to determine the length of time since death. Many factors influence the rate of decay; some have received only initial interest and many others have not been investigated at all. My experience with the Colonel Shy case points out the need to investigate factors involved in determining the time interval since death.

You may have wondered what happened to Colonel Shy. This summary would not be complete unless we conclude the scenario surrounding the events of his disturbance and final burial.

The police investigation indicates that Colonel Shy's grave was vandalized by individuals seeking Civil War items such as buttons, swords, etc. No one has ever been held accountable for disturbing the grave, and Dowd (1980:69) states:

> Many of the local residents are sure that they know the identity of the vandal but this does not necessarily mean that they are correct. The vandal may have escaped punishment from the law but he will probably have nightmares for the rest of his life over this gruesome deed.

After reconstructing the fragmentary skull (Fig. 11-1), Colonel Shy's remains were gathered from labs across the state, and plans were made for his reburial. Dowd (1980:66–67) says:

> Shy had not married and had no living descendants but other relatives were contacted and told of the upcoming ceremony. Mrs. W. J. Montana, a great-great-granddaughter of Colonel Shy's brother came to Franklin from Silsbee, Texas, to represent the family. The following is a newspaper article, in part, that describes the ceremony:
>
>> On Monday the 13th day of February, 1978, a cold rain was falling. The weather was probably much like as it was at the original burial, 114 years ago. The service was brief. There was no drumroll or rifle salute. Six civilian-dressed members of the Sons of the Confederacy carried the gray coffin to its resting place. Members of the D.A.C. were also on hand with Confederate flags, and one was placed on the grave. The Rev. Charles Fulton of St. Paul's Episcopal Church said a short eulogy over the Shy coffin, donated by the Franklin Memorial Chapel. Mrs. Montana praised Franklin's historical community for its warmth and sincerity. She remarked, "I guess he could have been put back in the ground in a pine box, but the people of Franklin gave a very warm ceremony". (Lyons 1978)
>
> The cast iron coffin that had originally contained the body of Colonel Shy had been severely damaged by the grave-robbers. Mrs. Montana graciously donated the cast iron coffin to the Carter House, a prominent home that was at the center of the heaviest fighting during the Battle of Franklin. The Carter House is now run by the Association for the Preservation of Tennessee Antiquities and has been turned into a famous Civil War Museum.
>
> Cast iron coffins were very expensive and only people of some prominence could have afforded them; most people in 1864 were buried in pine boxes. This cast iron coffin weighs almost 300 pounds and has a glass plate over the face area for viewing the remains. It has an oval iron plate that fits over the glass just before burial. The coffin was sealed and bolted with steel screws and has four handles on each side. It had been painted white when originally used.

REFERENCES

Dowd, John T. (1980). The Investigation of the Vandalized Graves of Two Historic Personages: Osceola, Seminole War Chief, and Colonel William M. Shy, Civil War Hero. *Tennessee Anthropologist*, 5:47–72.

El-Najjar, Mohmoud Y. and K. Richard McWilliams (1978). *Forensic Anthropology*. Charles C Thomas, Springfield, Illinois.

Gilbert, B. Miles and William M. Bass (1967). Seasonal dating of burials from the presence of fly pupae. *American Antiquity, 32*:534–535.

Krogman, Wilton M. (1962). *The Human Skeleton in Forensic Medicine.* Charles C Thomas, Springfield, Illinois.

Lyons, David (1978). *Nashville Banner*, February 14, 1978, Nashville, Tennessee.

Marshall, Park (1912). *The Confederate Veteran.* Vol. 20, No. 11, Nashville, Tennessee.

Marshall, T. K. (1968). Changes After Death. In F. E. Camps (Ed.): *Gradwohl's Legal Medicine,* 2nd ed. Bristol: John Wright and Son, Ltd.

Morse, Dan and James W. Stoutamire (1980). Determination of the time of death by the degree of deterioration of associated material. Abstract, Program American Academy of Forensic Sciences, 32nd Annual Meeting, New Orleans, Louisiana.

Motter, Murray G. (1898). A contribution to the study of the fauna of the grave. A study of one hundred and fifty disinterments, with some additional experimental observations. *Journal of the New York Entomological Society, 6*:201–231.

Payne, Jerry A. (1965). A summer carrion study of the baby pig *Sus Scrofa Linnaeus. Ecology, 46*:592–602.

Payne, Jerry A., Frank W. Mead and Edwin W. King (1968). Hemiptera associated with pig carrion. *Annals of the Entomological Society of America, 61*:565–567.

Payne, Jerry A., Edwin W. King and George Beinhart (1968). Arthropod succession and decomposition of buried pigs. *Nature, 219*:1180–1181.

Payne, Jerry A. and Edwin W. King (1970). Coleoptera associated with pig carrion. *Entomologist's Monthly Magazine, 105*:224–232.

———— (1972). Insect succession and decomposition of pig carcasses in water. *Journal of the Georgia Entomological Society, 7*:153–162.

Payne, Jerry A. and W. R. M. Mason (1971). Hymenoptera associated with pig carrion. *Proceedings of the Entomological Society of Washington, 73*:132–141.

Reed, Horace B., Jr. (1953). Ecological Studies of Dog Carcass Communities Near Knoxville, Tennessee, With Special Reference to the Insects. Doctoral Dissertation, University of Tennessee, Knoxville.

———— (1958). A study of dog carcass communities in Tennessee, with special reference to the insects. *American Midland Naturalist, 59*:213–245.

Stewart, T. D. (1979). *Essentials of Forensic Anthropology.* Charles C Thomas, Springfield, Illinois.

Sublett, Audrey J. (1966). Seneca Physical Types and Changes Through Time. Ph.D. Dissertation, State University of New York at Buffalo.

———— (1967). Anthropological information derived from known Seneca burials. *Abstract, American Journal of Physical Anthropology, 27*:237–238.

Ubelaker, Douglas H. (1974a). Reconstruction of Demographic Profiles from Ossuary Skeletal Samples. Smithsonian Contributions to Anthropology, No. 18. Smithsonian Institution Press. Washington, D.C.

———— (1974b). Demographic reconstruction from ossuary skeletal samples: a case study from southern Maryland. *Abstract, American Journal of Physical Anthropology, 40*:154.

Ubelaker, Douglas H. and P. Willey (1978). Complexity in Arikara mortuary practice. *Plains Anthropologist, 23*:69–74.

Warren, Charles P. (1980). Plants and related decomposition vectors of human skeletal remains. Abstract, Program American Academy of Forensic Sciences, 32nd Annual Meeting, New Orleans, Louisiana.

Chapter 12

BURNED REMAINS

RODGER HEGLAR

Cases involving burned remains demonstrate the utility of forensic anthropology in forensic science. Thermally affected human remains that require an opinion on identification, history, or condition demand the use of routine methodology from forensic anthropology, frequently in association with forensic pathology and forensic odontology. As is often the case in forensic sciences, however, standard methodology must be modified to meet the needs of a specific situation or case and autopsy.

After considering some general observations that can be made concerning burned bone, the discussion of two types of cases demonstrates cooperative efforts in forensic anthropology as well as methodological applications. The cases represent (1) mixed fragmentary remains remaining after deliberate disturbance, and (2) identification of a fire victim's burned body.

COMMENTS ON BURNED BONE

Burned human skeletal remains present specific problems in investigation and evidence gathering. Their condition can range from whole body regions and bone elements to highly fragmentary remains. In these states the most apparent alterations of bone are in color, weight, surface texture, and anatomical continuity.

Burned bone color varies from yellow–light brown, black–blue–grey, to white. These color ranges and combinations generally indicate temperature, time of exposure, and location to direct or indirect heating or burning. The entire range of color can sometimes be found in the bone fragments of a single thermal incident.

If bone is merely exposed to heat, it may show only soot or smoke streaking, but its color of yellow to brown often is due to fat and body oils. Such fat and oil-containing bone or fragment will be similar to fresh bone both in feel and weight, as there is little dehydration in ranges of heating. Charred and blackened bone can also contain oils, but more often it is considerably lighter in weight due to dehydration. With prolonged heating or direct flame, bone will usually reach the white stage. This results in very lightweight fragments and ash.

Skeletal segments that have undergone high heat with prolonged dehydration show this history in complete calcination. Calcination results in a fired-pottery appearance with the feel, weight, and sound of unglazed ceramic. In addition to the color considerations, degrees of calcination can be found with a range of colors if the bone is dehydrated to the residual calcium matrix.

In surface configuration, long bones and flat bones respond differently to a variety of heat exposures. While the articular surfaces of long bones will often show reticulated cracking patterns, their shaft fragments present typical "wet bone" transverse or oblique ring fractures in lineal sequence (Ubelaker, 1978). It is not uncommon to find warping in these fragments as well.

Of the flat bone elements of the body, the earliest to be affected by fire are the bones of the cranial vault. Here direct burning and dehydration can result in fire cracking of surface patterns and the isolated release of large portions of cortical outer table bone. Charred exposed cancellous (diploe) cranial vault areas are not uncommon. Likewise, the external iliac surface of the hip will appear similarly in highly charred burned remains (see Chap. 13).

In addition to the above changes, shrinkage in burned bone may take place. Although rare, this size change can be as much as 25 percent. In differential burning of regions of the body this could affect sex and age opinions based on size-related observations (Ubelaker, 1978). Bone shrinkage determinations related to temperature have been summarized by Stewart (1979).

If remains are not disturbed during the fire incident, then fragile and exposed skeletal areas will keep their general continuity. Shifting structural debris or removal can, however, cause breakage and disorientation of body and skeletal parts. It is helpful to know the characteristics of the fire site and victim location so as to sort out artifactual changes from possible antemortem trauma (see Chaps. 11 & 13). The disturbance factor plus those previously discussed must be considered when attempting to "match" body parts or fragments of several individuals in a multiple death situation.

In a high temperature and prolonged exposure incineration, such as in a commercial mortuary gas flame cremation, an estimated 2 to 3 pounds of white calcined bone fragments and ash are recovered (Spitz and Fisher, 1973). Even under these conditions it has been observed that the cranial base, lumbar spine, pelvic areas, and some long bone shaft segments are recognizable if not disturbed.

CASE PRESENTATIONS

Case 1

A rural family of four (father, mother, teen-age son and young daughter) had supposedly left their farm on a planned vacation trip to the southern part of the state. The farmhand attested to this fact when approached by several neighbors who were well acquainted with the family and their habits. They became concerned when signs of household duties not completed, appointments not kept, and failure of expected appearances of the children or parents accumulated. In spite of their being told that a planned trip had been taken, after two weeks uneasy friends filed a missing persons report at the County Sheriff's Office. This stimulated a visit to the farm and a questioning of the farmhand by Sheriff's deputies. Two findings from that initial visit initiated a thorough search of the buildings and grounds: suspicious responses by the farmhand, and a blood-stained inside wall of the combination barn and hog pen.

The search of the house, a shack built for the help, barn and hog pen flooring, plus farmyard produced little to satisfy the local authorities. The only findings that could have value as evidence were items in and around a 3 by 7 foot trash-burning pit to the south of the barn. Here expected kitchen garbage such as cans, bottles, and animal bones plus burned luggage hardware was recovered. Two belt buckles, suspender clasps, a woman's watch, and a wedding ring were recovered on further search of the trash pit. From the grass surrounding the pit area investigators noted several child's stuffed animals.

It was after this initial search that a forensic anthropologist (Heglar) was invited to continue the search with the deputies. Although the barn and hog pen were most suspect in the minds of the authorities, concentration on the trash pit seemed essential due to the previous finding of personal effects. Upon approaching the pit, which was now surrounded by ash and garbage tossed out from the first search, a charred human lower jaw fragment (mandibular left ramus) was in clear view atop a small ash pile. The response to this find was a full removal and screening of the remaining pit contents and a screening of the marginal grass containing ash from the pit. All resulting material was bagged and labeled according to designated pit margin areas. Quite soon it was realized that the remains being recovered did not show a pattern of either body placement or count in relation to the pit areas. The remains were highly fragmentary, few, and sporadic in their occurrence in the search area.

The field bags of human skeletal fragments were taken to the coroner's office, emptied onto a sorting table, flouroscoped for metal, and further sorted into dental and skeletal fragment categories. Two small metal fragments that resembled "shot" were sent to the crime laboratory. The anthropologist and odontologist found it advantageous to work and sort together. This facilitated control of information and provided a situation in which each expert could support the other's initial findings as chain of evidence. Dental remains, tooth or alveolar bone, were collected by both investigators and finally signed over to the odontologist. An inventory of the recorded fragmentary remains that served as evidence is given in Table 12-I. Also, a summary of the evidence allowing an opinion that the remains represented at least three persons besides a child is presented in Figure 12-1. This opinion that four individuals were involved and the finding of personal effects was enough evidence for the district attorney to charge the farmhand with multiple homicide. To show that the remains were indeed those of the particular missing family members was another matter.

If the remains did represent the missing family, proof would have to be given that the father (age 36), mother (age 27), son (age 14) and daughter (age 4) were specifically indicated. The combined anthropology and odontology report submitted to the coroner contained the opinion and findings given in Table 12-II. This table can best be appreciated by refering back to the inventory of remains in Table 12-I.

Although this information is generally consistant with the descriptions of these missing persons, solid identification was possible only for the mother and teen-age son. The mother was identified through a comparison of tooth root and trabecular alveolar bone points of similarity noted in antemortem and postmortem dental radiographs. The son was also identified through x-ray comparison. A year prior to this incident the son complained of hip joint discomfort and routine AP and oblique radiographs of both hips were taken at the local hospital. With these hospital films in hand, x-rays of burned proximal femora fragments were taken in like position to the clinical films. The antemortem films and the postmortem coroner's films were regionally scanned simultaneously from superior to inferior limits through a ½-inch slit in black cardboard. This procedure allowed one more quickly to recognize similar visual patterns of bone density that could be missed in the total film view. Identical bone cortical, trabecular, and epiphyseal images or margins were recorded as "matching" areas and points of similarity. Thirteen such areas or points of morphological match were found (right femur: AP = 2; oblique = 3; left femur: AP = 4; oblique = 4). For example, the left femur fragment in its AP view and four matching patterns are schematized and shown in Figure 12-2.

Two circumstances concluded this investigation prior to a jury trial. An accomplice turned state's evidence and testified in deposition to his knowl-

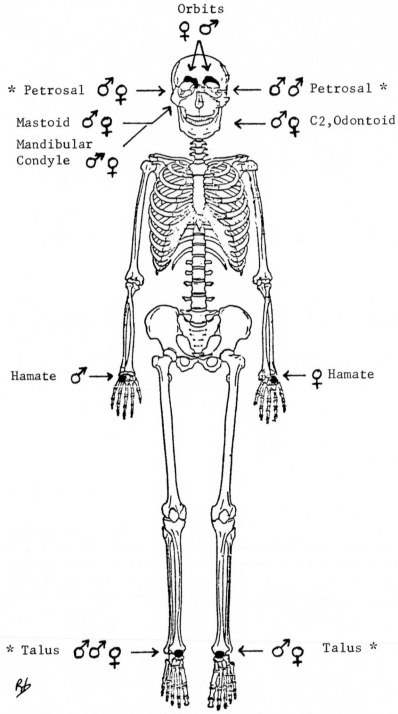

Figure 12-1. (Case 1) Composite demonstrating evidence of two and three (*) persons (child not included).

TABLE 12-I
CASE 1: INVENTORY OF BURNED SKELETAL FRAGMENTS

A. Craniofacial, Dental, Postcranial Fragments of a Child.

B. Craniofacial Fragments:
  —Posterior occipital to foramen magnum.
  —Occipital, temporal, and parietal.
  —Mandibular body, cortical bone of buccal surface.
  —Anterior maxillary with three teeth.
  —Maxilla, two sections with tooth sockets.
  —Misc. tooth roots and crowns.

(RIGHT)	(LEFT)
Mastoid process (2)	*Petrosal (2)
*Petrosal (2)	Orbital border, postorbital
Zygoma	*Occipital condyle
Frontal, postorbital ridge.	Mandible, reconstructed body
*Occipital condyle	with tooth roots.
Temporo-zygomatic arch	
Mandibular condyle (2)	

C. Postcranial Fragments
  —Femur shafts
  —Lumbar posterior vertebrae
  —Misc. carpals and long bones
  —Cervical (C_1) condyle and neural arch.
  —Cervical (C_2) two odontoid process with body.

(RIGHT)	(LEFT)
Humerus, trochlea and capitulum	Humerus, trochlea and capitulum
Radius, proximal shaft	Radius, ½ head
*Carpal, hook of hamate	Ulna, distal ½
Femur, proximal 1/5	*Carpal, hook of hamate
Femur, lateral border, lateral condyle	Femur, proximal 1/5
Tibia, mid-shaft	Talus, two articular surfaces
Fibula, malleolus	
Talus, three trochlear surfaces	

Note: * = Not same person.

edge of the time and manner of the crime. He described a gunshot homicide of all four family members, incineration of the bodies after a short storage in the barn, a collecting and crushing of the recognizable burned remains taken from the trash pit burn site with subsequent scattering of the fragments in unspecified locations along a nearby foothill road. The accused, when confronted with the above facts, plus the knowledge that four persons had been documented from the pit with two identified, confessed.

Case 2

There are occasions when single or multiple deaths from thermal origin require the aid of a forensic anthropologist for specific identification of the

TABLE 12-II
CASE 1: OPINIONS ON THE SEX AND ESTIMATION OF AGE

Sex Determination	*Age Estimate*
ADULT MALE	—40 years. (30–40)
Craniofacial size & muscularity.	Joint margins, cranial sutures.
Left orbit, superior and lateral borders.	Bone muscularity.
Upper & lower limb fragments.	
ADULT FEMALE	—40 years (early 30s)
Craniofacial fragments.	Joint margins.
Supraorbital area.	Tooth root and alveolar
Mandible, left body.	Mandibular features.
ADOLESCENT MALE	14–15 years.
Size & muscularity, unexpectedly large skeletal system.	Visual and x-ray epiphyseal status of femoral head
	Lesser trochanter and greater trochantric epiphyseal status.
CHILD	4–5 years.
————	Deciduous tooth status.

victims. This input usually is descriptive in nature and includes an estimate of age at the time of death, living stature estimation, and an opinion on biological population or race of an individual.

This opinion was asked when, following a multiple residence building fire, a charred body was recovered from the street level rubble of the collapsed upper floors. One female resident had not been accounted for by the Red Cross. She was a 46-year-old Caucasian woman approximately 5 feet 7 inches tall. Dental records were not available for her, but the family physician did have a two-year-old chest film of her that was made available to the coroner's office.

The body was typical of high thermal destruction, since the cranial vault displayed the exploded results of intercranial pressure and the limbs were retracted into the "pugilistic position" with shortened and charred forearms and legs. As a point of procedure, forensic odontology examinations can be greatly aided by the routine bagging of the head at the scene. If this could be done at removal of the body, both tooth and alveolar bone fragments would be better preserved for identification. Artifactual changes are difficult to avoid from handling such remains at the scene as well as at the time of autopsy in that head and limbs are fragile.

Age estimation was obtained by the removal and examination of the left pubic symphysis. Here an incision, as an extension of the pathologist's autopsy incision, was made inferior to the midline down and around the external genitalia. This allows a lateral retraction of the genitalia and a clear view of the anterior pubic surface. Palpation of the dorsal or internal symphysis area, with reflection of the bladder, provides an orientation to the symphysis cartilage. The cartilage is centrally incised, and the pubis articu-

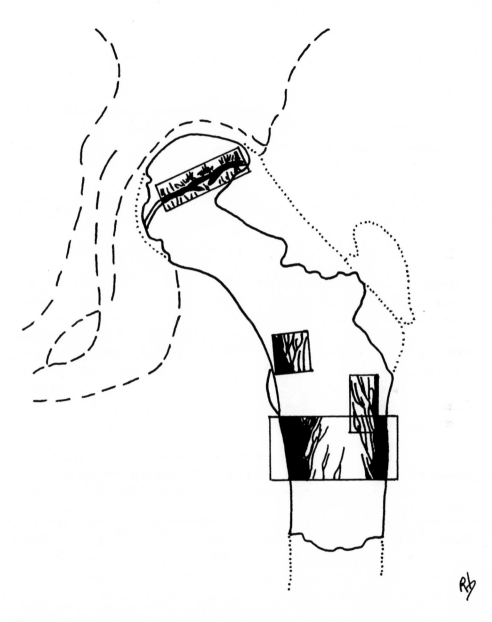

Figure 12-2. (Case 2) Left femoral fragment superimposed over antemortem x-ray showing four areas of trabecular morphological similarities.

lar surface with about ¾-inch of the bone is sawed free. One removed, the pubis face can be transversely sectioned into six sections with a fine blade high speed saw. The contours of the dorsal, ventral, and cartilage of the articular surface margins can be morphologically interpreted. This interpretation is then used as the shape and surface "Component I, II, & III" judgements routinely used as criteria for pubic symphysis aging. Such criteria are in the forensic literature for males (McKern and Stewart, 1957) and females (Gilbert and McKern, 1973) (see Chap. 20). Further general age range estimates can be had by palpating the vertebral margins and available joint areas for arthritic changes. If an elderly person is suspected, a cross section of the femur at mid-shaft will result in an impression of cortical bone thickness related to bone shaft width. Likewise, a radiographic view or direct measurement of cortical thickness, total width, and medullary width of the second metacarpal of the hand may support an age range opinion on burn cases. If a direct exposed bone measurement is used, 0.5 mm must be added to reflect the slight enlargement included in the radiographic base date and table (Lusted and Keats, 1972). It is assumed, however, that any incisions should be made after the pathologist's examination and with specific permission from the coroner or medical examiner.

Skeletal or body stature estimates more accurately reflect living height if the thigh (femur) and leg (tibia) bone lengths are determined. In this case, the femoral length was estimated through two incisions. One was made 2 inches superior to the hip joint prominence (trochantric) as a 4 inch deep muscle cut down to the superior hip joint area. A second incision is necessary at the knee joint to expose the lateral femoral condyle. Femoral length can be measured from the palpated superior acetabular-femoral head margin down to the most distal point on the lateral condylar surface. Here, though, one must add 1 cm to the obtained length to account for the portion of femoral head covered by the superior acetabular articulation. This long bone measurement is then taken to the formula or table based on the Trotter and Gleser data for living stature estimation (Trotter and Gleser, 1958).

This particular female body was recorded as a pubic symphysis "Component Score" of 13 = 47.75 ± 3.59 years of age. Her living height was estimated at approximately 5 feet 7 inches through her estimated femur length of 47 cms = 170 cm stature.

As indicated above, there was a chest film available. This film was compared to a similar routine chest film taken of the burned torso. A regional comparative scan of both films showed morphological similarities in the upper chest (thorax) and shoulder regions. Unique individuality was apparent in the general bone size and shape of the right rib 4 image. Further image similarity was noted in the asymmetry and pattern of the inferior borders of both clavicles and their acromioclavicular joints. These radiographic features were superimposable and specific enough to support the opinion that it would be highly unlikely that two persons of the same sex, age, and stature would display the same morphological features. Therefore, this fire victim was identified on the basis of the chest x-ray. Figure 12-3 schematically presents the necessary areas dealt with in the description and identification of this person.

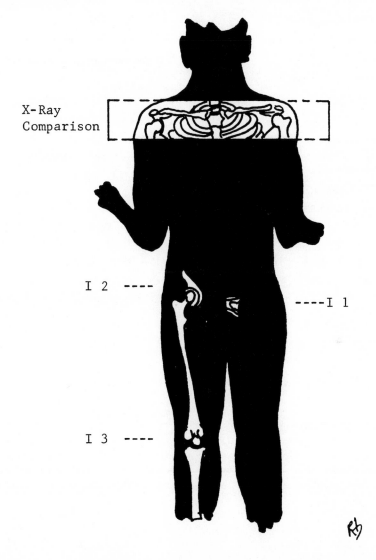

Figure 12-3. (Case 2) Identification approach to a burned body through incisions and x-ray comparison. I 1 = pubic sumphysis; I 2 = acetabular margin; I 3 = knee.

CONCLUSIONS

The team approach to human identification and death investigation between forensic pathology, forensic odontology, and forensic anthropology has increased in recent years. This approach is a valid and advantageous use of expertise and methodology basic to reliable forensic science evidence and opinion.

Although the techniques and cases presented in this and Bass's contributions are oriented toward human burned remains, similar methods have been designed to obtain medicolegal information from whole or fragmentary remains in a variety of conditions. There is the reliance on direct examination, anthropometrics and osteometrics, radiographics, and microscopic observation plus the knowledge of the site and circumstances of a death involved in a forensic anthropological report to the coroner or medical examiner's office.

As the three fields (pathology, dentistry, and anthropology) generate evidence and opinions in a specific case, each is independently supporting the final findings in identification and/or death investigation. Usually the odontological and anthropological examination and input follow that of pathology. In effect the anthropologist performs an "osteo-autopsy" with the majority of the reported information and description arising from skeletal system evidence.

REFERENCES

Gilbert, B. M. and McKern, T. W. (1973). A method for aging the female os pubis. *Am J Phys Anthropol, 38*:31–38.

Lusted, L. B. and Keats, T. E. (1972). *Atlas of Roentgenographic Measurements*. Chicago: Year Book Medical Publishers.

McKern, T. W. and Stewart, T. D. (1957). *Skeletal Age Changes in Young American Males.* Technical Report P-45, Quartermaster Research and Development Command, U.S. Army, Natick, Mass.

Spitz, W. U. and Fisher, R. S. (1973). *Medicolegal Investigation of Death.* Springfield: Charles C Thomas.

Stewart, T. D. (1979). *Essentials of Forensic Anthropology.* Springfield: Charles C Thomas.

Trotter, M. and Gleser, G. C. (1958). A re-evaluation of stature based on measurements taken during life and of long bones after death. *Am J Phys Anthropol, 16*:79–123.

Ublaker, D. H. (1978). *Human Skeletal Remains.* Chicago: Aldine.

Chapter 13

IS IT POSSIBLE TO CONSUME A BODY COMPLETELY IN A FIRE?

WILLIAM M. BASS

INTRODUCTION

Forensic anthropologists are often asked, "Is it possible to consume a body completely in a house or building fire?" The answer is no. Even though no soft tissue may remain, there are always pieces of the skeleton, and if a careful search is made by well-trained osteologists, fragments of bones can be recovered and subsequently identified.

One of the earliest reports involving burned bone was the "Furnace Murder Case" in which Wilton M. Krogman (1949) experimentally burned human remains to document the changes that occur when a skeleton is burned in a furnace. Krogman was able to identify the fragmentary pieces of the skeleton that remained as human and diagnosed some features of the individual. Although reports on burned bone are scattered in the literature, a good summary can be found in Stewart (1979). Early research on archaeological cremations (Adena and Hopewell Cultures) was done by Baby (1954), and more recent experiments have provided empirical evidence of bone burned under controlled conditions (Binford 1963, 1972; Buikstra and Goldstein 1973; Thurman and Willmore 1981). Other useful information on cremations has been reported by Gejvall (1963), Herrmann (1977), Merbs (1967), and Wells (1960).

Even when bodies are commercially cremated, the skeletal fragments can be identified if they are not ground too finely. Most people do not realize that a cremated adult human body produces approximately a half bushel or more of fragments and ashes. Usually only a small portion of the ashes is returned to the family in an urn while the major portion of the bony remains is ground and disposed of in various ways. Maples (1982) reported the analysis of a commercial cremation involved in a forensic case.

159

SPECIAL PROBLEMS

The aid of the forensic anthropologist is usually requested in cases where the body is extensively burned. I have previously reported on the special contributions of a forensic anthropologist in fire investigations (1979), and more recently Angel (1982), Rhine (1982), and Suchey (1982) have reported on the identification of burned bone. We, as forensic anthropologists, are seldom needed in cases involving death by smoke inhalation or in analyzing bodies on which much of the tissue remains. Burned bodies often assume the so-called pugilistic pose. As illustrated in Figure 13-1, this is a typical boxer's posture with the arms drawn up and the fists clenched in a defensive position. It is caused by heat coagulation and shrinkage of muscle bundles, predominately the stronger flexer muscles. Watanabe (1968:139) states, "This change can occur in bodies that are alive or dead and is only an indication of exposure to intense heat." In a hot fire the arms and legs usually burn and fall from the body, and the skull explodes because of the rapid expansion of fluids within the brain. Thus, the typical burned case seen by most forensic anthropologists consists of the torso (and if even more extensively burned, only the pelvic area) or a skeleton completely reduced to bone fragments and ashes.

It should be remembered that in burn cases where only the torso or pelvic area has been recovered (usually by the rescue squad or fire department), the best evidence for a positive identification still remains at the scene of the fire in the form of burned bone fragments of the skull and limb bones. Care should always be taken to search the fire scene for teeth, cranial fragments, dentures, orthodontic and orthopedic devices, jewelry, and items contained in or on the clothing worn by the victim.

ILLUSTRATING CASES

Case 1

A few years ago I was asked to identify some burned bones that had been identified by a physician and a forensic pathologist as being those of a dog. I first saw the material about 12 days after the fire. The bones submitted consisted of the fragmentary pelvis, the lower lumbar vertebrae, and about 4 inches of the proximal portions of both femora of a human male of approximately 38 years. The bones were held together by burned tissue. Age was based on an assessment of the pubic symphysis. Realizing that the fragmentary skull probably was still at the scene of the fire, I asked the sheriff if we could return to the burned house and search for teeth and bone from which

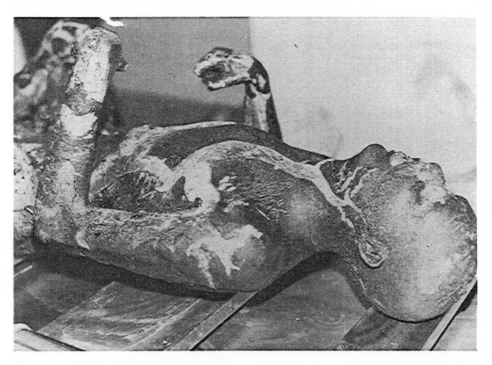

Figure 13-1. A good example of the pugilistic pose. This adult male fell into a brush fire. Note the typical boxer's posture, caused by contraction and shrinkage of muscle bundles, predominately the stronger flexer muscles.

we could make an estimation of race and, I hoped, a positive identification. Arrangements were made, and when we arrived, the sheriff took me aside and said the individual suspected to have burned to death in the fire always carried a .32 caliber pistol and always wore blue jeans. Even though we visited the fire scene some five weeks after the fire, we were able, through a careful search by well-trained osteologists using systematic archaeological techniques, to discover much new information. We found (1) the .32 caliber pistol near where the torso was recovered, (2) the type of metal rivets often found in blue jeans, (3) enough teeth and cranial fragments to make a positive identification through comparative records, and (4) enough evidence to prove the house fire was arson. Though there was a deceased suspect in this case, it was important to make a positive identification of the body or bodies, because there could be other possible victims of the fire. Therefore, we carefully excavated the entire house. Aside from the skeletal remains and items mentioned above, we also recovered three charcoal lighter cans on which labels were still legible (no charcoal grill was present). There were no coat hangers in the closets, no dishes or silverware in the

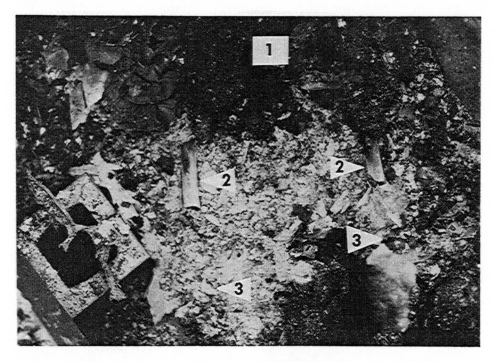

Figure 13-2. Because the legs and arms are smaller and surrounded by air, they usually burn to a greater degree than the torso. Above, the badly charred pelvis (1) is in the upper center of the picture. The proximal 4 to 6 inches of the femora can be seen (2) where the soft tissue has been burned away. The distal portions of the femora and the rest of the legs have been reduced to bone fragments, which can be recovered by careful excavation (3).

kitchen, and no furniture in the house at the time of the fire. It was obvious from our investigation that all items of value had been removed from the house prior to the fire. This illustrates that fire scenes contain much evidence even long after the fire, and much can be recovered for interpretation by using careful archaeological techniques.

Case 2

Another case illustrating how much information a forensic anthropologist can retrieve occurred in mid January of 1981 in Hawkins County, Tennessee. The sheriff's office called one Friday to request aid in locating a missing person, a 36-year-old male, who had been missing some 12 days and possibly could be in a house that recently burned. I arrived at the scene around 9:00 Saturday morning, along with three graduate students experienced in osteology and forensic anthropology.

The two-story brick home was on the outskirts of Kingsport, Tennessee,

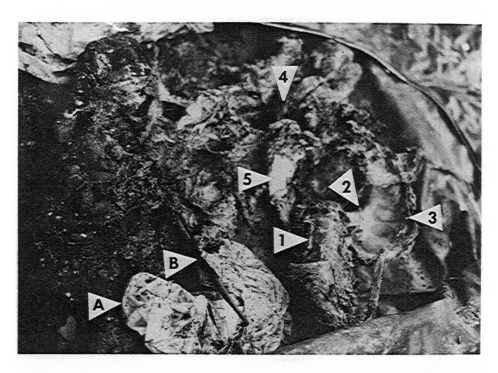

Figure 13-3. At first glance, this material recovered from a fire and submitted for identification appears to be of amorphous character. The above picture is the first view of material in a disaster bag, much of which is partially burned. The nonhuman material is (A) a sheet and (B) a stick. The human material is (1) lower lumbar vertebra covered by burned tissue, (2) right sacroiliac joint, (3) right ilium, (4) proximal portion of the left femur, and (5) remaining portion of the burned left ilium.

about 100 yards south of the Holston River and approximately 500 yards from its nearest neighbor. The sheriff related the following story. The house had recently been purchased by a Virginia man (J.G.) who was in the process of remodeling it. He usually spent the week working on the house with the help of a locally hired man and returned to Virginia on the weekends. One weekend the owner of the house did not return to Virginia, and by Sunday his family contacted the Hawkins County Sheriff's Office. A check was made, and for the first time the officials were aware that the house had burned. They had not been notified of the fire even though subsequent investigation in the neighborhood revealed that an explosion had preceded the fire.

The fire department had not been called, and the house was a total loss. Only the lower portion of the brick walls remained. Two large brick chimneys as well as part of the walls had fallen inside the structure. Because the house was being remodeled, no furniture was present to indicate the location of bedrooms. Our interview with the police revealed that the new owner had been sleeping in a sleeping bag on a wooden cot at one end of the house. Our forensic excavation was begun in that area.

An hour after we began, we discovered human foot bones. Further intensive search revealed an extensively burned skeleton with no soft tissue remaining. A small portion of the left buttock was found adhering to the floor, but not enough tissue remained to obtain a blood sample. The skeletal material recovered was similar to what is left from a commercial cremation, i.e. small charred or calcined fragments.

Careful excavation revealed that when the fire started the body was unnaturally contracted and lying on its back. The legs were folded back on top of the body with the femora on top of the thoracic region and the feet in the head area. A major complication, however, was that no skull or upper limb bones were present. This case was entirely different from the pugilistic pose discussed earlier. The pugilistic position can only be determined when the arms are still attached to the body. In the present case little tissue remained, and the entire skeleton was cremated. Even though cremated, the unnatural anatomical position of the thorax, pelvis, and legs suggested some unusual circumstances surrounding the death of J.G. Concentrated examination of the thorax, pelvis, and legs allowed us to prove that the body was in the basement when the fire started and had not fallen through from an upper floor. There was no debris between the skeleton and the concrete floor. Had the body fallen through from an upper floor, debris and burned particles would have been between the skeleton and the concrete basement floor.

In addition, the fire had been so hot that the body had cooked onto the basement floor. The left buttock (which had been reduced to a cinder) was removed. A small unburned portion of jockey shorts and dark green work pants lay immediately on top of the concrete floor. Three inches to the left of the fragmented spinal column was a chunk of lead (possibly a bullet) with an impression of fabric on the side next to the floor. The ribs had burned to ashes, so it was impossible to state definitely that the individual had been shot, but the proximity of the bullet to the spinal column and the fabric impression suggested such an event.

Numerous photographs were taken of every phase of excavation and recovery. After removal of the lower portion of the skeleton, the excavation was expanded, and the fragmented skull and upper arms were found about 8 feet south of the postcranial skeleton. We were able to collect most of the teeth and cranial bones as well as the bones of the upper limbs even though they were in hundreds of pieces. We were, again, able to show that the body lay on the basement floor prior to the fire and had not fallen from the floor above.

The field recovery being completed and the lead slug turned over to the

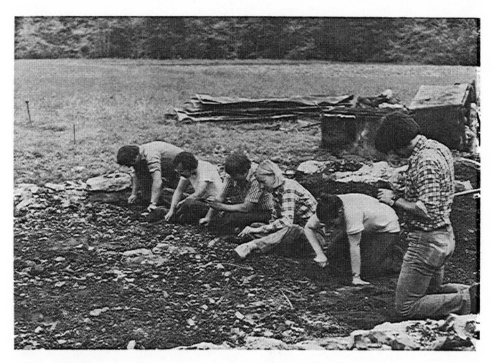

Figure 13-4. Graduate students in forensic anthropology are conducting a careful excavation of a two-story house that has burned a few months before. An elderly woman who lived in the house could not be found after the fire. The forensic excavation revealed no evidence of the woman, suggesting that she was not in the house at the time of the fire.

police for ballistics tests, we returned to the laboratory for the long and careful reconstruction of the face and dental regions from the small fragments. It was known that the suspect, J.G., had extensive dental work, and records from his dentist were obtained by the time we had pieced together the facial skeleton. Radiographs of the recovered burned material revealed a sufficient number of similar traits for positive identification. The missing person, J.G., was indeed the victim recovered from the fire.

Disposition of Case

Why had the skull and upper limb bones separated from the rest of the body? Had this body been blown up? The neighbors had reported an explosion prior to the fire. I had no previous experiences with explosions, and the extensive fragmentation of the entire skeleton did not allow much insight, since fragmentation and disintegration to ashes do occur in fires this hot.

After our recovery and positive identification, the law enforcement officers began an extensive investigation, which led to the arrest of the man hired to help in the remodeling. A court trial was held in October of 1981, and the defendant was found guilty and sentenced to die in the electric chair. Court testimony helped fill in some of the missing details.

J.G. had been shot and robbed. His truck and some of the materials purchased for the remodeling were sold. Two dogs were brought into the house to destroy the body. When that did not occur after a day, a decision was made to blow up the body and burn the house to cover up the murder. In this case, I suspect, both the explosion and the very hot fire contributed to fragmentation of the skull and arms. Certainly the explosion caused the unnatural anatomical position of the thorax, pelvis and lower limbs and their separation from the head and arms.

This fragmentary skeleton would not have been found and the subsequent interpretation could not have been made without the training and expertise of a forensic anthropologist. Thus, with careful investigation by trained experts we can answer the question proposed as the title of this chapter—in the average house or building fire, it is not possible to burn a skeleton completely beyond recognition!

REFERENCES

Angel, J. Lawrence (1982). Identification from burnt bones. Abstract of a paper presented at the 34th Annual Meeting of the American Academy of Forensic Sciences, Orlando, Florida. Program Abstract H24, p. 101.

Baby, Raymond S. (1954). Hopewell cremation practices. Ohio Historical Society, *Papers in Archaeology, 1*:1–7.

Bass, William M. (1979). The Forensic Anthropologist in fire investigations. Abstract of paper presented at the 31st Annual Meeting of the American Academy of Forensic Sciences, Atlanta, Georgia. Program Abstract H14, p. 124.

Binford, Lewis R. (1963). An analysis of cremations from three Michigan sites. *Wisconsin Archeologist, 44*:98–110.

———— (1972). An analysis of cremations from three Michigan sites. Reprinted in L. R. Binford: *An Archaeological Perspective*, pp. 373–382, Seminar Press, New York and London.

Buikstra, Jane E. and Lynne Goldstein (1973). The Perrins Ledge Crematory, Illinois State Museum, Report of Investigations, No. 28.

Gejvall, Nils-Gustaf (1963). Cremations. In Don Brothwell (Ed.): *Science in Archaeology*, pp. 379–389. Thames and Hudson, London.

Herrmann, B. (1977). On historical investigations of cremated human remains. *Journal of Human Evolution, 6*:101–105.

Krogman, Wilton M. (1949). The human skeleton in legal medicine: Medical aspects. In S. D. Levinson (Ed.): *Symposium on Medicolegal Problems. Ser. 2*:1–90. J. B. Lippincott, Philadelphia, Pennsylvania.

Maples, William (1982). Ashes to ashes, dust to dust. Abstract of paper presented at the 34th Annual Meeting of the American Academy of Forensic Sciences, Orlando, Florida. Program Abstract H30, p. 102.

Merbs, Charles (1967). Cremated Human Remains from Point of Pines, Arizona. *American Antiquity, 32*:498–506.

Rhine, Stanley (1982). Destruction of bodies by fire. Abstract of a paper presented at the 34th Annual Meeting of the American Academy of Forensic Sciences, Orlando, Florida. Program Abstract H26, p. 101.

Stewart, T. Dale (1979). *Essentials of Forensic Anthropology.* Charles C Thomas, Springfield, Illinois.

Suchey, Judy Myers (1982). Forensic Anthropological analysis of burned human remains. Abstract of a paper presented at the 34th Annual Meeting of the American Academy of Forensic Sciences, Orlando, Florida. Program Abstract H25, p. 101.

Thurman, Melburn D. and L. James Willmore (1981). A replicative cremation experiment. *North American Archaeologist,* 2:275–283.

Watanabe, Tomio (1968). *Atlas of Legal Medicine.* J. B. Lippincott, Philadelphia, Pennsylvania.

Wells, Calvin (1960). A study of cremation. *American Antiquity, 34*:29–37.

Chapter 14

DEATH BY STRANGULATION
A Forensic Anthropological Case from Wilmington, Delaware

J. Lawrence Angel and Peggy C. Caldwell*

SCENARIO

During the first week of January, 1978, a maintenance man from a local chemical company found a skull without mandible near the eighteenth hole of the Hercules Golf Course in Newark, Delaware. This was handed over to the Newark Police Department and, in turn, to Dr. A. Z. Hameli, Chief Medical Examiner in Wilmington, Delaware. Although the police officers who initially received the specimen suspected that it had been removed from a nearby cemetery, Dr. Hameli determined that it had not been buried because of the soil stains and sun bleaching on the bone. He requested a list of young white females (with dental restorations) missing from the area and eventually contacted a local dentist who had records that initially compared favorably with the dentition of the skull. Further inspection of the dental restorations in the maxilla (amalgam-filled caries in the crowns of RM^2, RM^1, LM^1, and an incompletely erupted LM^3) matched the recorded information obtained from the dentist and established the identity of S.S., who had been missing for the previous fourteen months. Dr. Hameli's request for a search to be conducted for additional remains subsequently yielded almost all of the rest of the skeleton, which had been dispersed over an area of some 2,000 square feet, apparently by dogs whose owners had homes bordering the golf course. Bones missing from the skeleton included only the left humerus and ulna; the right scapula, foot and clavicle; both hands; the first and third left ribs; the third thoracic vertebra; the seventh and eleventh right ribs; the sternum, hyoid, and a portion of the mandibular corpus from the left canine alveolus to the right M3 alveolus. The margins of the preserved mandibular fragments were beveled and suggested clean fractures apparently made close to the time of death. Other materials recovered

*The authors wish to express their gratitude to Katharine Holland for typing the manuscript. J.L.A. wishes to thank P.C.C. for revising and expanding the first draft of the chapter and for finding the relevant references on strangulation and the role of the expert witness.

168

during the search of the golf course area included a broken handgun butt, a bra, found in the vicinity of the cervical vertebrae, and a (cut) double noose of insulated wire that was found with a side loop around a piece of wood. The latter artifacts were found in proximity to each other.

ANALYSIS

After making sure that the partial skeleton and the previously discovered skull without mandible came from the same individual, S.S., (once again by comparative odontology, in addition to information provided by a mop of wavy brown hair and a set of contact lenses recovered at the scene—one in an orbit, the other near a part of the postcranial skeleton), the remains were sent to the senior author with Dr. Hameli's request for information on (1) possible indications of pathology; (2) an assessment of the skeletal areas that showed extensive carnivore chewing marks; (3) whether the margins of the preserved mandibular fragments suggested antemortem fracture; and (4) an analysis of other possible sites of antemortem fracture in the nasal, maxillary, and other areas that might have been related to the cause of S.S.'s death. Dr. Angel sent in a standard report on January 26, 1978, including statements on the general characteristics of individuality (e.g. age: 19 to 21; sex: female; ethnic background: white; stature: 62 to 65 inches) and answering Dr. Hameli's specific questions.

Although there were minimal indications of pathology in the classic sense (i.e. slight tooth enamel development arrest lines on the premolars and a trace of fine porosity at vertex on the skull vault), two skeletal areas presented signs of behavior-related stress. In the pelvic region, both acetabula had new bone growth extending the superior weight-bearing part of the joint medially, and both sacroiliac articulations showed extensions of the caudal surfaces and ligamentous "spikes" on the ilium. The latter apparently developed from the individual's active participation in college athletics. In the oral region, sharp tubercles were present on both the medial and lateral aspects of the anterior surfaces of both mandibular condyles (Fig. 14-1). These suggested habitual strong use of the external pterygoid muscles in thrusting the jaw forward. Much later, at the first trial of D.A.D. (a man in whose company S.S. had last been seen alive leaving a local singles' bar in West Chester, Pennsylvania on a November evening in 1976), the senior author asked S.S.'s mother what wind instrument the deceased had played. Somewhat surprised, the mother responded that S.S. had played the clarinet ever since she was eleven years old. The mother also confirmed Dr. Angel's inference that S.S. had been active in school sports.

Dr. Angel supported Dr. Hameli's assertion that dogs had damaged much

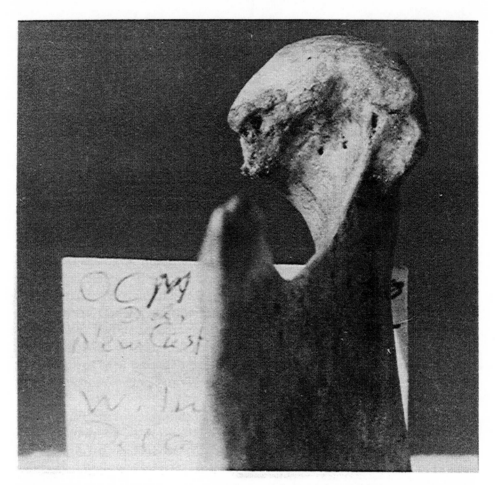

Figure 14-1. Anterior view of the left mandibular ramus, illustrating sharp tubercles on the medial and lateral surfaces of the condyle caused by habitual forward thrusting of the jaw, as in the playing of a musical wind instrument.

of the skeleton postmortem. The epiphyses of all of the bones of the upper extremities had been mostly chewed away (except those of the left clavicle), in addition to the upper left and lower right tibae; the left pubis and ischium; both anterior spines of the ilia; the costal ends of the left sixth and tenth and right fourth, sixth, eighth, and eleventh ribs; and the body of the fifth thoracic vertebra. Postmortem damage by dogs was also evident in the mastoid and maxillary regions.

The senior author agreed with Dr. Hameli on the indications of antemortem fracture on the preserved margins of the mandibular corpus. These margins (at the left canine and right M_3 alveoli) presented almost vertical surfaces showing "stepped" fracture lines and bevelling, fitting the pattern of fractures resulting from a very strong blow to the living chin (Fig. 14-2). The left M$_1$'s mesiolingual cusp had a semicircular crack, and there was pressure damage on the back of the left condyle, which were also consistent with the same pattern.

The only other antemortem fractures visible on the skeleton of S.S. were on the sixth cervical vertebra. Its left transverse process showed a vertical hinge fracture through the anterior lamina, and there was a hairline crack

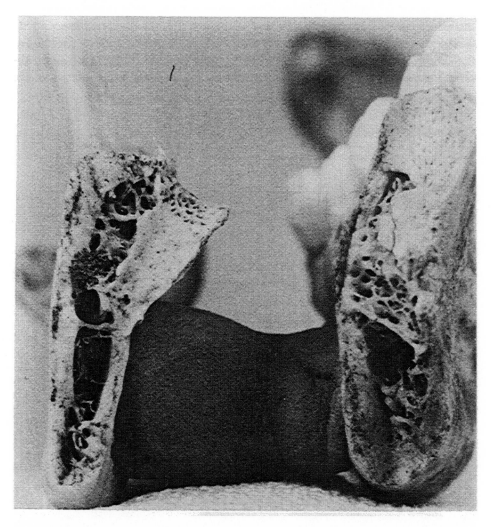

Figure 14-2. Anterior view of the mandibular fragments' margins at the sites of breakage, illustrating "stepped" fracture lines and bevelling, resulting from an antemortem blow to the chin area.

on the posterior lamina (Fig. 14-3). The former is a part of the origin for the anterior scalene muscle and ends in a bony lump referred to as the carotid tubercle because it is the pressure point for the carotid artery either in clinical testing or in strangulation, as was apparent in the present case. Since the wire noose alleged to have been used by D.A.D. was tightened enough to produce the hinge fracture in C6, with reasonable certainty it would have compressed the carotid sheaths enough to cut off the blood flow to and from the brain. The arrangement of the wire noose at the golf course recovery site (looped around the stub of a dead branch) explained why the force applied to S.S.'s neck had fractured only a single transverse process lamina, because a sufficiently severe back and crosswise wrench of the head against the contraction of the anterior scalene usually tears or loosens the anterior tubercles of the fourth through the sixth cervical vertebrae. The latter have been observed in two of Dr. Angel's previous cases. Because cervical vertebrae six and seven tilt diagonally at an angle of 5 to 10 degrees, pressure applied to the carotid tubercle from the front of the neck with reference to C6 has a slight caudal as well as posterior force.

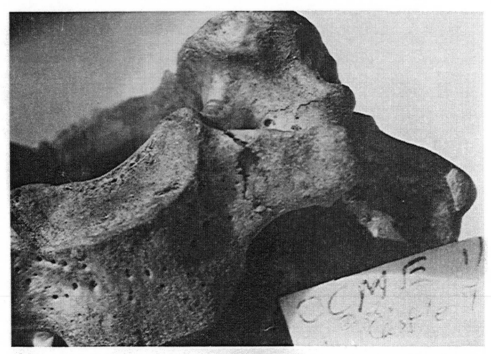

Figure 14-3. Left side of the sixth cervical vertebra, illustrating an antemortem hinge fracture through the anterior lamina and a hairline crack in the posterior lamina, resulting from "Spanish windlass" strangulation.

Previous references to strangulation as a cause of death noted in skeletonized remains suggest that it is only detectable in ossified material from the front of the throat (Dutra, 1944; Smith, 1939, 1942; Spitz and Fischer, 1980). To our knowledge, this is the first forensic anthropological case where strangulation has been determined as the cause of death from posterior neck bones. This is undoubtedly attributable to the unique strangulation procedure alleged to have been followed by D.A.D. The prosecution later used the term "Spanish windlass" to describe the strangulation arrangement of applying a double wire noose to an individual's neck with a side loop around a solid object so that by twisting the loop, the noose is tightened.

THE TRIALS

During the late spring of 1978, the senior author was contacted by both the deputy attorney general and the assistant public defender for the state of Delaware, each requesting pretrial conferences on the findings in the case of S.S. This is normal procedure in many forensic cases, and the literature strongly recommends that lawyers for the prosecution (and sometimes the defense) contact any expert witness involved in a given case (Cook, 1964; Hawkinson, 1948 (p. 38); Kogan, 1978; Philipps, 1977; Stewart, 1979; Tanay, 1981). The "assistant," who accompanied the defense lawyer to the second meeting, later (and surprisingly) turned out to be the defense counselor at both trials. In both pretrial meetings, the evaluation of the remains was reviewed, stressing opinions regarding the antemortem injuries to the jaw and the cause of death. Additionally, in the conference with the counselor for the prosecution, basic strategy for presenting testimony in court was discussed. The subject of payment was also raised, as it should be (Byrd and Stults, 1976; Tanay, 1976); however, as a government employee, the senior author could not accept any money except for travel expenses.

The first trial took place in October, 1978, and ended in a hung jury. Apparently, one of the jurors was prejudiced against the prosecution because of a grudge against a local jurisdiction. During the progress of the trial, the defense counselor conscientiously attempted to bar as much of the senior author's expert testimony as possible by arguing that only an M.D. can certify the cause of an individual's death. However, the question of the legal competence of an anthropologist to render an opinion on the cause of death was not directly tested in this trial, and the anatomical and physical evidence concerning observations on this issue (as previously explained in this chapter) was presented.

The second trial was held in late January to February, 1979, and resulted in a conviction of D.A.D. During this trial, the defense counselor did not stress the argument that only an M.D. can legally certify the cause of an individual's death. Expert testimony was permitted to include (without interruption, at the judge's request) the distinction between antemortem fractures in living, fresh bone and postmortem ones in dry bone; in the former, the softness and flexibility of the tissue with intact collagen fibers allows bending (especially in the trabeculae) and fractures with beveling and overlapping along the edge of the broken compact bone. It was the senior author's opinion that the mandibular fracture, even with the tearing of the right inferior alveolar artery, would not have caused immediate death. It was clearly testified that the wire noose, tightened around the neck at the level of C6 on the left, could have cut off both the circulation to and from the brain (except perhaps via the right vertebral vessels) and the airway to the lungs. A lunch break conference with a detective, the counselor for the defense, and Dr. Angel examining the wire noose further strengthened this view. However, it could not definitively be proven that this was indeed the actual cause of death. Nevertheless, expert testimony by an anthropologist, circumstantially reconstructing the attack on S.S., contributed to the conviction of D.A.D. in addition to the most damaging evidence of the broken handgun butt abandoned by the accused at the scene. The jury believed the truth of inference concerning the death of S.S. A commonsense description of the "weapons" recovered, linked to the postmortem anatomy of the deceased (not going beyond the physical evidence in any way), is more credible and persuasive to a jury than an aggressive expert opinion on the cause of death. No anthropologist lacking direct experience in the examination of bone fractures at death, in addition to a detailed knowledge of anatomy, should ever take on a skeletal case of this kind.

REFERENCES

Byrd, G. J. and T. Stults (1976). "The Expert Witness: A Dilemma." *Journal of Forensic Sciences,* 21:4:944–948.

Cook, C. M. (1964). "The Role and Rights of the Expert Witness." *Journal of Forensic Sciences,* 9(4):456–460.

Dutra, F. R. (1944). "Identification of Person and Determination of Cause of Death from Skeletal Remains." *Archives of Pathology 38*:339–349.

Hawkinson, O. (1948). "The Medical Witness in Court: Expert Testimony." In S. A. Levinson (Ed.): *Symposium on Medico-Legal Problems.* Philadelphia: J. B. Lippincott, pp. 1–42.

Kogan, J. D. (1978). "On Being a Good Expert Witness in a Criminal Case." *Journal of Forensic Sciences, 23(1)*:190–200.

Philipps, K. A. (1977). "The 'Nuts and Bolts' of Testifying as a Forensic Scientist." *Journal of Forensic Sciences, 22*:457–463.

Smith, S. (1939). "Studies in Identification: No. 3." *The Police Journal, (London) 12*:274–285.

———— (1942). "Studies in Identification and Reconstruction: No. 13." *The Police Journal, (London) 15*:32–39.

Spitz, W. U. and R. S. Fisher (1980). *Medicolegal Investigation of Death*, 2nd edition. Springfield: C. C Thomas. Chapter 12: Asphyxia, pp. 320–350.

Stewart, T. D. (1979). *Essentials of Forensic Anthropology*. Springfield: C. C Thomas. Chapter 2: Role of the Expert Witness, pp. 18–29.

Tanay, E. (1976). "Money and the Expert Witness: An Ethical Dilemma." *Journal of Forensic Sciences, 21*:4:769–774.

———— (1981). "The Expert Witness." Breakfast Session Presentations at the 33rd Annual Meeting of the American Academy of Forensic Sciences, Los Angeles, California, February 17–20, 1981.

Addendum: the October 1983 issue of the *Scientific Sleuthing Newsletter (7(8):*3–4) of M.A.A.F.S. reports that the Delaware supreme court, in response to D.A.D.'s appeal, upheld in 1982 the deductions made from skeletal material by Dr. Hameli and Dr. Angel and affirmed the murder conviction.

Chapter 15

MANNER OF DEATH
Skeletal Evidence of Blunt and Sharp Instrument Wounds

NORMAN J. SAUER

It is only rarely that forensic anthropologists are asked to testify about the manner or cause of death of a particular individual. In the majority of forensic anthropology cases, the partial or complete decomposition of soft tissue and organs obliterates the most obvious evidence for death-related injuries. The position of a body or the location of some artifact may suggest manner of death, but organic modifications are rarely detectable on badly decomposed remains. The analysis of completely skeletonized or "dry" specimens often presents the added complication of clouding one's ability to associate the occurrence of a bony lesion to the death event. It is frequently impossible to distinguish between premortem and postmortem changes and those which may be associated with death. To be sure, modifications that occurred several weeks prior to or a significant time after death may be revealed by evidence for healing or differential staining, but many cases are unclear. Consequently, the contribution of the forensic anthropologist often terminates after the positive identification of a set of remains.

It is my purpose here to report upon two sets of injuries to a single individual that, because of the special circumstances surrounding his death and subsequent testimony, were accepted as evidence for homicide. The case involves a person who was reportedly taken to a wooded area by two associates, murdered, and left behind on the surface of the ground. The reported manner of death in this case was directly supported by modifications that were later identified on the victim's skeleton.

This example illustrates that the potential exists for detecting death-related sharp and blunt force injuries from skeletonized remains and outlines a procedure for the detection and diagnosis of such lesions. I also include a short discussion of the distinction between the meaning of the phrases *cause of death* and *manner of death* and its relationship to this case.

THE CASE

In August, 1979, the partially skeletonized remains of a young adult male were delivered to me at a local morgue along with a request to verify a positive identification and to examine the remains for signs of trauma that might be related to the person's death. The remains had been deposited in a heavily wooded area, allegedly about twelve weeks prior to their discovery. Before they were sent to me, they were examined by a local medical examiner who reported that he found no evidence for cause or manner of death. The decomposition of the soft tissue of the skull was almost complete, while there was a considerable amount of skin, internal organ tissue, muscle, and fascia associated with the postcranial skeleton. Much of the first day of our investigation involved dissecting and macerating the specimen for osteological analysis. Clothing was still in place at the time of discovery, and a knotted length of cloth encircled the skull.

Examination of the bony surface of this specimen revealed two important features: an unusual fracture of the mastoid process of the right temporal bone and small cut marks on the opposing borders of two adjacent ribs. The mastoid process displayed a comminuted fracture at its apex (Figs. 15-1 & 15-2). The fragments were clearly displaced medially and appeared to reflect a blunt force injury directed from the lateral aspect of the temporal towards the middle of the cranium.

One of the two cut marks was actually a notch on the inferior border of the second left rib about 10 mm lateral to the sternal extremity (Figs. 15-3 & 15-4). This mark suggested that some crushing took place along with incision. The notch had a flat base, and the displaced fragments of bone appeared to have been pressed up toward the body of the rib. This lesion was accompanied by a dark stain, suggesting that a vital reaction had possibly occurred and that a hematoma may have formed beneath the adjacent periosteum.

The second cut was a small tear or uplift that extended between 10 mm and 15 mm lateral to the sternal extremity of the third left rib on its superior border (Fig. 15-5). The uplifted segment appeared to have been sliced away from the body of the bone by the edge of a sharp instrument. No signs of a vital reaction were detected in the area of this lesion. It was our conclusion that these latter two opposing injuries may have represented a single blow to the chest by a knife blade with one sharp edge and one backed or flat edge. Such an instrument might explain why the superior injury appeared to have been compressed while the lower mark displayed more obvious signs of cutting.

While we were conducting the analysis, it was revealed that witnesses had confessed to taking part in the murder of this victim and also described the manner in which he was killed. The victim was apparently taken by two

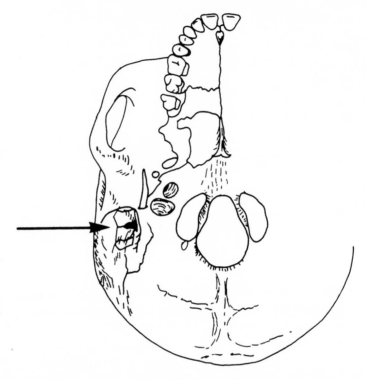

Figure 15-1. Right side of the base of the skull. Note the location of the lesion on the apex of the mastoid process (not to scale).

associates to a wooded area. He was then blindfolded and struck from behind with a tree limb. This blow, which was reportedly directed to the head, caused him to fall to the ground, where he was stabbed with a knife in the throat and chest. As mentioned earlier, the cranium, which had been almost completely skeletonized at the time of discovery, was found with a piece of cloth tied around it, which is consistent with the witnessed blindfold.

DIAGNOSIS

Our conclusion that the described lesions reflected the manner of death recounted by the witnesses to the homicide was initially made by direct diagnosis. The most reasonable interpretation for the lesion on the skull was that it reflected a blunt force injury to the side of the head, while the marks on the ribs with evidence for a vital reaction appeared to represent a sharp force injury to the chest. Nonetheless, such evidence would be valuable only if alternative explanations could effectively be ruled out. In other words, it was necessary for us to confront the possibility that the lesions were caused

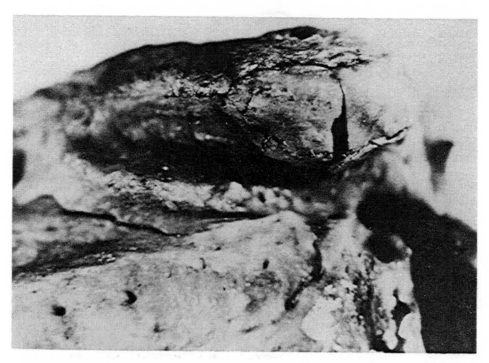

Figure 15-2. Lesion on the apex of the right mastoid process.

by events completely unrelated to the individual's death.

Two premortem changes that potentially could mimic signs of death on a skeleton are bone development and past injuries. A partially fused epiphysis, an irregularly developing flat bone, or an anomalous bony structure might erroneously suggest perimortem trauma. The forensic anthropologist should have a basic understanding of and familiarity with the skeleton and skeletal morphogenesis, which would allow him/her to rule out the majority of such developmental features. There are no characteristics of developing ribs or the mastoid process that resemble the lesions discussed herein.

To evaluate the possibility that the marks reflected old injuries, the surface discontinuities were studied macroscopically, microscopically, and with radiographs. Following the fracture of bone in a living individual, signs of healing are reflected in the smoothing or rounding off of the rough, broken edges or by the radiopacity of the tissue adjacent to the injury. According to Morse (1978:8), such changes may become apparent in dried bone after a month to six weeks. There were no signs of healing associated with any of these lesions. If the victim had received severe injuries within several months prior to his death, the event would likely have come to light during the trial.

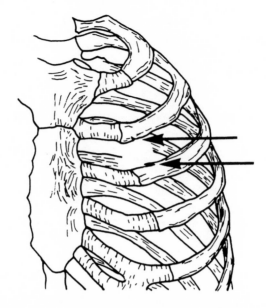

Figure 15-3. Left side of the human bony thorax. Note the location of the lesions on the inferior border of the second rib and superior border of the third rib (not to scale).

Postdepositional events that might result in discontinuities of bony surfaces include the activity of scavenging animals, the weight of large animals passing over the specimen, and human activity, most likely during recovery. The marks left by scavengers (particularly rodents and domestic or wild canids) are quite distinct and are usually easy to identify (Stewart 1979:79). Besides not being consistent with the lesions described here, animal marks were not detected anywhere else on the skeleton or soft tissue, nor had any body parts been significantly displaced or carried away from the initial area of deposition. It is similarly unlikely that the weight of a passing animal would have left the rib lesions or fractured the mastoid in the manner described.

If any of the marks were incurred at the time of discovery or during recovery, then the ground water staining on the newly exposed surfaces and the adjacent bone should be quite distinct. Most of the bony surfaces examined displayed a light brown stain that suggested exposure to the elements for many weeks. The exceptions to this were those surfaces protected by adherent soft tissue. The second and third left ribs and the right temporal displayed no significant color discontinuities that could be related to differential weathering.

Thus, the best explanation for the injuries to the ribs is that they reflect blunt and sharp force damage, while the lesion on the mastoid process appears to represent a severe blow to the side of the head. These injuries

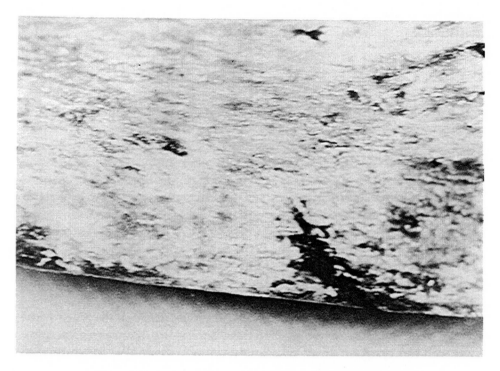

Figure 15-4. Lesion on the inferior border of the second left rib.

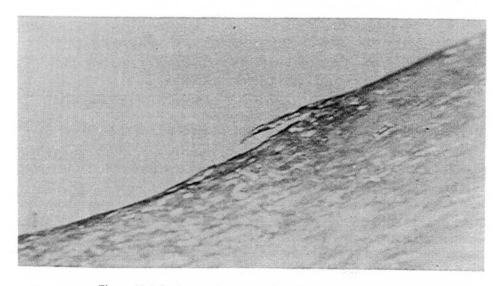

Figure 15-5. Lesion on the superior border of the third left rib.

were apparently inflicted at or near the time of death, and both sets are consistent with and support the testimonies of alleged assailants.

THE TRIAL

During the course of the trial that followed our investigation, the goal of the prosecutor was, in part, to establish that the manner of death in this case was by violent and malicious means. The bulk of his evidence rested upon the testimony of eyewitnesses, who not only reported the way in which they delivered the lethal injuries but also described in detail one of the weapons that was employed. The instrument that was allegedly used to stab the victim has never been recovered, but one of the witnesses produced a detailed description and drawing of a large hunting knife (with about a 7-inch blade) that had one sharp edge and an opposing squared-off or backed edge.

I testified that both the injury to the temporal bone and the cut marks evident on the ribs were consistent with the manner of death recounted by the witnesses. An obvious cross-examination query was directed at whether or not these modifications actually reflected some other agents. Since I had already dealt with alternative explanations during the diagnosis procedure, I was well prepared for this kind of questioning. Essentially, the testimony involved describing the considerations and conclusions that were discussed in the diagnosis section of this paper.

It is important to note that this evidence was used to support the testimony of eyewitnesses. Had there been no witness to the crime, then it seems unlikely that the marks detected on the skeleton would have been sufficient grounds to establish manner of death.

A most important aspect of my testimony involved the distinction between the determination of manner of death and of cause of death. Adelson and Hirsch (1980:91) characterize the two as follows:

> The *cause of death* is the disease or injury responsible for initiating the train of events, brief or prolonged, that produced the fatal end result.
> The *manner of death* is the fashion in which the cause of death came into being. . . .

The accurate assessment of the cause of death would rarely if ever be possible for a forensic anthropologist. A pathologist working on well-preserved remains might typically list cause of death as a gunshot wound to the heart or to the brain and support that diagnosis with a host of soft tissue changes. Nonetheless, although a bullet may be discovered in the region of a skeletonized thorax or in the endocranium of a skull, it would probably be impossible to demonstrate that a gunshot was the "injury responsible" for death. As the decomposition of human remains proceeds, the cause of death usually becomes obscure. On the other hand, it may be possible in a homicide, for example, to judge the manner of death by the disposition of a skeleton, the position of clothing, or the association of certain artifacts. Thus, while it is the responsibility of the pathologist to establish cause of death (Adelson 1974), the anthropologist may make a valuable contribution by determining manner of death or providing supporting evidence.

In the case described herein, after piecing together the testimony of the eyewitnesses, police reports of the discovery of the corpse in an out-of-the-way wooded area, and the evidence on the skeleton for perimortem injuries, it was established to a jury's satisfaction that the manner of death was by homicide. My testimony was restricted to providing evidence that was used to support that contention. When asked about the likelihood that the injuries to the skull and chest would have been sufficient to cause death, I deferred to a forensic pathologist.

The distinction between manner and cause of death may seem to be a semantic one. Nevertheless, it underlies a need for clarity with respect to the duties and capabilities of forensic anthropologists both as investigators and as expert witnesses.

SUMMARY

The case described here is one in which an anthropological investigation revealed evidence that was used by a prosecutor to support an argument that the manner of the death of an individual was by homicide, specifically by blunt and sharp force injuries. The diagnosis of the suspected lesions was supported by eyewitness testimony. In the absence of such support, it is possible that the skeletal evidence would have been of little or no value in the courtroom. Nevertheless, the case does demonstrate that both sharp force and blunt force injuries can be detected on human skeletal remains and that forensic anthropologists can make valuable contributions beyond those of a medical examiner or forensic pathologist.

Even if evidence of such a nature is never admitted in a court of law to establish "the manner of death," it can be extremely important in alerting investigators to the possibility that the death of an individual occurred by violent or unnatural means.

Keeping in mind the potential value of the kind of diagnosis described in this chapter, the forensic anthropologist should, as part of a routine investigation, examine the entire skeleton for unusual discontinuities in cortical surfaces. When suspected lesions are discovered they should be carefully scrutinized for important attendant signs:

1. They should be examined under magnification for signs of remodeling.
2. They should be radiographed to reveal signs of remodeling and evidence of associated foreign particles.

3. They should be examined for signs of vital reactions, since effused blood around a bony injury may become entrapped and preserved underneath the periosteum.

4. The displacement of bone should be studied for distinguishing between cuts and compression injuries and to determine the direction of force.

5. The color of all exposed surfaces should be examined for the differential effects of ground water and weathering, which may help to differentiate between recent and perimortem events.

6. The entire skeleton should be examined for signs of animal activity, including toothmarks, broken bones, and the displacement of body parts, which could mimic cut marks or blunt force injuries.

Finally, as soon as possible after their discovery on the skeleton, suspicious cortical discontinuities should be described in detail and photographed. With the passage of time, as the skeleton dries out, once clear marks may become obliterated. On the other hand, since such marks are occasionally enhanced as accumulated ground water and body fluids disappear, the specimen should be reexamined and possibly rephotographed after an interval of several hours or days. Obviously, good photographs can be crucial in the courtroom.

This case illustrates the important distinction between *cause of death* and *manner of death*. Forensic anthropologists can provide invaluable assistance by determining the way in which potentially lethal injuries were delivered to a victim. In many cases we are undoubtedly the specialists best prepared to do so. Nevertheless, determining the lethal consequences of a lesion is the responsibility of the forensic pathologist, regardless of the discoveries of the anthropologist. Such a distinction between manner and cause of death can be useful in the testimony of both experts.

REFERENCES

Adelson, L. (1974). *The Pathology of Homicide*. Springfield, Charles C Thomas.

Adelson, L. and Hirsch, C. S. (1980). Sudden and unexpected death from natural causes in adults. In W. U. Spitz and R. S. Fisher (Eds): *Medicolegal Investigation of Death*. Springfield, Charles C Thomas, pp. 88–117.

Morse, D. (1978). Ancient Disease in the Midwest. Reports of Investigations No. 15. Springfield, Illinois State Museum.

Stewart, T. D. (1979). *Essentials of Forensic Anthropology*. Springfield, Charles C Thomas.

Chapter 16

FORENSIC BIOMEDICAL AND ENGINEERING INVESTIGATIONS OF FATAL TRAUMA ATTRIBUTED TO SEAT FAILURE AND ROTATIONAL ACCELERATION IN A LIGHT AIRCRAFT CRASH

RICHARD G. SNYDER, SATHYA V. HANAGUD, ALLEN M. JONES,
THOMAS GRUBBS, AND PATRICIA MCFEELEY*

United States civil general aviation aircraft accidents are rarely subjected to the combined in-depth biomedical engineering and forensic medical investigation often associated with major air carrier disasters. During the past decade (1971–1980) over 14,259 fatalities (16.1%) occurred among the 100,000 occupants of general aviation aircraft involved in the 42,644 accidents reported during this period (National Transportation Safety Board, 1981). Despite this significant number of deaths, relatively few accidents have been subjected to thorough biomedical engineering crash injury analysis (Hasbrook and Dille, 1964), and only an estimated one in 2,000 accidents has been investigated by a human factors specialist (Snyder, 1981a). Most in-depth investigations have occurred after the fact, as a result of product liability litigation. While challenging interpretive problems are often presented at the scene, reconstructions are more difficult later in time. Among the problems one encounters may be removal of the wreckage, which may cause postaccident changes, or it may be destroyed or missing entirely; difficulty in locating witnesses, and dim memory of the event; physical

*The authors interacted with a number of other individuals in working on this forensic case and in particular would like to acknowledge Gaylord Harvey, U.S. Air Force seat expert, of San Antonio, Texas. The crash sequence illustration was drawn for trial by James Longacre of Austin, Texas, and subsequent medical illustrations for this chapter were drawn by Kathleen Richards, University of Michigan, Ann Arbor. Photographs were provided by Dr. Patricia McFeeley, Office of The Medical Investigator, Albuquerque, New Mexico. Particular acknowledgment should be given to Pat Maloney, George LeGrand, and Pat Maloney, Jr., of the law firm of Pat Maloney, San Antonio, Texas, plaintiffs attorneys, who provided the environment for the scientific team effort to develop and interact and skillfully used the experts' findings. This federal jury case resulted in award of $2.2 million to the plaintiffs, the largest award to date in a light aircraft case based upon crashworthiness theory. On July 13, 1983, the Supreme Court of Texas upheld the lower courts' decision on the liability issues.

changes in the accident site; and unavailability of other important pieces of evidence. Accident reconstruction can take place many years after the occurrence: The senior author in 1962 participated (some 52 years later) in a detailed medical-engineering accident reconstruction of a 1910 fatal crash (Garrido-Lecca Frias, 1963).

The following civil litigation case, investigated intensively some three years after the accident occurred, illustrates how multidisciplinary expert forensic effort can scientifically reconstruct crash injury mechanisms. This effort required the combined study of a forensic anthropologist-biomechanics scientist, specializing in human impact trauma; an aeronautical engineer, specializing in crash dynamic reconstruction; two forensic pathologist-medical examiners; and a mechanical engineer specializing in aircraft seat structures. The legal issue concerned how the two occupants received their fatal injuries and what role, if any, defective aircraft design played in contributing to these fatalities.

The role of the forensic anthropologist in this case developed from expertise in human impact trauma mechanisms in deceleration or crash conditions and knowledge of aircraft seating environments. While any one of the medical or engineering team could approach the critical questions as a highly qualified expert in a specialized area, the forensic anthropologist, who was also an experienced pilot, was the only member of the team who could apply a broad knowledge from actual experience gained in several pertinent areas. This included field investigation of accidents, the conduct of impact tests and autopsies of human surrogates in controlled laboratory injury studies, participation in and analysis of dynamic crash tests, in-depth study of pertinent federal regulations, knowledge of accident statistics and the technical state of the art both of occupant protection and human tolerances. This broad base of experience enabled him to bridge the gap between disciplines to integrate and apply the basic medical findings to the reconstructed engineering crash dynamic environment of the aircraft structure and seat, on the one hand, and, on the other, to determine occupant kinematics and probable injury causation and survivability.

BACKGROUND

A student pilot and his instructor departed a southwestern airport about noon on a clear October day for the student's fourth instructional dual flight. Three hours later the wreckage was found about 6 miles south of the airport in a field of high maize. The Hobbs flight recorder showed .5 hours on this flight, indicating that the crash occurred about 12:45 MST. The crash site was at 4,200 feet elevation. Both pilots received fatal injuries. There were no witnesses.

A routine postcrash accident investigation, focused on the probable cause of the accident, was conducted by an investigator from a regional office of the National Transportation Safety Board (NTSB), assisted by a local Federal Aviation Administration (FAA) maintenance inspector. They were joined by an accident investigator representing the airframe manufacturer, who flew directly to the scene from the factory in Wichita, Kansas. Apparently, no human factors, biomedical, or accident reconstruction was conducted during this investigation, and no sketch of the wreckage distribution, principal impact points, and reconstructed flight and ground paths was attempted. However, thorough gross autopsies were conducted on both bodies by the Office of the Medical Investigator for the State of New Mexico (by P.J.M. and reviewed by A.M.J.). State and federal laboratories independently conducted toxicological analyses on both bodies.

The accident was classified by the NTSB as a "stall spiral" accident; that is, the aircraft was considered to have stalled and entered a nose-down spiral. The probable causes of this accident were attributed to the pilot in command: "improper operation of flight controls," "failed to obtain/maintain flying speed," "inadequate supervision of flight" (National Transportation Safety Board, 1976; 1977).

The aircraft was a 1975 high wing single engine side-by-side two passenger trainer, manufactured in 1975 and incorporating 1973 model seats. Both seats were equipped with shoulder harnesses. This aircraft has a maximum cruising speed of 122 mph and stalling speed (flaps down, power off) of 48 mph. First produced in August, 1958, over 21,771 of this series had been produced by the time of this accident (Taylor, 1977), and it remains the most numerous U.S. light aircraft in operation.

The instructor pilot, in the right seat, had 2,100 total flight hours and had previously been a military flight instructor. He was rated as a Certified Flight Instructor (CFI), with Commercial and Instrument single-engine land privileges. The student pilot, in the left seat, had a total of 2.8 dual hours and had previously practiced slow flight, stalls, and turns about a point. Forced landings were also practiced on the two previous flights.

The NTSB accident report described the wreckage as coming to rest in an upright position with the inverted tail section beneath the right wing (NTSB Form 6120.4, 1976). Ground impact was 99 feet in length and direction of travel south to north (350°). It was noted that maize stubble was imbedded between the top surface of the wing and the leading edge of the wing flaps. The leading edge of both wings had impact damage from the wing tips inward a few feet on each wing. Both seats were reported to have separated from the seat tracks, and the shoulder harnesses were not thought to have been worn by either occupant. The NTSB investigator also reported that "the ground scar at the accident site was compatible with ground impact on the right wing, right main gear, nose gear, and power plant, followed by a cartwheeling of the aircraft before it came to rest upright" (NTSB Form 6120.4, 1976). The company investigator, who reports directly to the legal rather than engineering areas of the manufacturer, provided a more detailed description, noting that the impact with the ground appeared to be with the aircraft's right wing low and the nose down approximately 20 degrees.

The position of the defense experts was that the crash had occurred at an impact velocity exceeding 130 mph; it was nonsurvivable; the lap-belted occupants, who were not wearing the shoulder harnesses provided, hyperflexed forward into the instrument panel, resulting in the fatal injuries; the crash forces exceeded federal seat design requirements and human tolerances; failure to wear the shoulder harnesses provided by the manufacturer was a contributing cause. A superficial observation might support this conclusion, since jackknifing of the unrestrained head and upper torso into the instrument panel has long been shown to be the most common mechanism for fatal and serious head and chest trauma. However, it was not the mechanism responsible in this accident, as the in-depth analysis that follows reveals.

On-scene photographic coverage in the original investigation was extremely limited. Figure 16-1 shows a close-up view from the rear right quarter of the upright aircraft. The fuselage has separated at the rear of the cabin, and the two occupants were found in this position, strapped to their seats but hyperextended on their backs partially outside the open rear of the cabin. Note the flat terrain, the fairly intact wing, and the straw lodged in the top of the wing.

Figure 16-2 is a left front quarter close-up view of the cabin area. The nose has been distorted downwards, and the windshield is missing. The cabin area itself is relatively intact with no intrusion into the pilots' area. The wing struts are not deformed, the wing is relatively intact, and neither door or side window is broken, although the left door was distorted (which may be partly attributed to postcrash rescue attempts).

An interior view of the front left instrument panel is shown in Figure 16-3. Note that while the glass in the artificial horizon (second instrument from left, top row) is broken, the distortion is exaggerated by the panel plastic overlay. The control wheel shows no impact damage, and no evidence of pilot head impact could be found on the panel.

MEDICAL ANALYSIS OF OCCUPANT INJURIES

Both occupants were autopsied 16 hours postmortem (P.J.M.). The site and nature of external trauma found during gross autopsy examination are shown in Figures 16-4 and 16-5.

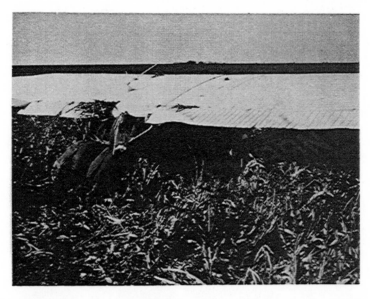

Figure 16-1. Polaroid® on-scene view from the right rear of the upright aircraft postimpact showing the separation of fuselage at the rear of cabin and the two occupants still strapped in the seats but hyperextended out the open rear of the aircraft.

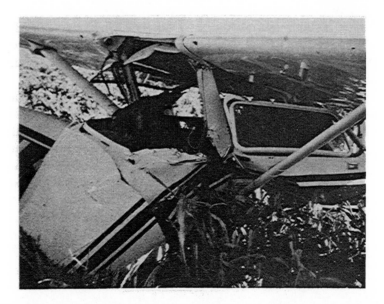

Figure 16-2. Close-up of the front left quarter view of the cabin area postcrash.

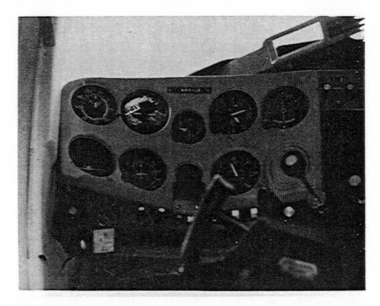

Figure 16-3. Front left instrument panel and control wheel, showing no evidence of pilot head impact.

The instructor pilot was a male age thirty-one and measured 6 feet in stature and weighed 210 lbs. He was wearing a lightweight jacket, short-sleeved shirt, double knit pants, and well-worn cowboy boots. Wet red bloodlike and tissuelike material was present around the collar and entire posterior aspects of his jacket and left sleeve, which had an irregular tear. Examination of his pants showed red bloodlike material mixed with red brown dirtlike material in a 15 by 12 cm area over the left back extending from the pocket upwards. There were multiple external lacerations, discolorations, and denudations.

The primary findings include lacerations to the head and face, aorta, septum pellucidum, and left hemidiaphragm; contusions to the head and face, anterior thorax, and lungs bilaterally; abrasions to the head and face (Fig. 16-4), abdomen, and lower extremities, bilaterally; and fractures to both femurs. Examination also revealed a right thyroid adenoma, which was microscopically reviewed. Immediate cause of death was a consequence of "multiple injuries."

Several injuries were significant. The aorta was completely transected at the junction of the arch with the thoracic aorta. The lungs bilaterally revealed multiple contusions primarily on the superior-posterior aspects with hemorrhage into the underlying parenchyma. The septum pellucidum of the brain was ruptured. The left hemidiaphragm was lacerated within a 15 by 19 cm area, and portions of the stomach, pancreas, and spleen were

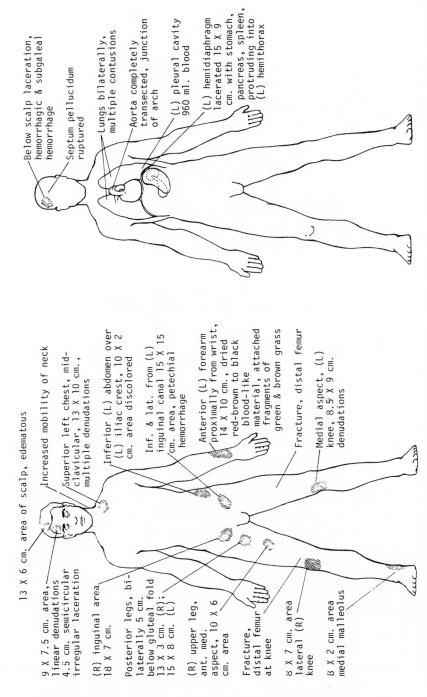

Figure 16–4. Location of the external evidence of injury found during autopsy examination of the pilot in the right seat. Areas of red brown hard, crusted denudations and discolorations are present.

Figure 16–5. Illustration of the site and nature of fatal internal trauma found during necropsy of the pilot in the right seat.

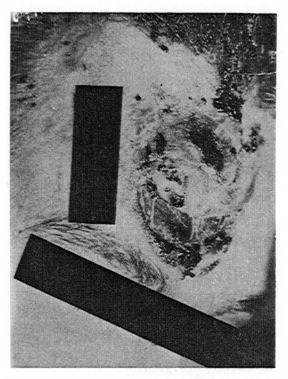

Figure 16-6. Area of trauma (9 × 7.5 cm) to the forehead of the right front seat pilot, showing multiple red brown superficial linear denudations and a semicircular irregular laceration with 4.5 cm flap. The scalp is edematous superior to this within a 13 × 6 cm area.

protruded into the left hemithorax. The left plural cavity contained 960 mls of sanguinous material. The soft tissue beneath the scalp laceration of the right forehead was found to be diffusely hemorrhagic, superiorly and laterally, with diffuse underlying subgaleal hemorrhage.

Toxicological analysis was independently conducted at the School of Medicine, University of New Mexico and at the Aviation Toxicology Laboratory of the FAA's Civil Aeromedical Institute in Oklahoma City. Tests were negative for ethyl alcohol, acidic and neutral drugs, and carbon monoxide.

The aortic rupture and transection is of particular interest from a biomechanics viewpoint and is reported to occur in about 10 percent of all automobile fatalities involving blunt chest trauma (Mulligan et al., 1976). Several mechanisms have been advanced to explain this injury, including heart compression or the hydrodynamic effects of acceleration causing an increase in intra-aortic pressure sufficient to cause an explosive outburst. Another theory is that the heart and arch remain fixed by the depressed sternum while the descending aorta continues forward. A third, probably most widely accepted theory, based largely on experimental evidence, is that the descending aorta remains fixed to the posterior thoracic wall while the heart and arch undergo large displacements, thereby causing failure at the isthmus. No matter which mechanism was involved, this injury is consistent with blunt chest trauma.

The student pilot, a male aged thirty-three years, was also 6 feet in stature and weighed 212 lbs. He was wearing a long-sleeved button shirt, T-shirt, Levi® blue denim pants, and moderately worn cowboy boots. The pants and shirt revealed multiple tears and areas of dried blood and dirt. Immediate cause of death was determined to be as a consequence of multiple injuries. These included lacerations to the head and face, liver, mesocolon, and corpus colosum; contusions to the head and face (Fig. 16-7), anterior (Fig. 16-8) and posterior thorax, abdomen, upper extremities bilaterally, lungs, posterior mediastinum, liver, right perirenal soft tissue, mesocolon, and soft tissue of the left lower quadrant of the abdomen. In addition, there were fractures to the right ribs 1–5, left ribs 1–2, sternum, right tibia and fibula, and bilaterally to the radius and ulna. Abrasions were found on the face and head (see Fig. 16-5), anterior (see Fig. 16-6) and posterior thorax, upper extremities bilaterally, and left lower extremity. There was a right hemothorax (50 ml).

Significant internal necropsy findings, shown in Figure 16-9, involved 50 ml of sanguinous material in the right pleural cavity, fractured sternum and ribs 1–5 on the right side, and fractured ribs 1 and 2 on the left. There was irregular laceration of the mesocolon and soft tissues surrounding the sigmoid colon in the left lower quadrant of the abdomen; the posterior superior mediastinum was hemorrhagic, as were the fat and soft tissue in the right retroperitoneal area, the liver, and the internal scalp surface, with mild to moderate diffuse subarachnoid hemorrhage on the brain surface. The corpus collosum of the brain was lacerated throughout most of its length. The lungs revealed multiple contusions bilaterally. The capsule of the superior surface of the right lobe of the liver at the diaphragmatic attachment was lacerated within a 10 by 1.5 cm area.

Toxicological analysis was negative for ethanol, and no carbon monoxide was detected in the specimens submitted to the university. In specimens sent to the FAA aviation toxicology laboratory a 9 percent saturation of carbon monoxide was reported in a specimen containing 12.3 gm/100 cm of hemoglobin. This does not exceed the normal upper limits of a smoker.

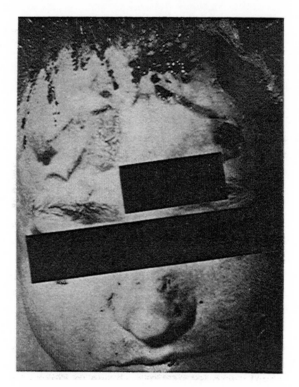

Figure 16-7. Areas of trauma to the forehead of the left seat pilot.

ACCIDENT SEQUENCE RECONSTRUCTION

The crash dynamics of this accident can be separated into three stages, each having several steps. Due to the complexity of aircraft and occupant motion, Figure 16-10 provides a step-by-step analysis and comparison. During the first stage of the crash, the high wing aircraft approached the ground, nose down, at approximately 20 percent pitch angle, and banked with right wing down. The right wing tip, the nose wheel, and the surrounding areas made the initial contacts with the ground. During this stage of the crash the instrument panel was damaged, and the control wheel and the supporting column (push-pull rod) also buckled. The fuselage also failed at the baggage compartment and separated into two sections. However, the separated part of the fuselage, aft of the wing, remained attached to the rest of the aircraft through connecting cables. By the end of the first stage of the crash, the area behind the seats of the pilot and the passenger was exposed to the outside because of the tail failure.

The second stage of the crash involved the impact of the nose wheel, its

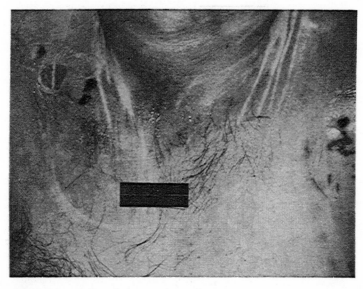

Figure 16-8. Areas of denudation on the anterior upper thorax of the left seat pilot.

surrounding areas and the left wing, in a flip (forward rotation). The forward rotation was initiated as a result of the initial impact, and the flipping motion was mostly in the pitching mode (that is, motion of the nose about the X axis). At this point, the aircraft lifted above the ground and rotated about the tip of the nose of the aircraft by about 180 degrees to an upside down position. The center of gravity continued to move in a forward direction. The second stage ended with the aircraft contacting the ground on the top of the wing and the cabin in an upside-down position. By this time the seats had come loose from their floor attachments. The clips and the canted legs had failed.

The third stage of the crash occurred when the aircraft bounced back from its upside-down position and continued to flip in a pitching mode. The next contact with the ground was on the bottom of the aircraft on its main landing gear. The aircraft then came to a stop in an upright position.

EFFECTS ON OCCUPANTS

The approach angle with the ground was approximately 20 degrees with the right wing down. The speed and the angle were determined, to a reasonable degree of engineering certainty, from the available information and observations from the NTSB report, failure data available on this model aircraft, and comparison of the damage with known crash tests. In addition,

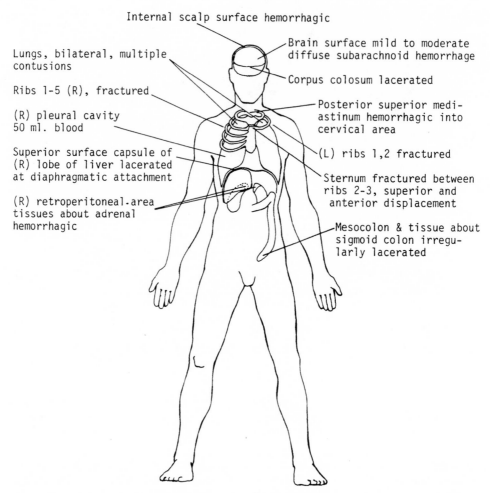

Internal scalp surface hemorrhagic

Brain surface mild to moderate diffuse subarachnoid hemorrhage

Lungs, bilateral, multiple contusions

Corpus colosum lacerated

Ribs 1-5 (R), fractured

Posterior superior mediastinum hemorrhagic into cervical area

(R) pleural cavity 50 ml. blood

(L) ribs 1,2 fractured

Superior surface capsule of (R) lobe of liver lacerated at diaphragmatic attachment

Sternum fractured between ribs 2-3, superior and anterior displacement

(R) retroperitoneal area tissues about adrenal hemorrhagic

Mesocolon & tissue about sigmoid colon irregularly lacerated

Figure 16-9. Location of the fatal internal trauma found during necropsy of the pilot in the left seat.

high-speed (1,000 fps) films of NASA experimental crash tests were reviewed (NASA, 1979; Vaughan and Hayduk, 1980) as well as the films and data on a previous crash test of this model by the manufacturer (Bloedel and Lee, 1973; Wittlin and Gamon, 1976).

The velocity of the aircraft changed during the various stages of the crash from initial velocity, in the range 52 to 59 MPH, to zero at the end of the third stage of the crash. The various changes in the velocity of the aircraft and the time durations in which the changes took place determined the forces on the occupants and their motion. The motion was also influenced by their lap belt restraints, the occupant space available in the cabin, and the

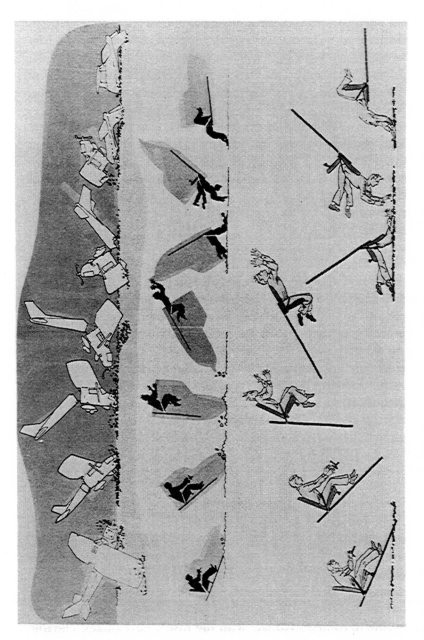

Figure 16-10. Due to the complicated crash dynamics of this accident, the impact sequence has been illustrated from three levels at seven points in time. The top sequence shows the crash dynamics of the aircraft subsequent to impact, the middle shows the motion of the occupant relative to the aircraft, and the bottom sequence reconstructs the kinematics of the occupants, whose motion during the impact sequence was essentially the same. The occupants in this accident were subjected to rotational acceleration, forward, lateral, rearward, and vertical accelerations, with rotational forces and forward ($-Gx$) loads of primary significance. (Drawing courtesy of James Longacre.)

failure of certain structural components such as the seat, seat supports, and fuselage.

Once the initial conditions of the approach of the aircraft were established, various engineering computations were applied, and appropriate impulse-momentum relationships were determined. Additional equations necessary to determine the unknown linear and angular velocities were obtained by establishing the appropriate coefficient of restitutions on the basis of crash tests, other field tests, and materials that were involved. A second method was to use the subsequent history of the motion of the aircraft. Information that was used in establishing the path of the center of gravity included the available photographs, NTSB report, observations on the ground scar, crash tests, and physical examination of the aircraft wreckage. After computing the changes in velocity of the aircraft during the different steps of the three stages of the crash, the forces on the occupants were computed. These forces were computed by using the changes in velocity and the duration of time over which the changes took place. The duration of time was obtained from a knowledge of crash tests and other computations involving the motion of the aircraft.

Some of the significant forces were as follows. During the initial impact the maximum force on the occupants was in the range of 12 G. The forward forces were in the range of 8 to 10 Gs. During the rotation there was a force of 7 Gs into the seat and a force of 2 to 3 Gs directed toward the seat back. The force toward the back was the result of the centrifugal forces due to rotation. It should also be noted that the absolute velocity of the aircraft at the first step of the second stage was 39 miles per hour. The horizontal and vertical velocity were in the range of 31 feet per second (fps) and 17 to 20 fps. If the occupants had remained in their seats, if the seats had not failed, and if there had been no exposure to the outside due to fuselage failure, the maximum force on the occupants would have been 6.6 Gs when the aircraft hit the ground in an upside-down position.

OCCUPANT MOTION

From a knowledge of the forces and other observations, the motion of the occupants was established. Some of the significant aspects of the motion are shown in the second sequence included in Figure 16-10.

During the first stage of the crash, the occupants moved forward to the right. Contacts were made with the control wheel, but rotation was initiated *before* they were able to come in contact with the instrument panel. During the first step of the second stage the occupants were forced into their seats because they were subjected to an abrupt vertical velocity of 17 to 20 fps.

Prior to the initiation of the second step of the second stage, the seats and seat supports failed. During the second stage, the G forces, directed to the seat back, caused a motion of the occupants toward the rear of the aircraft. The occupants continued to move rearward because the seats and their floor attachments had failed. As the occupants fell backward, their upper torsos were exposed to the outside at the rear of the cabin, caused by the separation at the baggage compartment. When the aircraft hit the ground in an upside-down position at the end of the second stage, the upper torsos of the occupants struck the ground on their face and chest areas. *This impact caused the fatal injuries.* Their legs were inside the cockpit, and the seat belts were still on. The seat and its supports had failed, however, permitting the rearward motion of the upper torsos. When the aircraft came back to upright position, the occupants were lying back facing the sky (see Fig. 16-1).

It was determined that the force on the occupants was not severe enough to cause serious injury when they hit the control wheel and buckled the control column. This was established by computing the buckling load of the column, which was less than 700 pounds. It was also found that other forces during the first stage of the crash and impact did not cause the serious injuries. It was during the second impact, at the end of the second stage of the crash, that the most serious injuries occurred.

A number of dynamic crash tests or sled tests have shown by use of high-speed motion picture photography (1,000 fps) the occupant motion relative to time in various impact environments (Swearingen et al., 1962). A typical sequence of kinematics shows that even for low velocity forward impacts, the structure forward of the pilot collapses and absorbs considerable energy prior to the occupant decelerating. The seated occupant, restrained by a lap belt only, would remain upright for about 80 milliseconds (ms) even though the peak belt loads occurred earlier (Armstrong and Waters, 1969). The occupant continues in the direction of impact until the seat belt is stretched tight, sometimes involving 5 to 12 inches of belt stretch. At approximately 80 ms, the pilot will start to jackknife forward (or in the direction of the aircraft motion) over the belt and may arc upwards as well, most typically hitting his chest on the control wheel and head on the instrument panel. In this case at least one pilot came in contact with the control wheel, but did not flex further, before the rotation of the centrifugal force overcame the forward movement.

IMPACT STRUCTURES RECONSTRUCTION

Few photos were taken of the accident site during the on-scene investigation, and after several years of storage, the condition of the aircraft wreckage had deteriorated. Components had been disassembled; many parts had been removed, and not all were found. Figures 16-2 and 16-3 show the best views available of the cabin area, and Figure 16-3 shows the instrument panel area in front of the left seat occupant postcrash.

An important problem to resolve when reconstruction is attempted after wreckage has been moved from the site is to determine any damage that may have subsequently occurred postimpact. In addition to the visible damage to the aircraft, the reconstruction was aided by the original investigators' report that there was an initial ground contact area some 99 feet from the final resting point. It was not reported how long the earth scar was at either the initial point or at the final point. Hence, the length of the rebound path through the air would be some finite number less than 99 feet. The analysis of the rebound path was necessary to arrive at a length of time the aircraft was airborne following the initial impact and indicated that in all probability the aircraft was in the air for at least 1.04 seconds but not more than 1.39 seconds.

Damage to the main landing gear and the fuselage tear (at station 71.44) strongly indicates that the first impact was fairly flat with the ground. The presence of dirt and vegetation in the trailing edges of the wings and top of the exposed cabin indicated that the second impact occurred with the longitudinal axis of the aircraft pointing vertically.

The analytical formulation under the flight path recreation was based on basic laws of parabolic or projectile motion. In essence, if one knows the length of the flight path (99'–A–B) and the rebound angle, then the aircraft speed can be approximated. The calculated speed of 40 mph places the aircraft in the stall regime, which is consistent with a flat angle of attack with a moderate vertical velocity. (This is in contrast to the defense experts' estimate that the aircraft was traveling at 130+ mph at a high angle of incidence to the ground.)

With an approximation of rebound time, it is possible further to estimate angular velocity of the cabin. This angular velocity was based on 270 degrees rotation of the cabin during the approximated 1.04 to 1.39 seconds of rebound, resulting in an angular velocity of 3.4 to 4.5 rad/sec. A dimensional examination of the crew member position relative to the most likely point on the forward portion of the aircraft to pivot about the ground reveals that while the aircraft is spinning up to 3.4 to 4.5 rad/sec. angular velocity, the radius of rotation is approximately 7 feet. Therefore, the expelling centrifugal forces on the crew members are computed to be between 2.5 and 4.5 Gs. A comprehensive summary of human tolerances to rotary acceleration is given in Fraser, 1974.

The seat failure was attributed to several factors: the loads that were imposed on the legs and the manufacturer's two product "improvements," which resulted in a seat with far less load-carrying capability than its "unimproved" predecessor. The seat frame is the primary structural member of the seat system. The seat frame is attached to the seat rails by *C*-shaped shoes, which ride on top of the rails via a small roller. The *C*-shaped shoes encompass the cap of the seat track so as to restrain any upward movement. The rear rollers are mounted directly to the seat frame; therefore there are no rear legs. Legs do exist for the forward rollers. The inboard (medial) legs are straight (vertical) and contain the locking pin for fore/aft seat adjustment. This pin resists all fore/aft movement after seat adjustment by locking into the seat rail. The pin is approximately 2 inches below the frame so that the leg behaves as a short cantilevered beam with a moment arm of 2 inches.

Earlier models of this aircraft also contained an angle brace, which extended from the front roller to the rear roller. This feature is shown in Figure 16-11. The angle brace therefore became a compression and tension member and relieved the leg of its cantilevered loads. Our analysis showed that the braced leg was capable of withstanding 1,538 lbs. of force, while the "improved" cantilevered leg was only capable of withstanding 165 lbs. of force. Thus the earlier seat leg was 9 ⅓ times stronger than the installed "improved" leg. In this accident both inboard locking legs failed by means of a moment type of structural overload.

Another factor involved the forward outboard (lateral) leg. In this instance, the manufacturer's "improvement" involved moving the seat track slightly inboard. To maintain constant seat width, the leg was angled to allow the lower portion of the leg to ride on the track and to allow the upper portion to attach to the seat frame in about the same location as the earlier straight leg. The leg was offset 1 inch. Since there is no locking pin in the outboard leg, this leg is insensitive to longitudinal forces. A conservative analysis showed that the leg would fail at 704.6 lbs. of force. The absence of detailed data on the straight leg prevented a comparative straight leg analysis, but there is little doubt that such a leg would have been several times stronger than the canted "improved" leg.

The first impact imposed downward and forward forces on the legs. Both front legs on both seats failed through independent mechanisms, one due to forward loading and the other due to downward loading. As the legs failed, the vertical restraints provided by the front legs through the *C*-shaped shoe were negated, and the seats were free to pitch backward about the back roller under the influence of the expelling centrifugal forces. Had either leg maintained its integrity, then the rearward expulsion would not have taken place. It was documented that the manufacturer had equipment available in its inventory (the brace) or in its previous design experience (the straight leg) that would have prevented separation.

Much of the early analytical investigation centered on failed and unfailed

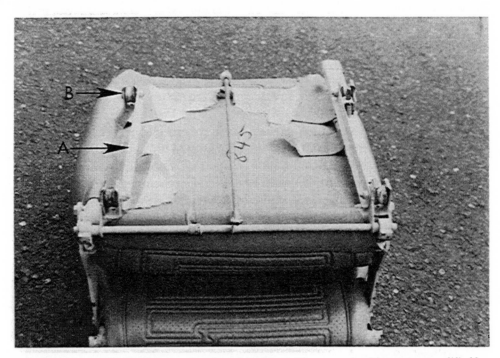

Figure 16-11. Earlier models than the aircraft in this accident contained front seats modified by an angle brace (A) from the front roller to the rear roller, which was 9-1/3 times stronger than the later seats having the angled leg (B) without the brace.

components in an attempt to bracket the severity of the impacts. The seat tracks all showed signs of structural overload. A relatively simple analysis revealed that only 7 Gs vertical load is required to buckle the seat rails. For the 200 lb. occupants, the forces at approximately 7 Gs were found to have caused the failure of the seat legs.

Undoubtedly, the airframe saw considerably higher forces than 7 Gs acceleration; however, once the floor began to fail, the occupants were spared any higher G loadings until the floor came in contact with other parts of the aircraft or earth. An analysis of the bent control column suggested that the acceleration to the pilot's upper torso was between 4 and 9 Gs. Hence, one can conclude that the vertical and horizontal accelerations were 7 and 9 Gs or greater, respectively.

If the loads required to produce a failure (buckling, brinelling, bending, or fracturing) in a component are calculated and it is then demonstrated that the failure is not present, then this load, in terms of G forces, would represent the upper limit for the inertial forces. The wing and wing strut were examined in detail. All structural attach fittings were found to be undamaged. None of the mounting hardware was available, but all of the close tolerance attach holes were found to be round within allowable specifications and with no hint of structural overload. Perhaps most surprising of all is that the wing strut has not failed, i.e. not buckled.

An analysis was performed on the wing structure, consisting of the wing strut and aft and forward wing attach fittings. The wing/fuselage/strut assembly was formulated as a finite element pin-connected truss structure with individual masses. The masses were obtained either through published data or from actual measurements of the accident aircraft. The wing was considered to be infinitely rigid in torsion.

From this analysis it is apparent that the structure did not exceed 90 Gs in either the horizontal or vertical direction; in all probability, the G forces did not even approach these levels.

Further evidence of cockpit survivability was gathered from the control column, the control wheel, and the instrument panel. Damage to these areas was clearly within the range of survivability based on comparison with staged and actual crashes of similar aircraft.

Various documents obtained during discovery and expert testimony revealed that the manufacturer had made several modifications to the seats in this model aircraft, which had an important bearing on occupant protection (crashworthiness). Significant points included the following:

1. 1969 model seats were used in a 55 mph dynamic full-scale crash test conducted by the manufacturer in 1971. This seat had straight legs mounted to the seat frame at 90 degree angles, and there was no seat failure reported (Bloedel and Lee, 1973; Wittlin and Gamon, 1976).

2. Beginning with 1970 model 150 series aircraft, reinforcement of the seat bottom frame by means of a steel brace between the front and rear legs was initiated on production aircraft, and a Service Kit (SK 150-35) was developed for installation updating in-service aircraft (Cessna Service letter, 1970).

3. In the 1973 model year the manufacturer redesigned the seat but did not incorporate a brace such as that added to the 1969 seat by Service Letter SE 70-30 (Cessna Test Reports dated 6/23/72). The outboard front leg of the new design was no longer attached to the seat frame at a 90 degree angle, but instead was canted at a 55 degree angle towards the inboard side of the seat to compensate for narrowing of the space between the seat rails. The 1973 Parts Manual shows this brace.

4. The aircraft in this accident was a 1975 model 150M (serial #15075844), manufactured and sold in 1975. It incorporated factory installed 1973 model seats with the angle leg and no braces.

5. On 17 July 1975 the manufacturer ran further static tests on its 1973 model seat and determined a need for the brace between front and rear legs. The brace was subsequently incorporated into production of all model 150s and Aerobat Model 150s.

6. On 31 October 1977 the manufacturer sent out notice of a seat frame modification (Service Kit SK-150-548) by means of a Service Letter (SE 77-40), adding the reinforcing braces and a heavier shaft to the seat frame "to provide additional seat strength" to all Aerobat Model 150s produced between incorporation of the 1973 seat design and production of the brace addition as a result of the 1975 tests. However, no letters were sent to owners of regular model 150s produced during that time period.

The certification of the seats of this aircraft was related to twenty-four-year-old standards (at the time of its manufacture), Part 3.390 and 3.390-2 (proof of strength) of the Civil Air Regulations (CAR) of 1950 (Civil Aeronautics Administration, 1950). This allowed a choice of structural analysis alone, static tests alone, or a combination. Minimum performance standards were further specified in TSO-C39a and National Aircraft Standards Specification 809, established in 1956.

Although this aircraft was manufactured in 1974, it was certified under twenty-four-year-old federal standards for occupant protection established in March 1950 (CAR 3.386 Protection and 3.386-1 Crash Protection CAA interpretations) rather than the more recent FAR Part 23 requirements established in 1964. The ultimate design accelerations on the occupants were 3 G upward, 9 G forward, and 1.5 G sideward. This regulation also required that if an aircraft's (such as this high wing model) characteristics are such as to make a turnover reasonably probable, the fuselage of the aircraft in combination with other portions of the structures shall be designed to afford protection of the occupants in a complete turnover. For design purposes a vertical ultimate acceleration of 3 G and a friction coefficient of 0.5 at the ground is assumed. No evidence was presented that the manufacturer complied with this rollover requirement.

Testimony was given by the forensic anthropologist that these minimal standards (Snyder, 1981b) are far below our knowledge of human impact tolerances and the state of the art for occupant protection. Airman voluntary subjects in 1951 tests have been subjected to 32 G wearing a lap belt only with no significant injury (Stapp, 1971) and have been tested at 16 G with a lap belt only in National Bureau of Standards tests (Armstrong and Waters, 1969) with no injury. Lewis and Stapp (1957) reported no lasting injury at 26 G (at 850 g/sec for 0.02 sec). Levels at which severe injury may occur are probably much higher, with the fatal threshold still higher (Snyder, 1971; 1973; SAE, 1980). The chest impact loading was sufficient to cause aortic rupture in this case.

There are several methods used to relate thoracic impact tolerance (Mulligan et al., 1976; Hess et al., 1981). Federal Motor Vehicle Safety Standard 208 for occupant protection specifies thoracic tolerance as 60 Gs for not over 3 ms, but this is primarily extrapolated from head impact data. A common criteria is force deflection relationships; for example, a deflection of the chest of 3.5 inches for a 95th percentile male is equated to an AIS 3 injury (severe; not life threatening), while 1.75 inches deflection is considered below rib fracture level. Another way of interpreting chest injury is by impact loads; thus human tolerance is variously estimated as 1500 to 2500 lbs of force. Since the load on the one bent control column was calculated to be 700 lbs, it seems unlikely that this was the cause of the fatal chest trauma, which must have occurred at subsequent ground impact.

SUMMARY AND CONCLUSIONS

Integrating the crash dynamics, structural analysis, biomechanics, kinematics, and medical findings provided a relatively consistent reconstruction of this unusual accident and illustrates the importance of and need for forensic teamwork.

It was concluded that this accident occurred in a low speed stall impact attitude, right wing low at 20 degree pitch angle with the ground, at 52 to 59 mph impact velocity. The aircraft crash dynamics were broken into three stages, each having several identifiable steps. The total travel after initial impact was 99 feet. Subsequent to initial impact the fuselage separated. In a second stage the aircraft rotated forward, subjecting the occupants to a centrifugal rotational acceleration of between 2.5 and 4.5 Gs during the 1.04 to 1.39 seconds during which this occurred. The rotational forces were a critical factor, since following initial impact the occupants would have continued forward at the same velocity, hyperflexing over their lap belts, and would normally be expected to hit the instrument panel structure with their heads and upper body. However, in this case the initiation of the rotational forces was sufficient to prevent either occupant from actually coming in contact with the panel, although it was calculated that some 700 lbs. and 4 to 9 Gs force was expended against the bent control column. (It requires a load of 1500 to 2500 lbs. to cause significant chest injury, or 60 G at 3 ms.) During rotation it was calculated that the forces on the seat were 7 G and only 2 to 3 G to the seat back. By the time the cabin had rotated in an inverted position partially to expell the occupants out the rear, the velocity had been reduced to 39 mph, and if the seats had not failed the occupants would have only been subjected to 6.6 Gs. (Young healthy males protected by double shoulder harnesses have been tested to 47 Gs whole body acceleration in the +Gx seated orientation without serious injury.)

The proximal cause of the injuries in this case was the failure of the seat, which detached from the rail, allowing the occupants to rotate rearwards outside the separated fuselage. The medical investigation in this case was thorough, and the nature of the trauma was consistent with partial ejection and anterior blunt impact of the face and chest with the ground. No panel impact indentations or evidence of blood was found on the panel, and the injuries could not be matched with panel structural contact. The nature of the injuries was also consistent with the engineering analysis. There were no skull fractures, as would be expected in panel impact, but there was evidence of dirt on the body, in the wounds of the face, chest, and clothing. The biomechanics of the laceration of the corpus collosum of the brain (probably by sheer force), the transection of the aorta (attributed to blunt impact), and the location of the rib fractures higher than would be expected also supported this mode of impact. Ironically, although the aircraft was destroyed, the cabin remained relatively intact and was considered to be a survivable capsule.

This unusual forensic case illustrates the value of multidisciplinary in-depth teamwork in investigation and that the "obvious" subjective conclusion may not be supported in fact when scientifically analyzed. It also shows that the forensic anthropologist may play a significant role in civil as well as criminal litigation. This state court jury case resulted in a verdict of $2.2 million to the plaintiffs, the largest verdict to date in a light aircraft case based on crashworthiness theory.

REFERENCES

Armstrong, R. W. and H. P. Waters (1969). Testing Programs and Research on Restraint Systems. National Bureau of Standards, Washington, D.C. Society of Automotive Engineers Technical Publication 690247, January.

Bloedel, A. W. and D. Lee (1973). Model 150 Crash Test. Engineering Test Memorandum Report ET-73-2, 26 February.

Cessna Aircraft Company (1970). Service Letter: Seat Frame Improvement, SE-70-30, November 13.

Cessna Aircraft Company (1972). Cabin Accommodations Test Results, 23 June, p. 30.

Cessna Aircraft Company (1977). Service Letter: Seat Frame Modification. 1972 through 1976 Model 150 Aerobat Series Aircraft, SE-77-40, October 31.

Civil Aeronautics Administration (1950). Emergency Provisions. CAR 3.386 Protection; CAR 3.386-1 Crash Protection; CAR Interpretations which apply to section 3.386, previously 3.3811; 3.390 Seats and Berths Civil Aeronautics Manual 3. U.S. Department of Commerce, March 8.

Fraser, T. M. (1974) Rotary Acceleration. *Bioastronautics Data Book* (2nd ed) National Aeronautics and Space Administration, Washington, D.C. NASA SP-3006, Chapter 5. pp. 191–219.

Garrido-Lecca Frias, G. (1963). El accidente de jorge chavez. Instituto Perauano de Fomento Educativo, Lima, Peru.

Hasbrook, A. H. and J. R. Dille (1964). Structural and medical analysis of a civil aircraft accident. *Aerospace Medicine*, 35:958–961.

Hess, R. L., K. Weber, J. W. Melvin (1981). Review of Literature and Regulations Relating to

Thoracic Impact Tolerance and Injury Criteria. University of Michigan, Ann Arbor, Report UM-HSRI-81-38, December.

Lewis, S. T. and J. P. Stapp (1957). Experiments Conducted on a Swing Device for Determining Human Tolerance to Lap Belt Type Decelerations. 6571st Aeromedical Research Laboratory, Holloway AFB, New Mexico, Rept. ARMDC N-57-1.

Mulligan, G. W. N., G. S. Pizey, D. Lane, L. Andersson, C. English, and C. Kohut (1976). An Introduction to the Understanding of Blunt Chest Trauma. The Human Thorax-Anatomy, Injury, and Biomechanics. Society of Automotive Engineers, Inc. Warrendale, Penn. Publication P-67, pp. 11–36, October.

National Aeronautics and Space Administration (1979). Aircraft Crash Tests Composite Data Film, Serial L-1252. Langley Research Center, Hampton, Va., June.

National Transportation Safety Board (1976). Factual Aircraft Accident Report General Aviation. Cessna 150 M N66113, NTSB Form 6120.4, 19 October.

National Transportation Safety Board (1977). Aircraft Accident Reports. Brief Format U.S. Civil Aviation Issue Number 4 of 1976 Accidents, Washington, D.C., Report No. NTSB–BA-77-2, p. 1583.

National Transportation Safety Board (1981). Annual Report to Congress, 1980, Washington, D.C., p. 79.

Snyder, R. G. (1971). Occupant Impact Injury Tolerances for Aircraft Crashworthiness Design. Society of Automotive Engineers, Inc., New York, NY, Technical Paper 710406.

Snyder, R. G. (1973). Impact. *Bioastronautics Data Book* (2nd ed.) National Aeronautics and Space Administration, Washington, D.C., Chapter 6, pp. 221–295.

Snyder, R. G. (1981a). Human Factors—The Missing Link in General Aviation Accident Investigation. Proceedings, Fifth Human Factors Workshop on Aviations' Biomedical and Behavioral Factors in Aviation, U.S. Department of Transportation, Oklahoma City, 7 July.

Snyder, R. G. (1981b). General Aviation Aircraft Crashworthiness. An Evaluation of FAA Safety Standards for Protection of Occupants in Crashes. The University of Michigan, Ann Arbor, Report UM–HSRI-81-10, 15 May.

Society of Automotive Engineers, Inc. (1980). Human Tolerance to Impact Conditions as Related to Motor Vehicle Design. SAE J885 APR80, April.

Stapp, J. P. (1971) Biodynamics of Deceleration, Impact, and Blast. In *Aerospace Medicine*, H. W. Randel (Ed.). Baltimore, Md.: Williams and Wilkins.

Swearingen, J. J., A. H. Hasbrook, R. G. Snyder, and E. B. McFadden (1962). Kinematic behavior of the human body during deceleration. *Aerospace Medicine, 33*:188–197, February.

Taylor, J. W. R. (Ed) (1977). *Janes' All The Worlds Aircraft.* Cessna Model 150, London: Janes' Publishing Co., Ltd., p. 254.

Vaughan, V. L., Jr. and R. J. Hayduk (1980). Crash Tests of Four Identical High-Wing Single-Engine Airplanes. National Aeronautics and Space Administration, Langley Research Ctr, Hampton, Va. NASA Technical Paper 1699, August (Technical Film Supplement L-1265).

Wittlin, G. and M. A. Gamon (1976). A Method of Analysis for General Aviation Administration, Washington, D.C., Rept. FAA–RD-76-123.

Section III
SEX, AGE, STATURE, AND ANCESTRY

T he case studies in the following section illustrate methods for estimating sex, age, stature, and ancestry from human skeletal remains. Although these four key attributes alone are seldom sufficient to establish individual identity, they frequently serve to narrow the range of possible matches and thus allow investigation to proceed more efficiently. Weinker's case study illustrates one such instance. In his example, authorities had initially diagnosed unknown remains as male, based upon features of a dental apparatus. Weinker's determination, developed from the more reliable skeletal attributes, indicated that the remains were female, and led both to further, productive recovery work at the discovery site and to renewed concern that the case involved a crime. This example underscores the importance of estimating such parameters as sex and age, as well as ancestry, from the remains themselves. Associated items can be misleading, either due to chance ambiguity or because contradictory objects have been left intentionally at the crime scene.

The report presented here by Suchey and co-workers provides another example of anthropological estimates changing the course of and indeed leading to a breakthrough in police investigations. Their second case, termed by them "John Doe #2," had been described as a 40-to-60-year-old Caucasoid male in the pathologist's report. Forensic anthropological study, based upon pubic traits and microscopic examination, suggested a much younger age and eventually led to identification of the remains as those of a 27.5-year-old man. A murder conviction ensued. Testimony by the forensic anthropologist was an important part of the murder trial, and it had been essential in discovering the identity of the unknown skeleton.

Most determinations of age, sex, stature, and ancestry by the forensic anthropologist will be on unknown remains, essentially descriptive attempts to extract as much information from the skeleton as possible. Snow and Luke's Oklahoma child case provides an example of a different, more directed form of investigation—one in which the forensic anthropologist attempts to test a known identity against skeletal evidence. Here the determination was whether or not the remains are compatible with the known records of an individual: a 6 year old child. Snow and Luke's probability estimates, carefully drawn from developmental data, were an essential test of a preliminary identification based upon hair and clothing found with the remains.

Sex

In his west central Florida example, Weinker describes the range of morphological and metric techniques commonly used for sex diagnosis in skeletal remains. He emphasizes that observers should consider the pattern of dimorphism throughout the skeleton, carefully weighing ambiguous evidence and using both morphological and metric methods whenever possible. As noted by Stewart (1979), most experienced osteologists will feel satisfied with conclusions reached through visual inspection of skeletal morphology. However, metric confirmation can be important supportive evidence in the courtroom, since probability of error is presented numerically. In addition, the less experienced observer is more likely to develop accurate estimates through the use of metric techniques.

Reporting metric standards for the head of femur, head of humerus, and glenoid fossa of the scapula, Weinker illustrates that a broad range of skeletal elements can serve as a basis for sex diagnosis in metric study. Dimorphism in the bones of the feet, e.g. the tarsals as described by Steele (1976), can also be evaluated metrically. Given that footwear frequently protects and thus preserves the feet in mass disasters and in other contexts where other body parts are destroyed, familiarity with Steele's method is important in forensic study. Table III-I (Buikstra and Mielke, in press) illustrates the range of skeletal elements that can be used accurately to estimate sex. The table is not exhaustive, and the reader should consult Stewart (1979), Krogman (1962), Bass (1971), and Ubelaker (1978) for additional sources. However this table does include examples of the most reliable strategies and should serve as a reference source for persons faced with the necessity of generating estimates from ambiguous or incomplete remains.

Weinker correctly emphasizes that patterns of dimorphism are known to vary among populations, and it is therefore important that standards— morphological or metric—applied to unknown cases be derived from groups of similar ancestry, if at all possible. When ancestry is unknown, accuracy often is severely reduced. For instance, Stewart (1979) reports that ischiopubic ratios are much less precise estimators of sex for pooled black and white samples than when the two racial groups are considered separately. In his example, accuracy drops from 91% and 83% for the black and white samples, respectively, to 74% for the pooled grouping. Weinker's study also illustrates this point, his ability to determine that his unknown was Caucasoid markedly increased the accuracy of his morphometric estimates of sex.

Since Weinker's unknown was an adult, sex could be estimated with confidence. Had the remains been adolescent or younger, sex diagnosis

TABLE III-I
COMPARISON OF VARIOUS TECHNIQUES FOR SEX DETERMINATION IN SKELETAL REMAINS

Element	Form of Observation/ Analytical Procedure	Maturity of Sample	Population Sampled	Accuracy of Method	Series of Known Sex?	Observer(s)
Entire skeleton	Morphological observation	Adult	Todd Collection	90/95–100%	YES	Krogman (1962)
Entire skeleton	Morphological observation	Adult	Todd Collection	90–95%	YES	Stewart (1948, 1951)
Skull	Morphological observation	Adult	Todd Collection	82/87–92%	YES	Krogman (1962)
Skull	Morphological observation	Adult	Todd Collection	80%	YES	Stewart (1948, 1951)
Skull	Morphological observation	Adult	Todd Collection	80% (90% w/ mandible)	YES	Hrdlicka (in Stewart, 1948)
Skull	Morphological Observation and Univariate Comparison	Adult	Cape Coloured	85%	YES	Keen (1950)
Skull	Discriminant Function Analysis	Adult	Todd/Terry Collections	82–89%	YES	Giles and Elliot (1963)
Skull	Discriminant Function Analysis	Adult	Forensic cases	88%	YES	Snow et al (1979)
Skull & mandible	Discriminant Function Analysis	Adult	Japanese	89%	YES	Hanihara (1959)
Mandible	Discriminant Function Analysis	Adult	Todd/Terry Collections	85%	YES	Giles and Elliott (1963)
Face	Discriminant Function Analysis of measurements taken from radiographs	Adult	Midwestern Whites	91–94%	YES	Hunter and Garn (1972)
Pelvis	Morphological observation	Adult	Todd Collection	85/90–95%	YES	Krogman (1962)
Pelvis	Morphological observation	Adult	Todd Collection	90–95%	YES	Stewart (1948, 1951)
Pelvis	Morphological observation, measurements, ratios	Adult	Cadaver and Archaeological samples	95%	YES; NO	Genovese (1959)
Pelvis	Ischiopubic Index	Adult	Terry Collection Blacks	93.5%	YES	Thieme and Schull (1967)
Pelvis	Ischiopubic Index	Adult	Terry Collection Blacks	82–94%	YES	Richman et al. (1979)
Pelvis	Ischiopubic Index	Adult	Terry Collection Whites	91–95%	YES	Richman et al. (1979)
Pelvis	Ischiopubic Index	Adult	Howard University Blacks	95.8%	YES	Richman et al. (1979)
Pelvis	Ischiopubic ratio and sciatic notch width	Adult	Bushman	98%	NO	Washburn (1948)
		Adult	Bantu	98%	YES	Washburn (1948)

TABLE III-1 (*Continued*)
COMPARISON OF VARIOUS TECHNIQUES FOR SEX DETERMINATION IN SKELETAL REMAINS

Element	Form of Observation/ Analytical Procedure	Maturity of Sample	Population Sampled	Accuracy of Method	Series of Known Sex?	Observer(s)
Pelvis	Ratio of Sciatic Notch Width to vertical diameter of the acetabulum	Adult	Todd Collection	90%	YES	Kelley (1979)
		Adult	Prehistoric California Amerindians	90%	NO	Kelley (1979)
Pelvis	Acetabulum-pubis Ratio	Adult	Terry Collection Blacks	92%	YES	Schulter-Ellis et al. (1983)
Pelvis	Morphological observation of ischiopubic ramus	Adult	Terry Collection	96%	YES	Phenice (1969)
Pelvis	Morphological observation of ischiopubic ramus	Adult	Prehistoric California Amerindians	96%	NO	Kelley (1978)
Pelvis	Discriminant Function Analysis	Adult	Prehistoric Illinois Amerindians	98.8%	NO	Gustav *diss.* (1972)
Pelvis and Femur	Ischiopubic Index with sorting by femoral dimensions	Adult	Terry Collection Blacks	99%	YES	Thieme and Schull (1957)
Pelvis and Femur	Ischiopubic Index with sorting by femoral dimensions	Adult	Terry Collection Whites and Blacks; Howard University Blacks	92–99%	YES	Richman et al. (1979)
Pelvis and Femur	Acetabulum-pubis index with sorting femoral dimensions	Adult	Terry Collection Blacks	96%	YES	Schulter-Ellis et al. (1983)
Pelvis and Femur	Discriminant Function Analysis with sorting by femoral dimensions	Adult	Terry Collection Blacks	97%	YES	Schulter-Ellis et al. (1983)
Femur	Discriminant Function Analysis	Adult	Portuguese	94%	YES	Pons (1955)
Femur	Shaft diameter; Discriminant Function Analysis	Adult	Prehistoric Ohio Amerindians	85%	NO	Black (1978a)
Femur	Shaft diameter; Stepwise Discriminant Function Analysis	Adult	North American Whites (AMNH)	82%	YES	DiBennardo and Taylor (1979); Taylor and DiBennardo (1982)
Femur	Shaft diameter; Stepwise Discriminant Function Analysis	Adult	Terry Collection Blacks	76.4%	YES	DiBennardo and Taylor (1982)

TABLE III-I (*Continued*)

COMPARISON OF VARIOUS TECHNIQUES FOR SEX DETERMINATION IN SKELETAL REMAINS

Element	Form of Observation/ Analytical Procedure	Maturity of Sample	Population Sampled	Accuracy of Method	Series of Known Sex?	Observer(s)
Femur	Discriminant Function generated from measures with greatest univariate difference	Adult	Prehistoric Illinois Amerindians	87%	NO	Van Gerven (1971, 1972)
Femur	Stepwise Discriminant Function Analysis	Adult	Prehistoric Illinois Amerindians	93%	NO	Van Gerven (1971, 1972)
Sternum	Penrose size/shape statistic	Adult	Portuguese	89%	YES	Pons (1955)
Clavicle	Parson's (1912) formula	Adult	St. Bride's series	91%	YES	Steel (1967)
Clavicle	Parson's (1912) formula	Adult	Modern English	88%	YES	Parsons (1916)
Clavicle	Discriminant Function Analysis	Adult	Modern English	87%	YES	Steel (1967)
			St. Bride's series	96%	YES	Steel (1967)
Humerus, ulna, radius, femur, tibia	Discriminant Function Analysis	Adult	Japanese	97%	YES	Hanihara (1958)
Femur, humerus, clavicle, ischium, pubis, sternum	Discriminant Function Analysis	Adult	Terry Collection Blacks	98.5%	YES	Thieme and Schull (1957)
Femur, humerus, clavicle, ischium, pubis, sternum	Discriminant Function Analysis	Adult	Terry Collection Whites and Blacks; Howard University Blacks	88–98%	YES	Richman et al. (1979)
Talus/Talus & Calcaneus	Discriminant Function Analysis	Adult	Terry Collections Whites and Blacks; Pre- and Proto-historic Amerindians	79–89%	YES; NO	Steele (1976)
Sacrum	Univariate Comparison and Indices	Adult	Terry Coll Blacks Terry Coll Whites	84–91% 79–84%	YES	Flander (1978)
Sacrum	Discriminant Function Analysis	Adult	Terry Coll Blacks Terry Coll Whites	92% 96%	YES	Flander (1978)
Sacrum	Discriminant Function Analysis	Adult	Prehistoric Illinois Amerindians	85%	YES	Gustav (1972)

TABLE III-I (*Continued*)

COMPARISON OF VARIOUS TECHNIQUES FOR SEX DETERMINATION IN SKELETAL REMAINS

Element	Form of Observation/ Analytical Procedure	Maturity of Sample	Population Sampled	Accuracy of Method	Series of Known Sex?	Observer(s)
2nd Cervical Vertebra	Discriminant Function Analysis	Adult	European, Middle Ages	78–80%	NO	Helmuth and Rempe (1968)
2nd Cervical vertebra, scapula, radius, humerus & femur	Discriminant Function Analysis	Adult	Early 19th Century Dutch	95–98%	YES	Van Vark (1970)
Tooth Crowns	Discriminant Function	Adult	American Whites	65–81%	YES	Owsley and Webb (1983)
Tooth Crowns	Discriminant Function Analysis	Permanent Dentition	Protohistoric Arikara	80–85%	NO	Owsley (1981)
Tooth Crowns	Discriminant Function Analysis	Permanent Dentition	Prehistoric Tennessee Amerindians	78–88%	NO	Scott and Parham (1979)
Tooth Crowns	Discriminant Function Analysis	Permanent Dentition	Prehistoric Illinois Amerindians	80–100%	NO	Ditch and Rose (1972)
Tooth Crowns	Discriminant Function Analysis (canines only)	Permanent Dentition	Prehistoric Ohio Amerindians	79.4%	NO	Sciulli et al. (1977)
Tooth Crowns	Discriminant Function Analysis	Deciduous Dentition	Ohio Whites	64–75%	NO	Black (1978)
Hand/Wrist Epiphyses & M development	Comparison of Developmental stages	Juveniles	New England Whites	73–81%	YES	Hunt & Gleiser (1955)
Teeth	C-M_2 Maturation compared to sex-specific standards	Juveniles	New England Whites	58% (70% using C alone, age known)	YES	Hunt & Gleiser (1955)
Ilium	Auricular surface elevation	Fetal to 6 months	Mixed race (primarily black and white)	64–87%	YES	Weaver (1980)
Upper/Lower Limbs	Weights and lengths; Discriminant Function Analysis	Fetal	American Whites and Blacks	72%	YES	Choi & Trotter (1970)

would have been much more difficult, likely impossible, given the current state of our forensic art. Statistical analyses of dental measurements, however, hold promise for extending sex estimates to juvenile materials. As illustrated in Table III–I, multivariate methods for estimating sex from measurements of the permanent (Corruccini and Henderson, 1976; Garn et al., 1977; Ditch and Rose, 1972; Owsley, 1983; Potter, 1972; Scott and Parham, 1979) and deciduous (Black, 1978a) dentitions have led to accurate estimates of sex in immature remains. Most of this work, however, has used prehistoric population samples rather than contemporary individuals of documented sex. Further studies that develop standards appropriate for a broad range of modern populations would be useful and thus allow sex determinations in forensic cases to be standardly extended into the pre-adult years.

Age

The estimation of age at death from skeletal remains is a more complicated task than sex diagnosis. As the Krogman (1962) and Stewart (1979) forensic texts caution, individuals vary in their maturation rates, and limited point estimates of age at death are therefore inappropriate. Ranges of possible ages should be reported. In general, standards for estimation are more accurate for the younger ages, though varying by the nature of the materials available to the forensic anthropologist. A number of techniques exist for age estimation, depending upon the material available for analysis and the maturation stage that the individual had reached at the time of his/her demise. These are usually dichotomized as either features of development—appropriate to the juvenile and young adult years, i.e. fetal to c. 23–24 years—or those of degeneration, which are evident in older remains (Stewart, 1979). The forensic anthropologist, thus, in determining which techniques to use, will initially categorize the remains in terms of a broad age range, e.g. Perzigian and Jolly's general characterization of their unknown female as postpuberal and pre-adult, prior to selecting a method appropriate for rigorous analysis.

The most reliable criteria for estimating chronological age in pre-adult remains include (1) the appearance and fusion of ossification centers, (2) long bone growth, and (3) dental development. As noted by Stewart (1979), the recognition and identification of primary ossification centers in fully skeletonized remains is difficult, and in fact, their recovery is infrequent. Thus, for the pre-adult years most workers emphasize the importance of criteria for evaluating long bone length, epiphyseal fusion, and dental development—as illustrated here in the reports of Snow and Luke, Perzigian and Jolly, and Suchey and co-workers.

In juveniles, long bone length is generally considered a less accurate predictor of age than dental development because growth is affected more by extrinsic factors such as health status and diet than are tooth formation and eruption. Both long bone growth and dental development are known to vary by sex and between races, however, and one's precision is therefore enhanced by knowledge of ancestry and sex of the remains.

To establish the appropriate age range when working with dental development or epiphyseal union, the worker identifies two key variables: the most recent developmental event that has occurred and the next developmental stage as yet unachieved. The researcher usually begins with a rather broad range and then proceeds to narrow the limits, as do Snow and Luke, who progress from a 5-to-12-year age range, based upon vertebral traits, to 4.9 to 8.0 years and ultimately 5.6 to 8.0 years based upon the dentition. As illustrated by this and by other cases reported here, Perzigian and Jolly for example, it is important that the observer establish a full body maturation pattern for the remains, viewing as many developmental attributes as possible.

As reported by Stewart, long bone length is a key criterion for establishing age in fetal remains. He also reports standards, as do Krogman (1962), Fazekas and Kosa (1978), Hoffman (1979), Merchant and Ubelaker (1977), and Ubelaker (1978), among others, for estimating juvenile age based upon long bone length. In the case study reported here, Snow and Luke extrapolate a stature estimate based upon long bone length and then compare this figure against those expected in white girls at various ages. Given that their analysis is a directed one and that the stature estimate is also important in record comparison, this strategy was appropriate here. However, in the case of unknown remains, the best age estimates are taken directly from the long bones themselves rather than introducing further imprecision as a result of the imperfect relationship of stature to long bone length.

Various standards exist for the estimation of age from features of dental maturation. Snow and Luke apply the complex technique developed by Nolla (1959) in her longitudinal study of white girls. Other appropriate, simpler methods include those described by Moorrees et al. (1963a) for deciduous teeth and by Garn et al. (1958) and Moorrees et al. (1963b) for the permanent dentition. Stewart (1979) also reports that the familiar Schour and Massler (1944) chart is still useful, although it may lead to underestimates of age. Ubelaker (1978) has developed a chart patterned after that of Schour and Massler that is appropriate to Amerindian dentitions.

Perzigian and Jolly's age estimate, while referencing other methods, is developed primarily upon the basis of McKern and Stewart's (1957)

Segment III indicators of skeletal age. Also preferred by Stewart (1979), this technique is relatively simple, requiring the observer to score the stage of union for nine epiphyses on a five-point scale: proximal humerus, medial epicondyle, distal radius, head of femur, distal femur, iliac crest, medial clavicle, sacral bodies 3 and 4, and the lateral sacral joints. These scores are summed and then used to generate an age prediction through algebraic transformation. Given that these standards were developed from the study of male skeletons, one to two years should be subtracted to apply the estimate to females, as did Perzigian and Jolly whose predicted age of 16 to 17 years coincided with the probable age at death of their remains. It should also be emphasized that if the researcher chooses to use criteria developed from radiographic study, rather than dry bone observations, estimates will likely be systematically lower than if dry bone standards are applied (Stewart, 1979).

Although some workers (e.g. Acsadi and Nemeskeri, 1970; Lovejoy et al., 1977; Meindl, Lovejoy, and Mensforth, 1980, 1981; Mensforth and Lovejoy, 1980) favor the use of multiple indicators in estimating age in adults, most forensic anthropologists in the United States tend to rely upon a few key indicators, such as pubic symphysis morphology and microscopic observations of bone and teeth. The case studies reported here by Suchey and co-workers, by Cook, and by Kerley illustrate each of these three commonly used methods. Researchers are, however, well advised to consider total body patterns when estimating age and not to rely exclusively upon single indicators if these appear to conflict with all other criteria.

Promising results for estimation of adult age using morphological changes on the auricular surface of the pelvis have been reported by workers who have studied the Hamann-Todd Collection (Meindl, Lovejoy, and Mensforth, 1980). Only preliminary results have been published to date, however, and to our knowledge the technique has not received broad application in forensic contexts.

Suchey and co-workers provide here a good summary of the development and application of pubic symphysis aging techniques, along with an evaluation of their accuracy. They argue, based upon carefully controlled studies of documented autopsy cases, that pubic symphysis morphology provides accurate estimates for the young and middle adult years, being much less reliable in females than in males. Even the standards developed specifically for females by Gilbert and McKern (1973) are reported to be inaccurate. Older individuals of both sexes are difficult to age by means other than microscopic techniques, such as those illustrated here by Kerley and by Cook.

The report by Suchey et al. also provides strong evidence that skeletal analysis should not be limited simply to skeletonized remains, but should also become a standard part of all autopsies, especially of adult unknowns. Two of their cases had been incorrectly assessed by pathologists who based their determinations upon soft tissue features. Suchey's observations of the clavicle, the iliac crest, and the pubic symphysis yielded much more accurate results.

The case reports by Cook and by Kerley illustrate two commonly used microscopic techniques for the estimation of age. These have the advantage of being applicable in the older adult age ranges where no other reliable standards have been developed. As noted by both workers, there are several approaches to each type of analysis, and each is being refined through ongoing study.

As reported by Cook, the pioneer work in dental histological assessments of age is that of Gustafson (1950), published over 30 years ago. In general, workers today continue to code some or all of the attributes recorded by Gustafson: attrition, paradontosis, secondary dentine, cementum, transparency, and root resorption. Given that these can be influenced by disease and diet as well as by population-specific rates of aging, Cook is properly cautious and uses an array of evaluative standards before concluding that her unknown remains represent an age range centered at approximately 55 years. In so doing, she strikes a middle ground between an osteologist's estimate of 45 to 50 years and the radiologist's assessment of 60. Unfortunately, the case remains unidentified, and the validity of the alternative strategies cannot be evaluated at this time.

The Gustafson method and its refinements require longitudinal sections of the study specimen. As noted by Cook it is probably wise to use more than one tooth in a given dentition in generating an age estimate, particularly in instances where dental disease is obvious. It is therefore important, when using a destructive method such as this, that the tooth be studied, photographed, and preferably cast prior to sectioning. Thus, although dental histology does, in fact, require the destruction of evidence, this destruction is desirable when there is no other technique available for attaining accurate age estimates. Such techniques are particularly important in the analysis of older individuals when bone histology is not an option.

A different dental histological technique, newly applied to *Homo sapiens*, is the use of horizontal tooth root sections to estimate age. Cemental annulation, long used as predictors of age in nonhuman mammals, has recently been tested with promising results in a small sample of humans (Stott et al., 1982). A further test by Condon and Charles (1983) in a larger sample of documented adults suggests that the initial optimism of Stott and co-workers may be overstated, although after further refinement the technique may become an important addition to methodologies used by forensic anthropologists to estimate age.

As noted by Cook, dental histological age estimates carry ranges of ± 7 to 15 years, which is decidedly better than the "over 50" estimates possible on macroscopic grounds. Bone histology can afford slightly more precision than dental histology, as Kerley reports. Kerley himself has been a pioneer in this field, and his three cases well illustrate the application of bone histology to the problem of age estimation in adults, although it is appropriately applied in younger individuals as well.

Kerley's method requires observation of several sites on a single midshaft long bone section. Most other techniques, although slightly different from that of Kerley, also require relatively complete long bone sections (Ahlqvist and Damsten, 1969; Singh and Gunberg, 1970). (Singh and Gunberg also provide data on mandibular bone.) Thompson (1979) has demonstrated the less destructive use of bone cores, which do not require complete midshaft sections to be cut.

It is clear that a fully equiped forensic anthropology laboratory should include facilities for histological study of teeth and bones as a means for generating age estimates, particularly useful in assessing adult remains. Ubelaker (1974; 1978) presents a clear and detailed statement of the process and equipment necessary for this task.

Stature

Although this section does not include any case study specifically chosen to highlight the estimation of stature from skeletal remains, we must emphasize that this is an important technique in forensic anthropology and that stature estimates are a standard part of forensic reports. Many of the case studies in this volume include stature estimates generated from skeletonized materials, with Heglar also describing a method appropriate for fleshed remains. Krogman (1962) and Stewart (1979) both provide extensive discussions of the methods appropriate for estimating stature from skeletons, which Stewart dichotomizes as being either mathematical or anatomical. In general, mathematical methods are to be preferred, the most commonly used in the United States being that of Trotter and Gleser (1958). In this section, the case studies by Perzigian and Jolly and by Snow and Luke illustrate the application of the Trotter and Gleser method. Trotter and Gleser (1958) present a series of equations that allow the observer to predict statures based upon specified length measurements of the limb long bones. Given that the relationship of bone length to stature varies significantly among the races and between the sexes, different equations are presented for male and female adults, as well as for major racial groupings. Although these formulae are suitable for most forensic cases in the United States, there exist a few standards, generated from specific populations, that are occasionally more suitable. For instance if the deceased is of Mesoamerican origins, the formulae of Genovès (1967) would be more appropriate, since these were generated from Mesoamerican samples. Another important point made by Trotter and Gleser (1958) is that the error factor is lower, i.e. the relationship strongest, between bones of the lower limb and stature. Therefore, the observer should rely upon estimates based upon the femur, tibia, and/or fibula when these elements are present and measurable. With a significant reduction in precision, stature can be estimated from incomplete long bones (Steele, 1970).

Ancestry

Determining ancestry or "race" solely from skeletal remains is a difficult exercise, even for the experienced forensic anthropologist. There are few, if any, population-specific skeletal or dental features, and these may not be correlated with attributes of soft tissue anatomy, such as pigmentation, fat distribution, or hair morphology that have been used to designate an individual's race. Further, it must be recognized that in many instances, racial categories are not necessarily biological but instead reflect social or ethnic affiliations. Legal documents may define race through information volunteered by an individual, or they may designate a person as a member of a minority group in instances where there was only a single remote ancestor of that race. Descriptions of an unknown individual by friends and relatives and photographs are frequently more useful, but this information must be qualified by the fact that soft and hard tissue structures are not perfectly correlated. We are, in racial attribution studies, estimating ethnic and social categories from biological evidence that reflects both genetic background and the environment of the individual. It is scarcely surprising that such estimates are rather imprecise when compared with those of sex, stature, and age at death. The estimation of ancestry is, therefore, a task to be approached conservatively.

A further complication in contemporary society is that mating between persons of different racial backgrounds is common. Thus, in heavily populated environs, as reported by Weinker for the Florida suncoast, and even in the relatively remote regions where Gill works, one can expect to find individuals representing several different ancestral lines. Racial affiliation is therefore best considered to reflect an arbitrary truncation of a continuum of human variability, and forensic estimates of race should be evaluated in that light. Single skeletal and dental traits are seldom race specific, as noted here by Gill for the shovelled incisors commonly defined as Mongoloid characters. It is common in a specific case for a forensic anthropologist to observe features that are associated with more than one race. These should be reported as such, rather than for the observer to try to generate a single category when the skeleton is truly ambiguous. It may be better in these circumstances to emphasize categories that can be safely excluded rather than trying to define a single ancestral line.

The two most commonly used American forensic anthropology texts, Krogman (1962) and Stewart (1979), are appropriately cautionary about the success of racial determinations based upon skeletal remains. Krogman states that "it is difficult for me to evaluate *how* a single skull is classified as white, or Negro, or Mongoloid" (Krogman, 1962:195) and argues that multivariate statistical analyses of the cranium are more likely to generate reliable results than visual assessment of morphological traits. Stewart reports the traditional distinctions between black African and American white crania: that black skulls have lower orbits, wider interorbital distances, less salient nasal bones, pronounced alveolar prognathism, and a broad nasal aperture that is poorly defined at its inferior aspect (Stewart, 1979:231). He also indicates that, in general, femora from American blacks are straighter and flatter than those of American whites, though this does not distinguish whites from persons of Asiatic (Mongoloid) ancestry. The standard markers of Mongoloid heritage are listed by Stewart as extreme narrowing of the nasal bones at the nasal ridge, prominent cheekbones, and shovelled incisors. However, as noted above, shovelled incisors occur in racial groups other than Mongoloids, and the other features are difficult accurately to evaluate through visual inspection.

Recognizing the difficulty of assigning racial affiliation through visual inspection, several physical anthropologists have attempted to develop metric means for estimating ancestry. The most frequently used method is that of Giles and Elliot (1962), although Howells (1973) has also presented appropriate techniques. Partitioning their samples by sex, Giles and Elliot achieved between 80 and 88 percent accuracy in separating American blacks from American whites. Their formulae for separating American whites from prehistoric Indian remains is reported by them to have achieved greater accuracy (93–95%), although this level may not be reached in samples not closely related to the Indian Knoll series used by Giles and Elliot to generate their discriminant functions (Birkby, 1966).

In general, it appears that the most reliable estimates of racial ancestry are made from observations, preferably measurements, of the cranium.

Elaborating upon methodology initiated by Brues (1980) and Howells (1973), Gill reports here a case that required him to concentrate upon the problem of distinguishing American Indian remains from those of American whites. Focusing upon the midfacial region, Gill achieves considerable accuracy through the use of six measurements to obtain three discriminating indices, a relatively simple strategy if an appropriate instrument is available. His technique should be tested in additional contexts, given the population-specific nature of many features of skeletal morphology; however, his results are promising. Gill's case study also illustrates the difficulty in achieving accurate racial estimates, even using both visual and metric techniques and consultation with other trained observers of racial variation. The forensic anthropologist is well advised to adopt a flexible attitude toward racial designations and, when proven incorrect, as in Gill's case study, turn an evaluation of error into a contribution that will facilitate improved estimates in the future. Forensic anthropologists should never become so ego involved in their designations that they will not admit to a mistake, for ours is not—as noted by Stewart—"an exact science" (Stewart, 1979:228).

The following cases have been selected to provide examples of the applications of forensic anthropological methods to estimates of age at death, sex, stature, and ancestry. As such, they should be considered examples rather than as inclusive statements concerning the subject at hand. The interested reader should supplement this reading with information presented in forensic anthropology and human osteology texts, such as those by Bass (1971), Brothwell (1972), Krogman (1962), Stewart (1970, 1979), and Ubelaker (1978).

REFERENCES

Acsadi, G., and Nemeskeri, J. (1970). *History of Human Life Span and Mortality*. Budapest: Akademiai Kaido.

Ahlqvist, J., and Damsten, O. (1969). Modification of Kerley's method for the microscopic determination of age in human bone. *J Forensic Sci, 14*:205–212.

Bailit, H. L., and Hunt, E. E. (1964). The sexing of children's skeletons from teeth alone and its genetic implications. *Am J Phys Anthropol, 22*:171–174.

Bass, W. M. (1974). Human Osteology: A Laboratory and Field Manual of the Human Skeleton. Columbia: Missouri Archaeological Society.

Birkby, W. (1966). An evaluation of race and sex identification from cranial measurements. *Am J Phys Anthropol, 24*:21–28.

Black, T. K. (1978a). A new method for assessing the sex of fragmentary skeletal remains: Femoral shaft circumference. *Am J Phys Anthropol, 48*:227–231.

———— (1978b). Sexual dimorphism in the tooth-crown diameters of the deciduous teeth. *Am J Phys Anthropol, 48*:77–82.

Brothwell, D. R. (1972). *Digging Up Bones*, 3rd ed. London: British Museum.

Brues, A. M. (1980). Discussant's comments presented at the Forensic Anthropology Symposium, 40th annual meeting of the Society for Applied Anthropology, Denver, Colorado.

Buikstra, J. E., and Mielke, J. H. (1984). Demography, diet, and health. In R. I. Gilbert and J. H. Mielke (Eds.) *Techniques for the Analysis of Prehistoric Diet.* New York: Academic Press, in press.

Choi, C. C., and Trotter, M. (1970). A statistical study of the multivariate structure and race-sex differences of American white and Negro fetal skeletons. *Am J Phys Anthropol, 33*:307–312.

Condon, K. W., and Charles, D. K. (1983). An evaluation of the cemental annulation aging technique. *Am J Phys Anthropol, 60*:183 (abstract).

Corruccini, R. S., and Henderson, A. M. (1976). Odontometric discriminant function analysis of American whites and blacks. *J Dent Res, 55*:713.

DiBennardo, R., and Taylor, J. V. (1979). Sex assessment of the femur: A test of a new method. *Am J Phys Anthropol, 50*:635–638.

Ditch, L. E., and Rose, J. C. (1972). A mutivariate dental sexing technique. *Am J Phys Anthropol, 37*:61–64.

Fazekas, I. G., and Kosa, F. (1978). *Forensic Fetal Osteology.* Budapest: Akademiai Kaido.

Flander, L. B. (1978). Univariate and multivariate methods for sexing the sacrum. *Am J Phys Anthropol, 49*:103–110.

Garn, S. M., Cole, P. E., Wainwright, R. L., and Guire, K. E. (1977). Sex discriminatory effectiveness using combinations of permanent teeth. *J Dent Res, 56*:697.

Genovès, S. (1967). Proportionality of the long bones and their relation to stature among Mesoamericans. *Am J Phys Anthropol, 26*:67–77.

Genovese, S. (1959). L'estimation des differences sexuelles dans l'os coxal; differences metriques et differences morphologiques. *Bull Mem Soc Anthropol, Paris, 10*:3–95.

Gilbert, B. M., and McKern, T. W. (1973). A method for aging the female *os pubis. Am J Phys Anthropol, 38*:31–38.

Giles, E., and Elliot, O. (1962). Race identification from cranial measurements. *J Forensic Sci, 7*:147–157.

——— (1963). Sex determination by discriminant analysis. *Am J Phys Anthropol, 21*:53–68.

Gustafson, G. (1950). Age determinations of teeth. *J Am Dent Assoc, 41*:45–54.

Gustav, B. L. (1972). "Sexual Dimorphism in the Adult Bony Pelvis of a Prehistoric Human Population from Illinois." Ph.D. dissertation, University of Massachusetts, Amherst.

Hanihara, K. (1958a). Sexual diagnosis of Japanese long bones by means of discriminant function. *J Anthropol Soc Nippon, 66*:187–196 (English summary).

——— (1958b). Sex diagnosis of Japanese skulls and scapulae by means of discriminant function. *J Anthropol Soc Nippon, 67*:191–197.

Helmuth, H., and Rempe, U. (1968). Über den Geschlechtsdimorphismus des Epistropheus beim Menschen. *Z Morphol Anthropol, 59*:300–321.

Hoffman, J. M. (1979). Age estimations from diaphyseal lengths: Two months to twelve years. *J Forensic Sci, 24*:461–469.

Howells, W. W. (1973). *Cranial variation in man.* Papers of the Peabody Museum of Archaeology and Ethnology, vol. 67. Cambridge: Harvard University Press.

Hunt, E. E., and Gleiser, I. (1955). The estimation of age and sex of preadolescent children from bones and teeth. *Am J Phys Anthropol, 13*:479–487.

Hunter, W. S., and Garn, S. M. (1972). Disproportionate sexual dimorphism in the human face. *Am J Phys Anthropol, 36*:133–138.

Keen, J. A. (1950). A study of the differences between male and female skulls. *Am J Phys Anthropol, 8*:65–79.

Kelley, M. A. (1978). Phenice's visual sexing technique for the os pubis: A critique. *Am J Phys Anthropol, 48*:121–122.

_____ (1979). Sex determination with fragmented skeletal remains. *J Forensic Sci, 24*:154–158.

Krogman, W. M. (1962). *The Human Skeleton in Forensic Medicine*. Springfield, IL: Charles C Thomas.

Lovejoy, O., Meindl, R. S., Pryzbeck, T. R., Barton, T. S., Heiple, K. G., and Kotting, D. (1977). Paleodemography of the Libben site, Ottawa County, Ohio. *Science 198*:291–293.

McKern, T. W., and Stewart, T. D. (1957). Skeletal Age Changes in Young American Males. Headquarters, Quartermaster Research & Development Command, Technical Report EP-45.

Meindl, R. S., Lovejoy, C. O., and Mensforth, R. P. (1980). Multifactorial determination of skeletal age at death: a double blind test on a population of known age. *Am J Phys Anthropol, 52*:255.

_____ (1981). Skeletal age at death: accuracy of determination and implications for human demography. *Am J Phys Anthropol, 54*:252.

Mensforth, R. P., and Lovejoy, C. O. (1980). Anatomical, pathophysiological, and demographic correlates of the aging process: a confirmation of multifactorial age determination in the Libben skeletal population. *Am J Phys Anthropol, 52*:256.

Merchant, V. L., and Ubelaker, D. H. (1977). Skeletal growth of the Protohistoric Arikara. *Am J Phys Anthropol, 46*:61–72.

Moorrees, C. F. A., Fanning, E. A., and Hunt, E. E. (1963a). Formation and resorption of three deciduous teeth in children. *Am J Phys Anthropol, 21*:205–213.

_____ (1963b) Age variation of formation stages for ten permanent teeth. *J Dent Res, 42*:1490–1502.

Nolla, C. M. (1960). The development of the permanent teeth. *J Dent Child, 27*:254–266.

Owsley, D. W. (1981). Dental discriminant sexing of Arikara skeletons. *Plains Anthropol, 26*:165–169.

Owsley, D. W., and Webb, R. S. (1983). Misclassification probability of dental discriminant functions for sex determination. *J Forensic Sci, 28*:181–185.

Parson, F. G. (1916). On the proportions and characteristics of the modern English clavicle. *J Anat Lond, 51*:71–93.

Phenice, T. W. (1969). A newly developed visual method of sexing the os pubis. *Am J Phys Anthropol, 30*:297–302.

Pons, J. (1955). The sexual diagnosis of isolated bones of the skeleton. *Hum Biol, 27*:12–21.

Potter, R. H. Y. (1972). Univariate versus multivariate differences in tooth size to sex. *J Dent Res, 51*:716–722.

Richman, E. A., Michel, M. E., Schulter-Ellis, F. P., and Corruccini, R. S. (1979). Determination of sex by discriminant function analysis of postcranial skeletal measurements. *J Forensic Sci, 24*:159–167.

Schulter-Ellis, F. P., Schmidt, D. J., Hayek, L. A., and Craig, J. (1983). Determination of sex with a discriminant analysis of new pelvic bone measurements: Part I. *J Forensic Sci, 28*:169–180.

Sciulli, P. W., Williams, J. A., and Gugelchuk, G. M. (1977). Canine size: an aid in sexing prehistoric Amerindians. *J Dent Res, 56*:1424.

Schour, I., and Massler, M. (1944). Chart—Development of the human dentition, 2nd ed. Chicago: American Dental Association.

Scott, G. T., and Parham, K. R. (1979). Multivariate dental sexing: discrimination of the sexes within an east Tennessee Mississippian skeletal sample. *Tenn Anthropol, 4*:189–198.

Singh, I. J., and Gunberg, D. L. (1970). Estimation of age at death in human males from quantitative histology of bone fragments. *Am J Phys Anthropol, 33*:373–381.

Snow, C. C., Hartman, S., Giles, E., and Young, F. A. (1979). Sex and age determination of crania by calipers and computer: A test of the Giles and Elliot discriminant functions in 52 forensic science cases. *J Forensic Sci, 24*:448–460.

Steel, F. L. D. (1967). Further observations on the osteometric discriminant function: The human clavicle. *Am J Phys Anthropol, 25*:319–322.

Steele, D. G. (1970). Estimation of stature from fragments of long limb bones. In T. D. Stewart (Ed), *Personal Identification in Mass Disasters*, pp. 85–97. Washington, DC: National Museum of Natural History.

_____ (1976). The estimation of sex on the basis of the talus and calcaneus. *Am J Phys Anthropol, 45*:581–588.

Stewart, T. D. (1948). Medico-legal aspects of the skeleton. I: Sex, age, race and status. *Am J Phys Anthropol, 6*:315–322.

_____ (1951). What bones tell. *FBI Law Enforce Bull, 20*(2):2–5.

_____ (1970). Identification of the scars of parturition in the skeletal remains of females. In T. D. Stewart (Ed), *Personal Identification in Mass Disasters*, pp. 127–133. Washington, DC: National Museum of Natural History.

_____ (1979). *Essentials of Forensic Anthropology*. Springfield, IL: Charles C Thomas.

Stott, G. G., Sis, R. F., and Levy, B. M. (1982). Cemental annulation as an age criterion in forensic dentistry. *J Dent Res, 61*:814–817.

Taylor, J. V., and DiBennardo, R. (1982). Determination of sex of white femora by discriminant function analysis: Forensic science applications. *J Forensic Sci, 27*:417–423.

Thieme, F. P., and Schull, W. J. (1957). Sex determination from the skeleton. *Hum Biol, 29*:242–273.

Thompson, D. D. (1979). The core technique in the determination of age at death in skeletons. *J Forensic Sci, 24*:902–915.

Trotter, M., and Gleser, G. C. (1958). A pre-evaluation of estimation of stature based on measurements of stature taken during life and of long bones after death. *Am J Phys Anthropol, 16*:79–123.

Ubelaker, D. H. (1974). Reconstruction of demographic profiles from ossuary skeletal samples: A case study from the tidewater Potomac. Washington, DC: Smithsonian Contributions to Anthropology, Number 18.

_____ (1978). *Human Skeletal Remains*. Chicago: Aldine.

Van Gerven, D. (1971). "The Contribution of Size and Shape Variation to Patterns of Sexual Dimorphism of the Human Femur." Ph.D. dissertation, University of Massachusetts, Amherst.

_____ (1972). The contribution of size and shape variation to patterns of sexual dimorphism of the human femur. *Am J Phys Anthropol, 37*:49–60.

Van Vark, G. N. (1970). "Some Statistical Procedures for the Investigation of Prehistoric Human Skeletal Material." Thesis, Rijksuniversiteit de Groningen.

Washburn, S. L. (1948). Sex differences in the pubic bone. *Am J Phys Anthropol, 6*:199–207.

Weaver, D. S. (1980). Sex differences in the ilia of a known sex and age sample of fetal and infant skeletons. *Am J Phys Anthropol, 52*:191–195.

Chapter 17

SEX DETERMINATION FROM HUMAN SKELETAL REMAINS
A Case of a Mistaken Assumption

CURTIS W. WIENKER

When a forensic anthropologist has the luxury of dealing with the relatively complete and unfragmented skeletal remains of an individual, he or she can typically estimate three major demographic parameters from the bones: age, sex, and a major "racial" or ancestral stock. Of these three, the forensic anthropologist is usually able to assess the sex of the unidentified individual with the greatest degree of confidence and accuracy. The following provides a general summary of some of the frequently used methods and techniques for diagnosis of sex from the analysis of human skeletal remains. A particular case upon which the author served as a consultant to a medical examiner will be used to illustrate some of the osteological features that normally vary sexually and some of the methods of sex estimation.

Unfortunately, the skeletal features that typically serve to discriminate males from females do not usually manifest themselves until approximately the time of puberty. Therefore, the techniques by which one may accurately estimate the sex of a subadult skeleton are nearly nonexistent. Nevertheless, in special circumstances some strategies exist whereby estimation of sex may be made on subadult material; each, however, has a distinct limitation. For further information on these, the reader should consult Boucher (1957), Ditch and Rose (1972), and Hunt and Gleiser (1955).

Certain factors facilitate the estimation of sex from individual adult skeletal remains. Of positive value is that so many features of the human skeleton (and indeed the entire body) vary by gender. However, unlike many other mammals, humans are not particularly dimorphic sexually. That is, many (if not most) of the anatomical differences between the bones of men and women are not pronounced; they are differences of moderate degree rather than great degree, distinctiveness, or kind (Stewart, 1979). In terms of skeletal dimensions, adult males and females differ proportionally only by approximately 8 percent (Krogman, 1962).

Another limitation to the sex diagnosis of an individual from osteological remains is that few adults are "typically" male or female in their total osteological profile. Bones vary sexually in so many ways and often to such small degrees that it is infrequent, if not rare, to encounter a skeleton that is either typically male or female in absolutely every regard. More often, the total osteological pattern usually strongly suggests either masculinity or femininity, but it also includes a few skeletal features that may be slightly ambiguous or even contradictory.

A thorough and accurate estimation of sex for an individual skeleton is based upon an analysis and consideration of multiple skeletal features that compose the total osteological profile. An estimation of sex based primarily on a single diagnostic character or a particular set of diagnostic characters to the exclusion of information provided by other diagnostic characters is liable to yield mistaken results. Estimates based on morphological observation should be corroborated with assessments based on measurements and numerical analysis. The prudent professional should make use of all available techniques of analysis, including study of morphological features, specific measurements and osteometric indices, and analytical formulae.

Much of our knowledge regarding osteological variation in recent living humans is derived from two major osteological reference populations in the United States, the Todd Collection of Cleveland's Museum of Natural History and the Terry Collection of the National Museum of Natural History in Washington, D.C. Both collections consist of hundreds of skeletons of known sex, age, ethnicity, and other personal characteristics. Because of that, they have been excellent research resources for forensic anthropologists and other students of human skeletal variation. However, they also suffer from a few limitations. The collections are not demographically representative of the structure of modern human populations. Also, most of the individuals in these collections lived during the first half of the twentieth century. Thus, the collections may not be osteologically representative of contemporary humans. Modern human populations vary both in size and the amount of osteological sexual dimorphism evident in them (Calcagno, 1981).

Indeed, as El-Najjar and McWilliams (1978) have observed, some populations are typically robust and others typically gracile. To an inexperienced observer, skulls of both sexes derived from a typically robust population may appear to be male. Theoretically, techniques of sexual diagnosis for osteological materials change in both their accuracy and applicability when they are used on osteological materials that are not derived from the reference population upon which the diagnostic techniques were developed.

Despite the limitations noted above, it is possible to assess the sex of a set of individual adult skeletal remains with good accuracy if the remains are relatively complete and unfragmented. Techniques of evaluation include visual examination, measurement, and mathematical treatment of measurements of osteological features. Evaluation of the many osteological features that vary sexually should lead—in normal cases—to assessment with at least 90 percent accuracy (Giles, 1970; Krogman, 1962). A recent test of statistical techniques (Snow et al., 1979) demonstrated a success rate of over 88 percent. When making morphological observations of a case specimen, it is best to have typically male and female specimens available for comparison. Accuracy and confidence in the estimate usually decline in proportion to the completeness and fragmentary nature of the remains under scrutiny.

THE ILLUSTRATIVE CASE

Due to several natural and social factors, east central Florida is a particularly challenging place in which to practice forensic anthropology. The great amount of sunshine, high water table, abundance of annual rainfall, and acidity of the soil all contribute to the relatively rapid deterioration of flesh and bone, whether remains are deposited on the ground or are buried.

Moreover, the suncoast of Florida is the residential home of an extreme diversity of human populations. It is the winter haven of thousands of "snowbirds" and the permanent home of many retirees from the northern United States. Sizeable numbers of American blacks and Afro-American hybrid populations live in the area. Finally, because of extensive agricultural industry, it is the seasonal home of numbers of Mexican-Americans and other Latin American individuals who possess some American Indian ancestry. These factors—the ecological conditions that influence the preservation of osteological remains and the ethnic diversity of residents—serve to complicate the diagnosis of sex from individual skeletons found in the greater Tampa Bay area.

The human skeletal remains that will be used to illustrate the estimation of sex were discovered by construction workers clearing vegetation from the site of a growing residential development in east central Florida. Such an occurrence is not unusual in recent years, given the enormous population boom experienced in coastal metropolitan areas of Florida.

The workers discovered a nearly complete human skeleton beneath several centimeters of pine needles and sand in an area adjacent to a coastal waterway. The police were contacted; they exhumed the skeleton and took it to the office of the medical examiner, who called me to analyze the skeleton. The remains were nearly complete and devoid of any soft tissue.

There was no evidence of intentional interment. Available evidence indicated that a cadaver was deposited at the spot and that it decomposed prior to being covered by naturally occurring materials. The known tidal current patterns and two nearby hurricanes from the preceding summer indicated to authorities that the overburden (layers of pine needles and sand) had resulted from high tides and storms affecting the nearby marine waterway. During the initial site investigation, a heavily rusted zipper and a partial upper dental plate were discovered in association with the remains. While the police wanted any information that the consulting forensic anthropologist could derive from the bones, the ensuing discussion focuses solely on the attribute of sex.

MORPHOLOGICAL AND METRIC OBSERVATIONS

Indications of the sex of a skeleton can be gained by studying selected features of the skull and pelvis and by taking simple metric measurements from some of the other parts of the skeleton. The determinants of osteological sexual dimorphism are the relatively greater body size and muscularity of males and the childbearing capability of females. Normally, the pelvis is the area of the skeleton that yields the greatest accuracy in estimating sex by morphological observation alone, because the pelvis displays the most definitive, sex-related variation within the entire skeleton. Coleman (1969) discusses the development of pelvic variation during adolescence.

The Pelvis

Morphological differences between the pelves of adult males and females are primarily due to structural variations associated with childbirth. Stewart (1979) summarizes many of these dimorphic features. The pelvis of a male tends to be larger and more robust—especially in the areas of the iliac crest and ischial tuberosities. Also, the acetabula tend to be larger in males, while the obturator foramen, the large aperture in the ischio-pubic area, tends to be more triangulate and smaller in females. As Figure 17-1 shows, the obturator foramen and acetabulum of the case specimen pelvis appear more male in morphology. However, the case specimen appears to be female when the size and shape of the pubic bone are considered.

Smith (1938) first noted two aspects of the os pubis that differ by gender. Typically, the pubic bone, from the obturator foramen to the symphysis, is wider in females. Also, the relatively greater width of the pubic bone and other structural differences combine to make the body of the pubic bone more rectangular in females and more triangular in males. The shape of the pubic bone is one of six such features that are most useful in providing a rapid assessment of sex (Stewart, 1979). With regard to the width and shape differences of the os pubis, the case specimen (Fig 17-1C) is clearly more female in appearance.

Two other dimorphic features in the pubic area are most readily observ-

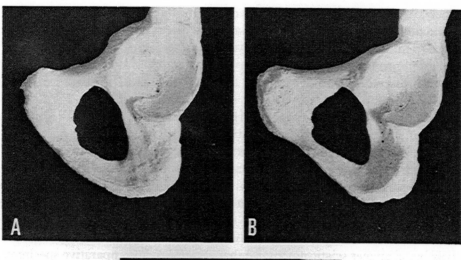

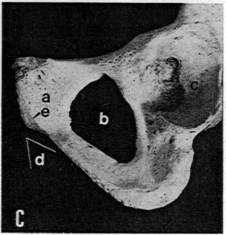

Figure 17-1. Left pelves, ventral view. A. Representative male. B. Representative female. C. Case specimen: a = pubic bone, b = obturator foramen, c = acetabulum, d = subpubic angle, e = ventral arc. (Photos by G. Ballo.)

able when the pelvis is viewed from the ventral aspect, as it is seen in Figure 17-1. Both features are described and discussed in greater detail by Phenice (1969). Stewart (1979) considers them as among the most helpful in the diagnosis of sex.

The subpubic or inferior border of the pubic bone tends to be slightly concave in females and slightly convex in males. When the pubic bones of a pelvis are articulated into the anatomical position, a male usually has a noticeably more acute subpubic angle than a female.

Another morphological indicator of the sex of a pubic bone occurs on the medial and inferior aspect of the bone, near the symphyseal rim. In females a moderate to well-pronounced line, the ventral arc, usually runs craniomedially from the approximate juncture of the pubic and ischial bones to the midpoint of the symphyseal rim. In females, when the ventral arc is well pronounced, it tends to isolate the medial, inferiormost aspect of the ventral pubic bone as a small triangle. In males, the ventral arc is usually absent and, if present, is typically barely visible. As Figure 17-1 illustrates, the case specimen is clearly female in the shape of the subpubic border and the presence of a well-defined ventral arc.

The greater sciatic notch lies ventral and inferior to the sacroiliac articular surface; generally it is a wedge-shaped indentation. In males, the notch is typically narrower than it is in females. A general rule is that if the thumb can be inserted into the greater sciatic notch and moved a bit through the plane of the iliac blade, then the individual represented is probably a female. As seen in Figure 17-2, the case specimen appears to have a relatively broad greater sciatic notch, like that of the female comparative specimen.

Other morphological variables of the pelvis may be useful in estimating the sex of a skeleton. St. Hoyme (1963) has noted that the posterior-inferior portion of the facet of the ilium that articulates with the sacrum tends to be slightly elevated or more pedestallike among females; in males that portion of the articular surface does not normally protrude.

Due to physiological changes associated with pregnancy, evidence of childbearing or parity may manifest itself in two areas of the pelvis (Houghton, 1974). Scars of parturition in the form of pits may occur on the dorsal aspect of the pubis, near the symphysis or in the preaurecular area of the ilium immediately inferior to the sacroiliac articular surface. Scaring may also be present on the adjacent aspect of the sacrum (Dunlap, 1979).

Suchey et al. (1979) have shown that "medium to large" dorsal pits are good indicators of sex. They studied 160 individuals who displayed "medium to large" dorsal pitting; only 4 (2.5%) were male. On the other hand, their data showed that the absence of dorsal pits was not nearly as powerful in estimating sex. Of 486 females studied, 66 (12.6%) had no dorsal pitting.

Suchey et al. (1979) have also demonstrated that, when present in females, dorsal pits are not good indicators of parity. A female may have been multiparous and evidence no or "trace" scars, or have been nulliparous and manifest "medium to large" scars. Parity pitting should only be used as a possible indication of childbearing.

Two indices of structural variation of the pelvis are relatively powerful discriminators of gender in humans. Each index is based upon the ratio between two different measurements of the pelvis and may be used even though the pelvic remains are incomplete or fragmentary. Whenever re-

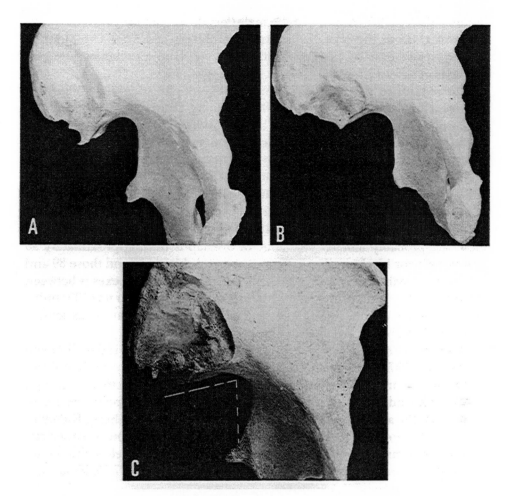

Figure 17-2. Left pelves, medial view of greater sciatic notch. A. Representative male. B. Representative female. C. Case specimen. (Photos by G. Ballo.)

quired measurements are taken from bilaterally symmetrical bones (those which are present in pairs, such as right and left femora), measurements from the right and left sides should be taken and an average calculated. This practice will minimize bias due to over– or underdevelopment of one or the other of the paired bones.

The sciatic notch/acetabular index can discriminate sexes of known ethnicity greater than 90 percent of the time (Kelley, 1979). The width (in mm) of the greater sciatic notch, measured from the base of the ischial spine to the pyramidal process of the ilium, is divided by the vertical diameter (in mm) of the acetabulum, the distance between the inferiormost and superiormost margins of the acetabulum. The measurements are easily taken with sliding calipers. Kelley (1979) found that the male/female separation point in American whites was an index of 87; for American blacks it was 86. The index of the case specimen is 87 (notch width 47 mm; acetabulum diameter 54 mm) and does not clearly indicate gender.

The ischium-pubis index (Washburn, 1948) is the length of the pubis from the acetabular juncture point of the ischium, ilium, and pubis to the medialmost portion of the superior border of the pubic symphysis, divided by the length of the ischium from the acetabular juncture to the caudalmost point of the ischium. This percentage is multiplied by 100 to yield an index. With this index it is frequently important to know the ethnic ancestry of the remains in question because the cutoff points that discriminate between females and males are markedly different for blacks and whites. With white individuals, indices of 90 and below are probably male, and those 95 and above are probably female; the range of overlap is from approximately 90 through 94. For blacks indices below 83 are probably male and those 89 and above are probably female; the area of overlap between the sexes is between 84 through 88. The ischium-pubis index of the case specimen was 105 (pubis length = 85 mm; ischium length = 81 mm), indicating that it was female with a high degree of probability, regardless of ethnicity.

Attempts have been made to improve the ischium-pubis index (Thieme and Schull, 1957), because the acetabular juncture point is usually obliterated in adults, and its location is therefore a matter of subjective judgment. The refined index includes consideration of ischium and pubis measurements from the acetabular border and the size of the femoral head. Richman et al. (1979) applied the technique to a reference population of American whites and obtained a section point of 91 (females lying below the value, males above). For the case specimen the index was 74.9 (7.75/10.35) and indicated a female.

The Skull

Krogman (1962) discusses sexual variation of the skull in some detail. The general morphological structure and configurations of adult male skulls tend to be more robust than those of females. Sexual variation in the skull does not usually become evident until puberty or even later in subadulthood. (Krogman, 1962). The various ridges, lines, and other protruberances of the cranium and mandible are usually slightly rougher and more pronounced in adult males. In the cranium this robusticity is usually most evident in three areas: the supraorbital tori or brow ridges, the nuchal area of the occipital bone (the most posterior aspect of the skull), and the mastoid process of the temporal bone, immediately posterior and inferior to the external auditory meatus. Figure 17-3 compares the case specimen and "typical" male and female skulls. The case specimen has less robust supraorbital tori, suggestive of "femininity"; however, its mastoid process (Fig 17-4) is not typically small as one would expect with a female.

Three features of the facial skeleton are sometimes helpful in the determination of sex. When palpated, the nasal bridge, which includes the union of the two small nasal bones with the inferiormost portion of the infraorbital

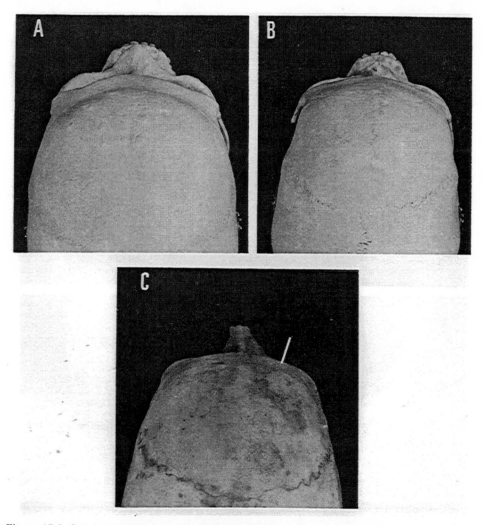

Figure 17-3. Crania. Top view showing relative pronunciation of supraorbital tori. A. Representative male. B. Representative female. C. Case specimen. (Photos by G. Ballo.)

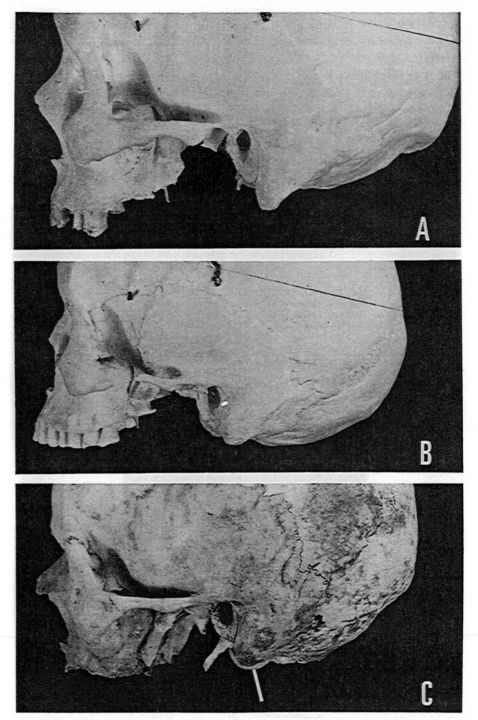

Figure 17-4. Left lateral view showing mastoid process. A. Representative male. B. Representative female. C. Case specimen. (Photos by G. Ballo.)

part of the frontal bone, tends to be sharper in males and rounder and smoother in females (Krogman, 1962). The superior borders of the orbital cavities display the opposite pattern when palpated; they are sharper in females and blunter in males (Bass, 1971). Among males, the mental protruberance or chin tends to be more squarish; in females it is usually rounder or more pointed when viewed from above or below (Stewart, 1979). The chin shape of the case specimen is clearly female.

It is often difficult to make morphological assessments such as those noted here if only a single specimen — the particular case in question — is available for scrutiny. It is easier and wiser to reserve such estimations and judgments based upon degrees of development and difference to cases when "typically" male and female specimens are available for comparison. If possible, the comparative specimens should be of an age range and ethnic background similar to that of the case specimen.

OTHER MORPHOLOGICAL INDICATORS

Although the pelvis and skull manifest the most numerous marked and accurate morphological indicators of sex, many other aspects of the skeleton are dimorphic to one degree or another. In most of these areas, however, the amount of male-female similarity is considerable. Accordingly, these indicators are most appropriately used as corraborative to the morphological features of the pelvis and skull, or when only isolated elements are present.

Two dimensions of the scapula are useful indicators of skeletal sex, as Thomas Dwight (1894) first demonstrated: the maximum length between the superior and inferior angles, and glenoid cavity length. As Stewart (1979) notes, the range of overlap in scapular length between males and females is 140 to 159 mm; for glenoid length it is from 34 to 36 mm. The case specimen scapular length measurements are right = 147 mm, left = 146 mm. Glenoid cavity lengths are right = 36 mm, left = 35 mm. In neither instance is the case specimen obviously female. However, these data do suggest a female rather than a male.

The proximal articular facets or heads of the humerus and femur are also easily measured and indicative of skeletal sex, as first reported (1894) and later published (1905) by Dwight. Refinements in sectioning points have been made on the basis of dry bone measurements, by Stewart (1979). With respect to the vertical diameter of the head of the humerus, the range of overlap between the sexes is 43 to 45 mm. Vertical humeral head diameters for the case specimen are right = 44.8 mm, left = 44.4 mm, slightly suggestive of a male.

Both Dwight (1905) and Stewart (1977, 1979) suggest that femoral head diameter is less accurate than the humeral head diameter as an indicator of skeletal sex. The sectioning points and common ranges for the femoral head have been revised (Pearson and Bell, 1919) and re-revised (Stewart, 1979) since Dwight's (1905) early publication. Moreover, data gathered from black skeletons by Thieme and Schull (1957) are considerably more variable by sex than those presented in the three studies cited above. Stewart's (1979) work on the Terry Collection revealed a common range for males and females of 44 to 46 mm. He estimates that a femoral head diameter of 42.5 to 43.5 mm is questionably female; 43.5 to 46.5 indeterminate, and 46.5 to 47.5 mm questionably male. Femoral head diameters of the case specimen are right = 45.2 mm, left = 44.8 mm. In this regard, the case specimen is of indeterminate sex.

DISCRIMINANT FUNCTION ANALYSIS

Some of the most powerful (in terms of accuracy and objectivity) methods of sexing skeletal material are based upon the application of statistical analysis to osteological materials. Discriminant function analysis is one such sophisticated mathematical approach. It is beyond the scope of this presentation to delve into either the theory or methods by which the mathematical formulae are generated. Giles (1970) discusses the basic aspects of formula generation, and Calcagno (1981) treats some of the problems inherent in the technique as it pertains to human identification. It is important to note that the formulae are theoretically only applicable to specimens from the reference populations that were studied to develop the formulae. Some of the differences between these reference populations, typically the Todd and Terry Collections, and contemporary living populations were mentioned earlier. Despite the criticism that discriminant function sexing has received, and Calcagno's (1981) assertion that estimates based upon it should be used as secondary, the techniques should be applied to forensic cases whenever possible. Discriminant function analysis can serve as a check on one's subjective impressions formulated during morphological analysis, as Stewart (1979) notes.

To use a discriminant function formula for sexing, one must have estimated or ascertained the racial ancestry of the case specimen. A set of specific measurements is taken from the skeleton. Each measurement is multiplied by its respective weight in the formula for discrimination of sex. A total number is obtained by summing the products. Each formula has its respective section point, or numerical value that separates the sexes; typically, values above the section point are male. Different formulae weights are used for skeletons of different racial groups.

Each discriminant function formula has its own reliability and accuracy. Most of them accurately assess the sex of a skeleton in at least 80 percent of the cases; some offer theoretical accuracy greater than 90 percent of the time (Giles, 1970). The greater the distance from the sectioning point the case specimen's value lies, the greater the probability that the assessment is accurate. There are many different formulae using different sets of cranial, mandibular, and postcranial measurements. Giles (1970) provides a summary of many formulae and a description of the appropriate measurements.

Table 17-I documents the application and results of three discriminant function formulae to the case specimen, which is Caucasoid. This method of analysis clearly suggests that the case specimen is a female, based on the cranium (Giles and Elliot, 1963), mandible (Giles, 1964), and femur (Pons, 1955). The formula based on femoral dimensions yields the highest accuracy (over 95% correctly sexed from the reference population) of the three formulae applied here. For the case specimen, its value fell only slightly on the female side of the section point.

TABLE 17-I
DISCRIMINANT FUNCTION ANALYSIS OF SEX OF CASE SPECIMEN*

Measurement	Metric Value (mm)	Formula Weight	Metric Value — Weight Product
Cranium			
Cranial length	170.0	1.236	210.120
Cranial breadth	140.0	− 1.000	− 140.000
Mastoid length	24.5	1.528	037.436
Bizygomatic breadth	127.0	3.291	417.957
Section Point =	536.93	TOTAL	525.513
Mandible			
Symphysis height	27.7	22,206	615.106
Body height	23.5	−30.265	− 711.228
Body length	79.0	1.000	79.000
Condyle height	64.8	19.708	1,277.078
Gonial diameter	93.5	7.360	688.160
Section Point =	1,960.05	TOTAL	1,944.05
Femur (Lt.)			
Oblique length	381.0	1.000	381.000
Head diameter	44.8	30.716	1,376.077
Min. Shaft Diameter (Trans.)	22.5	− 12.643	− 322.397
Epicondylar breadth	69.3	17.565	1,217.255
Section Point =	2,656.51	TOTAL	2,651.935

*See text for source of specific formulae.

DISPOSITION OF THE CASE SPECIMEN

A clear majority (but not all) of the cranial and pelvic features indicated that the case specimen was female, although the authorities had made an original assumption of masculinity based primarily upon the presence of a partial upper dental plate. The analysis by the forensic anthropologist revealed the remains to be female and caused the police to revisit the location where the skeleton was discovered. The police were of the opinion that because the remains were female, there was a much higher probability that a crime was involved. Accordingly, they scoured the location where the skeleton was discovered even more thoroughly than they had during their original investigation. The revisit of the scene brought to light additional evidence, including a cigarette pack (of a brand usually smoked by women) and enough of the remains of a pair of blue jeans to identify the manufacturer and the retail vendor. However, the subject remains unidentified at the time of this writing.

REFERENCES

Bass, W.: *Human Osteology.* Columbia, Missouri Archaeological Society, 1971.

Boucher, B. J.: Sex differences in the fetal pelvis. *Am J Phys Anthropol, 15*:581–600, 1957.

Calcagno, J. M.: On the applicability of sexing material by discriminant function analysis. *J Hum Evol, 10*: 189–198, 1981.

Coleman, W.: Sex differences in the growth of the pelvis. *Am J Phys Anthropol, 31*:125–152, 1969.

Ditch, L. E. and Rose, J.: A multivariate sexing technique. *Am J Phys Anthropol, 37*:61–64, 1972.

Dunlap, S. S.: Sex, Parity and the Preauricular Sulcus. Paper presented at 48th Ann Mtg, Am Assoc Phys Anthropol, San Francisco, 1979.

Dwight, Thomas: The range and significance of variations in the human skeleton. *Bost Med Surg J, 13*:73–76; *1* (4):97–101, 1894.

———— : The size of the articular surfaces of the long bones as characteristics of sex: An anthropological study. *Am J Anat, 4*:19–32, 1905.

El-Najjar, M. and McWilliams, K.: *Forensic Anthropology.* Springfield, Thomas, 1978.

Giles, E.: Sex determination by discriminant function analysis of the mandible. *Am J Phys Anthropol, 22*:129–135, 1964.

Giles, E.: Discriminant function sexing of the human skeleton. In Stewart, T. D. (Ed.): *Personal Identification in Mass Disasters,* pp. 99–109. Washington, National Museum of Natural History, 1970.

Giles, E. and Elliot, O.: Sex determination by discriminant function analysis of crania. *Am J Phys Anthropol, 21*:53–68, 1963.

Houghton, P.: The relationship of the pre-auricular groove of the ilium to pregnancy. *Am J Phys Anthropol, 41*:381–389, 1974.

Hunt, E. E., Jr. and Gleiser, I.: The estimation of age and sex of preadolescent children from bones and teeth. *Am J Phys Anthropol, 13*:389–487, 1955.

Kelley, M. A.: Sex determination with fragmented skeletal remains. *J Forensic Sci, 24*:154–158, 1979.

Krogman, W. M.: *The Human Skeleton in Forensic Medicine*. Springfield, Thomas, 1962.

Pearson, K. and Bell, J.: A study of the bones of the English skeleton, 1. The femur (Chapters 1 to 6). Drapers Co Res Mem (Biometric Ser. X), Dept. Applied Stat., Univ. London, Univ. College, 1919.

Phenice, T. W.: A newly developed visual method of sexing the os pubis. *Am J Phys Anthropol, 30*:297–301, 1969.

Pons, J.: The sexual diagnosis of isolated bones of the skeleton. *Hum Biol, 27*:12–21, 1955.

Richman, E., Michel, M., Schulter-Ellis, F., and Corruccini, R.: Determination of sex by discriminant function analysis of skeleton measurements. *J Forensic Sci, 24*:159–167, 1979.

Smith, S.: Studies in identification, No. 3. *Police J London, 12*:403–408, 1939.

Snow, C., Hartman, S., Giles, E. and Young, F.: Sex and race determination of crania by calipers and computer: A test of the Giles and Elliot discriminant functions in 52 forensic science cases. *J Forensic Sci, 24*:448–460, 1979.

Stewart, T. D.: An examination of selected post-cranial features recommended in the literature as good indicators of sex. Am Acad For Sci Book of Abstracts (Ann. Mtg, San Diego, CA), No. 125, Feb. 1977.

———: *Essentials of Forensic Anthropology Especially as Developed in the United States*. Springfield, Thomas, 1979.

St. Hoyme, L. E.: Human Skeletal Variation. Thesis, Oxford University, Lady Margaret Hall, 1963.

Suchey, J., Wiseley, D., Green, R., and Noguchi, T.: Analysis of dorsal pitting in the os pubis in an extensive sample of modern American females. *Am J Phys Anthropol, 51*:517–540, 1979.

Thieme, F. and Schull, W.: Sex determination from the skeleton. *Hum Biol, 29*:242–273, 1957.

Washburn, S.: Sex differences in the pubic bone. *Am J Phys Anthropol, 6*:199–207, 1948.

Chapter 18

SKELETAL AND DENTAL IDENTIFICATION OF AN ADOLESCENT FEMALE*

Anthony J. Perzigian and Paul N. Jolly

Human remains were discovered by hunters on October 22, 1977, in a rural section of Clermont County, Ohio. The body was sent to the Hamilton County Coroner's Office in Cincinnati for analysis and identification. The remains were badly decomposed. Viscera were no longer identifiable, and the integument was destroyed; however, ligaments, fascia, and tendons along with joint capsules were partially preserved. A large mass of straight light brown hair was also recovered. With the exception of two ribs and the right upper extremity, the skeleton was complete and in good condition. Of note, no dental fillings were observed. No clothing or identification was found in association with the remains.

State of preservation suggested that death had probably occurred within the past year. Postmortem examination was performed by the authors to determine sex, age, race, stature, and cause of death. The primary focus of this report will be the assessment of age at time of death.

ASSESSMENT OF RACE, SEX, AND STATURE

Racial attribution was based on the recovery of the straight light brown hair, which strongly suggested someone of predominantly European ancestry. Assessment of sex was based on both pelvic and cranial features. The pelvic bones were quite gracile and smooth; the subpubic angle was markedly *U*-shaped; the obturator foramina were small and triangular; the greater sciatic notch was extremely wide and shallow. From these criteria (Stewart, 1979) the strong indication is female. The pelvic inlet measured 11.0 cm in the anteroposterior direction and 12.0 cm in the trans-

*The authors wish to express their appreciation to Mr. Jack Leach, Special Investigator for the Hamilton County Coroner's Office. His assistance in the identification and in the preparation of this chapter was invaluable.

verse direction. Such an individual would be classified as mesatipellic, which is usually characteristic of females rather than males (Gruelich and Thoms, 1938; Krogman, 1962). Cranial features were highly corroborative. A gracile skull, small mastoid processes, absence of supraorbital ridges, and a smooth, rounded chin describe the feminine qualities of the individual. The authors were confident that the remains were those of a white female.

Trotter and Gleser's (1952) regression equations for the estimation of living stature from long bones were used. Maximum lengths of the femur, 43.0 cm, and tibia, 35.5 cm, were introduced into the following equation, which was empirically derived for white females:

$$\text{Stature} = 1.48\,(\text{Fem}) + 1.28\,(\text{Tib}) + 53.07$$

This yielded a stature estimation of 162.15 ± 3.55 cm or between 5 feet 3 inches and 5 feet 4 inches.

ESTIMATION OF AGE

Routine osteologic criteria were first used to estimate a general age at time of death. No ectocranial closure of either the vault or circummeatal sutures was observed; however, the spheno-occipital synchondrosis appeared fully fused. Gilbert and McKern's (1973) method for aging the female pubic symphysis was employed; an age in the range of fourteen to eighteen years was determined. Of note, Suchey (1979) has demonstrated a limited accuracy for the Gilbert and McKern method. The adult dentition with the exception of the third molars had erupted. Lower third molars were not observed; upper third molars appeared impacted. Fusion of the ilium, ischium, and pubis was complete and indicated an age over thirteen years. The degree of union of the epiphyses to diaphyses was quite variable from bone to bone. In sum, a preliminary analysis suggested that death had occurred sometime in the postpubertal, preadult period. With a nearly complete skeleton with which to work, an effort was made to estimate chronologic age more precisely on the basis of epiphyseal union.

Regardless of the physiologic criteria chosen to estimate chronologic age, the investigator must be aware of the extreme variability that characterizes human growth and development. A primary source of variability is, of course, sexual dimorphism. The well-known developmental advancement of females applies especially well to the appearance and subsequent fusion of epiphyses to diaphyses. Garn and co-workers (1961) report considerable anatomical difference in the magnitude of maturational dimorphism. For example, females average approximately 13 percent ahead of males chronologically in the fusion of epiphyses in the hand; yet, the difference reaches 19 percent for the knee; moreover, females are chronologically 26 percent ahead in the appearance of other epiphyses. The appearance of epiphyses and their later union are virtually uncorrelated either on a sequential basis or a timing basis. Krogman (1962) advocates the use of sex-specific schedules for the appearance and fusion of epiphyses. As a rough rule of thumb he views female skeletal advancement as approximately one year between ages five and ten, two years between ages ten and fifteen, and one year between ages fifteen and twenty.

Skeletal development is also influenced by other factors. Genetic sources of variation that affect the appearance and fusion of epiphyses have been amply demonstrated by Garn et al. (1961, 1963, 1969). Racial differences in skeletal development have also been reported (Garn et al., 1972; Roche et al., 1978). The impact of economic and nutritional factors has been well documented (Garn, 1973; Martorell et al., 1978). In sum, various factors associated with inheritance, diet, socioeconomic background, or health can interact and influence the time and sequence of skeletal maturation. Indeed, even samples of healthy children display considerable variation in both the appearance and fusion of epiphyses.

For forensic purposes it is customary to devote more attention to the major epiphyses of the long bones than to those of the smaller bones. The major epiphyses generally unite in the following sequence: elbow, hip, ankle, knee, wrist, shoulder (Stewart, 1979). Normal union can take place at any time within a range of ages; as a consequence, the above sequence may not apply in all individual cases. For example, McKern and Stewart (1957), in a study of fifty-five individuals, showed that complete union of the medial epicondyle can occur as early as seventeen years or as late as twenty years; in addition, the proximal humerus displayed a range from seventeen to twenty-four years.

The determination of complete, incomplete, or recent union can be difficult and ambiguous. Stewart (1979) and Krogman (1962) point out that radiographs can frequently give the appearance of complete union, while gross inspection indicates markedly incomplete union. Furthermore, the gross appearance of a securely attached epiphysis should not be mistakenly taken to mean complete union. The authors initially and mistakenly rated some epiphyses as completely united despite the persistence of a discernible line of demarcation between the epiphyses and diaphyses. Such epiphyses should not be considered completely united; rather, they should be classified as perhaps three-fourths united (McKern, 1957) or recently united (Stevenson, 1924). In this way the risk of overestimation of age can be minimized.

Schedules of epiphyseal union for females have been reported by Paterson (1929), Todd (1930), Flecker (1932, 1933), Modi (1957), and Johnston (1961). Summary tables are provided by Krogman (1962) and Stewart (1979). Most of the data are based on European populations. Flecker's work is especially valuable, since information for individual epiphyses is listed according to (1) earliest ages at which fusion occurs, (2) ages at which a majority have fused, and (3) latest ages at which fusion has not yet occurred. Epiphyses were evaluated by gross inspection and classified according to the following conditions: nonunion, partial union, complete union. Epiphyses were considered partially united if a relatively prominent line or "scar" of demarcation was present between the epiphysis and diaphysis. If the line was either absent or only barely discernible, i.e. a trace, the epiphysis was considered completely united.

In Table 18-I, epiphyses are grouped by anatomical regions, and their degree of union is recorded. Ages were determined from published standards cited above; a weighted age or age range is estimated for each of the anatomical regions. With complete union of the elbow epiphyses but with only partial union of the femoral head, an approximate range of 14 to 17 is indicated. When complete union of the distal fibula, proximal fibula, proximal tibia, and distal femur is considered, an age of 16 or 17 appears likely. With the presence of both nonunited and partially united epiphyses in the wrist and pectoral region, an age of approximately 17 is further substantiated.

Miscellaneous epiphyses and growth centers are listed in Table 18-II. Again, only partial union was observed for epiphyses of the ilium, ischium, sacrum, and vertebrae. These results are not inconsistent with those in Table 18-I and strengthen the claim that the female died sometime after her sixteenth birthday and possibly before her seventeenth birthday.

After evaluating the union of twenty-five separate growth centers along with the spinous processes and annular epiphyses of twenty-four vertebrae, one should be able to ascertain with some reliability and precision the age at time of death within the second decade of life. By pooling and weighing a large number of observations as provided in Tables 18-I and 18-II, the effects of any aberrant epiphyses should be minimized. McKern (1957) demonstrated that adequate age estimates can be made by sampling only a small number of critical growth areas. He has shown that the nine epiphyses listed in Table 18-III provide estimates as good as those from thirty-eight epiphyses and eleven sutures. Although based on male standards, McKern's approach was also adopted. The nine epiphyses were each ranked on a scale of one to five where one equals nonunion, two, three, and four equal increasing degrees of partial union, and five equals complete union. Summing the stages of union for the nine epiphyses yields a total score of twenty-six or a predicted age of 18.59 years (Stewart, 1979). Assuming that females are approximately one to two years in advance of males and subtracting the same from the predicted age places this female in a 16.6 to 17.6 year age range. These results clearly reinforce the conclusions based on Tables 18-I and 18-II. In sum, an estimated age range of 16 to 17 seems justified, though factors associated with her inheritance and/or environment may account for error.

TABLE 18-I
EPIPHYSEAL UNION OF THE MAJOR BONES

Region	Epiphysis	Nonunion	Partial Union	Complete Union		Estimated Age
Elbow	Distal humerus			+		>14
	Medial epicondyle			+		>14
	Proximal radius			+		>14
	Proximal ulna			+		>14
					Weighted age:	>14
Hip	Femoral head		+			<17
	Greater trochanter			+		14–17
					Weighted age:	<17
Ankle	Distal tibia		+			>14
	Distal fibula			+		>15
	Calcaneus		+			13–17
					Weighted age:	15–17
Knee	Distal femur			+		17
	Proximal tibia			+		15–17
	Proximal fibula			+		16–17
					Weighted age:	16–17
Wrist	Distal radius		+			<18
	Distal ulna		+			<17
					Weighted age:	<17
Pectoral	Proximal humerus		+			<17
	Inferior angle, scapula	+				<20
	Coracoid process		+			16
	Acromial process		+			13–16
	Medial clavicle	+				<20
					Weighted age:	<17

TABLE 18-II
UNION OF MISCELLANEOUS EPIPHYSES AND GROWTH CENTERS

Bone	Nonunion	Partial Union	Complete Union		Estimated Age
Iliac crest		+			<20
Ischial tuberosity		+			<21
Annular epiphyses (cervical, thoracic, lumbar)		+			<17
Vertebral spinous processes		+			<17
Lateral sacral epiphyses		+			<17
Sacral segments 1, 2		+			<17*
Sacral segments 2, 3		+			<17*
Sternal segments 1, 2	+				<17*
				Weighted age:	<17

*Based on males (McKern, 1970)

TABLE 18-III
ESTIMATION OF AGE BY MCKERN'S (1957) GROUP V EPIPHYSES

	Stages of Union*				
Epiphysis	1	2	3	4	5
Proximal humerus		+			
Medial epicondyle					+
Distal radius			+		
Femoral head		+			
Distal femur					+
Iliac crest		+			
Medial clavicle,	+				
Sacrum 3, 4 joint				+	
Lateral sacral joints		+			
SUM OF COLUMN SCORES	1	8	3	4	10
TOTAL SCORE 26					
PREDICTED AGE 18.59 years					

*1 = no union; 2 = 1/4 union; 3 = 1/2 union; 4 = 3/4 union; 5 = complete union

IDENTIFICATION AND DISPOSITION OF THE CASE

Our analysis indicated that the unidentified remains were those of a white teenage female approximately 5 feet 3 inches in height. With the help of Clermont County investigators, a female (D.S.M.) was located in missing persons files who fit the description. She had disappeared and was last seen in the area on July 17, 1977, or three months before hunters had discovered the human remains. Her parents supplied a recent photograph, which was compared to the unidentified corpse. Figure 18-I displays the maxilla and dentition of the unidentified specimen. Loss of the left lateral incisor had occurred postmortem. The right lateral incisor prominently displays a large carious lesion on the mesial border. Both the right and left central incisors are chipped in identical locations at the median sagittal plane. Of note, too, the right and left premolars were reduced to carious stumps. Figure 18-2 is that of the missing person. She, too, displays a large carious lesion on the mesial border of the right upper lateral incisor; she, too, displays the same approximal chipping of the central incisors. In addition, no upper first premolars are readily observable in the photograph. Their obscurity is ostensibly due to their severely reduced size as seen in Figure 18-1. Comparison of Figure 18-1 to Figure 18-2 provides almost certain identification.

The missing person is a white female born on October 10, 1960, but who probably never reached her seventeenth birthday. Indeed, her badly decomposed remains found on October 22, 1977, indicate death prior to two weeks before their discovery and, therefore, prior to her birthday. Her stature is reported to be 5 feet 3 inches as is the estimation of the corpse. Her hair is

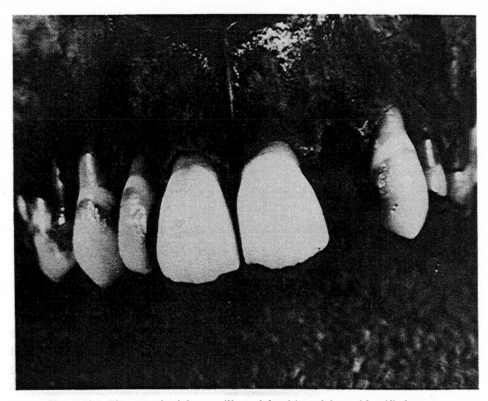

Figure 18-1. Photograph of the maxilla and dentition of the unidentified person.

described as brown as is that of the corpse. She was reported missing almost three months before her seventeenth birthday; extent of epiphyseal union would suggest approximately the same age. In sum, the particulars of the missing person, i.e. race, hair color, sex, stature, condition of teeth, and age consistently correspond to those of the corpse. The compelling conclusion, then, is that they are in fact the same person.

In 1978, a convicted murderer was brought to trial for the murder of D.S.M. He had earlier confessed to the murder. According to the confession, he had picked up D.S.M., who joined him voluntarily. They drove to a secluded, wooded area in Clermont County, where he forcefully disrobed her in preparation for intercourse. During the attack he "inadvertently" strangled her. He disposed of the body nearby, and her whereabouts was unknown until hunters happened upon her remains some months later. Chief Deputy Coroner Jolly testified during the trial that the skeletal remains were unequivocally those of D.S.M.

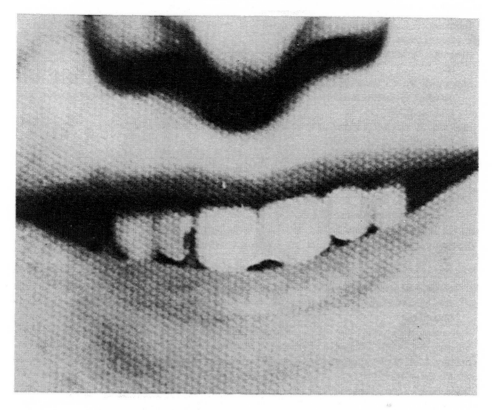

Figure 18-2. Photograph of a missing person (D.S.M.).

REFERENCES

Flecker, H. (1932–33). Roentgenographic observations of the times of appearance of epiphyses and their fusion with diaphyses. *J Anat, 67*: 118–164.

Garn, S. M., C. G. Rohmann, and B. Apfelbaum (1961). Complete epiphyseal union of the hand. *Am J Phys Anthropol, 19*:365–372.

Garn, S. M., C. G. Rohmann, and A. A. Davis (1963). Genetics of hand-wrist ossification. *Am J Phys Anthropol, 21*: 33–40.

Garn, S. M., C. G. Rohmann, and K. P. Hertzog (1969). Apparent influence of the X chromosome on timing of 73 ossification centers. *Am J Phys Anthropol, 30*: 123–128.

Garn, S. M., S. T. Sandusky, J. M. Nagy, and M. B. McCann (1972). Advanced skeletal development in low-income Negro children. *J Pediatr, 80*: 965–969.

Garn, S. M., S. T. Sandusky, N. N. Rosen, and F. Trowbridge (1973). Economic impact on postnatal ossification. *Am J Phys Anthropol, 38*: 1–4.

Gilbert, B. M. and T. W. McKern 1973 A method for aging the female *os pubis. Am J Phys Anthropol, 38*: 31–38.

Gruelich, W. W. and H. Thoms (1938). The dimension of the pelvic inlet of 789 white females. *Anat Rec, 72*: 45–51.

Johnston, F. E. (1961). Sequence of epiphyseal union in a prehistoric Kentucky population from Indian Knoll. *Hum Biol, 33*: 66–81.

Krogman, W. M. (1962). *The Human Skeleton in Forensic Medicine.* Charles C Thomas, Springfield, Ill.

Martorell, R., C. Yarbrough, J. H. Himes, and R. E. Klein (1978). Sibling similarities in number of ossification centers of the hand and wrist in a malnourished population. *Hum Biol, 50*: 73–81.

McKern, T. W. (1957). Estimation of skeletal age from combined maturational activity. *Am J Phys Anthropol, 15*: 399–408.

_____ (1970). Estimation of skeletal age: From puberty to about 30 years of age. In: *Personal Identification in Mass Disasters.* T. D. Stewart, Ed. Smithsonian Institution, Wash. D.C., pp. 41–56.

McKern, T. W. and T. D. Stewart (1957). *Skeletal Age Changes in Young, Analyzed from the Standpoint of Identification.* Headqu. Q. M. Dev. Command., Tech. Rep. EP-45, Natick, Mass.

Modi, J. P. (1957). *Medical Jurisprudence and Toxicology.* Tripathi Private, Ltd., Bombay.

Paterson, R. S. 1929 A radiological investigation of the epiphyses of the long bones. *J Anat, 64*: 28–46.

Roche, A. F., J. Roberts and P. V. V. Hamill (1978). *Skeletal Maturity of Youths 12–17 Years: Racial, Geographic Area, and Socioeconomic Differentials.* Vital and Health Statistics, Series 11, No. 167. DHEW Publication No. (PHS) 79-1654. National Center for Health Statistics, Hyattsville, Maryland.

Stevenson, P. H. (1924) Age order of epiphyseal union in man. *Am J Phys Anthropol, 7*:53–93.

Stewart, T. D. (1979). *Essentials of Forensic Anthropology.* Charles C Thomas, Springfield, Ill.

Suchey, J. M. (1979). Problems in the aging of females using the *Os pubis. Am J Phys Anthropol, 51*: 467–470.

Todd, T. W. (1930). The anatomical features of epiphyseal union. *Child Develop, 1*: 186–194.

Trotter, M., and G. C. Gleser (1952). Estimation of stature from long bones of American whites and Negroes. *Am J Phys Anthropol, 10*: 463–514.

Chapter 19

THE OKLAHOMA CITY CHILD DISAPPEARANCES OF 1967
Forensic Anthropology in the
Identification of Skeletal Remains*

CLYDE C. SNOW AND JAMES L. LUKE

In the summer of 1967, two children disappeared from the Oklahoma City area. The first was a five year old girl reported missing on the evening of Thursday, July 6. She was last seen playing near her home late in the afternoon. When she had not returned for supper, a search of the neighborhood was conducted by her family and friends. She was not located, and the police were notified. In the following weeks an intensive search was undertaken by local and state authorities. One of her sneakers, found in a vacant lot near her home, was the only clue recovered.

The second disappearance occurred on the afternoon of Thursday, August 3, exactly four weeks after the first. The missing child was a six year old girl from a suburban municipality several miles south of Oklahoma City. Like the first child, she disappeared in the late afternoon. That evening her bicycle was found in an alley behind a neighborhood grocery. Later, one of her playmates reported that he saw her in an automobile on the evening of her disappearance. He stated the driver was a dark complexioned young man with light blond hair. He did not remember the make or model of the car, and he did not recognize the driver.

Again, the efforts of a massive search were without result. The families of the girls were not related; their homes were several miles apart. Despite the

*Copyright, American Society for Testing and Materials, 1916 Race Street, Philadelphia, PA 19103. Reprinted/Adapted, with permission. *Journal of Forensic Sciences*, 1970, *15(2)*:125–153.

The authors are deeply grateful for advice and assistance from personnel of the three agencies involved in the investigation of this case: the Midwest City Police Department, the Oklahoma City Police Department, and the Oklahoma Bureau of Investigation. Each agency made its files and records pertaining to the disappearances freely available to the authors. In particular, Captain J. W. Forney, Midwest City Police, contributed generously by answering many questions concerning the background of the cases, cross-checking details, and also undertook the tedious job of reviewing the final manuscript.

Throughout the study, physicians, dentists, and teachers of the two missing girls cooperated generously in supplying background information. Dr. Robert Gaylord, Department of Orthodontics, Baylor Dental College, independently reviewed the dental evidence on which the identification was based and contributed many useful comments and suggestions.

coincidences in timing and the general similarity of circumstances, police discovered no evidence linking the two disappearances.

Throughout the remainder of this paper the first girl will be referred to by the pseudonym "Anna" and the second as "Barbara."

DISCOVERY

On November 19, 1967, approximately four and one-half months after Anna's disappearance, two quail hunters found some bones on an abandoned farm on the southeastern outskirts of Oklahoma City. Among them was a cranium, and while the hunters were not certain it was human, their curiosity was sufficiently aroused for them to take it home with them. At home, after comparing it with illustrations of human skulls in an encyclopedia, they recognized the importance of their find. The next day they notified law enforcement officers and led them to the site.

Upon arriving at the scene, the investigators searched the immediate area and found several more bones, mostly fragmented ribs and vertebrae, and a child's dress. These remains lay scattered in a thicket of underbrush about 150 feet south of the vacant farmhouse. In the sandy soil at the center of the thicket was a shallow depression. Upon excavation it yielded more bones, a tangled mass of hair, and a badly deteriorated piece of child's underwear. This grave was approximately 3 feet long, 2 feet wide, and only 1½ feet deep. Its depth was limited by an undisturbed layer of hard red clay that underlies the sandy topsoil of the area. Penetration of this clay would have required a pick or shovel and much effort. It appeared that whoever dug the grave had neither tools nor time to make it deeper.

IDENTIFICATION OF CHILD'S SKELETAL REMAINS

The soil of the grave was sifted through a ⅜-inch mesh screen in an attempt to recover fragments overlooked during excavation. Darkness precluded further search that evening.

The next morning officers reassembled at the scene, and a systematic search was conducted with the aid of approximately fifty volunteers from a nearby military base. The area surrounding the grave was marked off in rectangular plots measuring approximately 200 by 1,000 feet. Each plot was covered separately by aligning the searchers, equipped with rakes and probes, at one end of the rectangle and having them advance in line, carefully raking the thick clumps of prairie grass as they proceeded. Upon finding any sign of soil disturbance, a bone, or other unusual object, the line was halted until the find could be recorded. All bones and other items recovered were placed in plastic bags with tags indicating the location of the find. In this manner, approximately 100 acres were covered in a three-day effort.

After the surface search was complete, a small grader was used to skim the surface vegetation from a 40 by 40 yard area around the grave. The resulting piles of loose grass and weeds were inspected and areas of discoloration or soil disturbance noted. Test pits were sunk in such spots to see if they might mark the location of another grave.

Meanwhile, smaller parties were sent farther afield to examine ditches, culverts, creekbeds, outbuildings, wells, and other likely spots where bones might have been concealed by humans or deposited by animals. Local game conservation officials and farmers familiar with the location of the dens of badgers, coyotes, and other "varmints" of the region helped locate and search lairs within 2 to 3 miles of the grave.

The result of this effort was a collection of several hundred bones ranging in origin from field mouse to horse. Among them were found four additional human bones: two ribs, a left fibula, and a right femur. While the result of this massive search was meager, it eliminated the possibility of the area concealing more human remains or another grave.

From the start, it appeared most likely that the bones were those of Barbara. Not only was the grave located several miles closer to her home than to Anna's, but Barbara's mother also recognized the recovered hair and dress as those of her daughter. However, several considerations dictated the necessity of further osteological examination. First, of course, was the possibility that the bones might reveal some clue to the cause of death. Second, there was the remote but lingering chance that the recovered assemblage included the commingled remains of both missing girls. Finally, since positive identification would be a vital issue in any subsequent legal proceeding, it was imperative to collect all evidence to support or deny the preliminary assumption that the bones belonged to Barbara.

Description of Remains

In all, about one-third of a human skeleton was recovered. The most important find was the nearly intact cranium; the mandible was not found. The trunk was represented by several cervical and thoracic vertebrae, both clavicles, and almost all the ribs, but no lumbar vertebrae or pelvic bones. Each limb was represented by at least one long bone, but with the exception of two phalanges, the smaller bones of the hands and feet were missing. Thus, all the major body regions were represented skeletally except the lower trunk.

CRANIUM: (Fig. 19-1) The color of the cranium varied from rich grey cream on the left side to a darkly stained rusty brown on the right. No soft tissue residues were found on the exterior or within the cranial cavities, nor were any putrefactive odors noted. Spider webs were present in the cranial and nasal cavities. When cleaned, the cranial cavity yielded approximately 20 gm of dry debris consisting of loose sand, small seeds and other vegetable matter, egg and pupae cases, and the remains of adult insects.

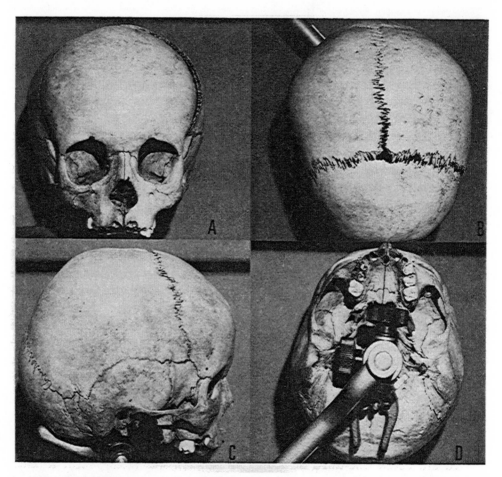

Figure 19-1. Cranium in (A) frontal, (B) superior, (C) right lateral and (D) basilar views.

In the frontal view, the cranium displayed the childhood configuration of a relatively large brain case and small facial skeleton. The orbits were rather square in outline, and the nasal aperture was of moderate breadth. Viewed laterally, the facial profile was orthognathous with a straight, well-developed nasal bridge. The frontal portion of sagittal contour was steep and bulged anteriorly. There was a pronounced disconformity in the posterior sagittal contour, with the squamous portion of the occipital contour being more strongly curved than the parietals, giving the occiput a somewhat "bun-shaped" appearance. From the posterior aspect, the cranium was tapeinocranic in contour with the axis of maximum breadth located high on the vault and passing through the well-developed parietal eminences. Measurements of the cranium are given in Table 19-I.

TABLE 19-I
MEASUREMENTS OF THE CRANIUM

Measurement	mm.	Measurement	mm.
Cranial length	167	Upper face height	51
Cranial breadth	145	Nasal height	39
Biauricular height	117	Nasal aperture height	23
Basion-vertex	131	Nasal aperture breadth	20
Biporion breadth	91	Orbital height	30
Bizygomatic breadth	109	Orbital breadth	32
Minimum frontal diameter	93	Basion-prosthion length	82
Interorbital breadth	22	Palate length	39
Biorbital breadth	93	Foramen magnum length	30
Bimaxillary breadth	52	Foramen magnum breadth	27

The four parts of the occipital bone were united without any persistent traces of union. The metopic suture was closed except for a 4-mm segment immediately superior to its juncture with the nasofrontal suture. The remaining facial and cranial sutures were patent.

The texture of the bone was sound and its surface smooth and glossy. There were no signs of chronic disease or poor nutrition. Anomalies were limited to a 4-by-8-mm intersutural bone in the right pars asterica of the lambdoid suture and transversely divided occipital condyles.

The coronal and sagittal sutures were widely separated. At bregma, the coronal separation measured 6 mm; it was more pronounced on the left side of the cranium. The sagittal separation measured 4 mm at bregma but diminished posteriorly so that in the region of the parietal foramina opposition appeared normal. There was also separation to a lesser degree of the left squamous suture with the parietal displaced about 3 mm superiorly. When viewed anteriorly, the inner table of the parietal was about the same level as the outer table of the frontal. That this was due to outward displacement of the parietal rather than depression of the frontal is shown by the normal sutural relationships between the latter and the other facial and cranial bones adjoining it. There were no fractures or other signs of trauma of the cranial vault.

The right lacrimal bone was missing; the delicate margins of the orbital bones surrounding it were intact. A 5-by-12-mm portion of bone was missing from the buccal surface of the right maxillary alveolus opposite the positions of the missing deciduous molars (dm^1, dm^2).

DENTITION: The maxilla retained four fully erupted teeth (Fig. 19-2): both left deciduous molars (dm^1, dm^2) and, bilaterally, the permanent first molars (M^1). The incisors, canines, and right deciduous molars were missing. The crowns of the unerupted lateral incisors (I^2) were visible in their sockets. The loss of the right deciduous molars exposed the crowns of the underlying permanent premolars (PM^1, PM^2).

The following descriptions are based on examination of the specimen and a dental cast. Table 19-II gives measurements (taken from the specimen) of the four erupted teeth.

Deciduous Dentention

1. *Central incisors* (di^1): Replaced bilaterally by permanents.
2. *Lateral incisors* (di^2): Missing bilaterally. Labial walls of sockets still present. Most probably present at death and lost postmortem, but possibly shed a few days or weeks premortem.
3. *Canines* (dc): Missing bilaterally but marked by deep, well-formed sockets with no signs of resorption.
4. *First molars* (dm^1):
Left: Small outgrowth of enamel on mesiobuccal surface.
Right: Circummortem loss. Mesiolingual wall of socket intact, buccodistal wall missing.
5. *Second molars* (dm^2):
Left: Carious defect of mesio-occlusal aspect. Slight Carabelli's cusp.
Right: Missing. Buccal wall of socket missing.

Permanent Dentition

1. *Central incisors* (I^1): Postmortem loss. Deep, well-formed sockets indicated that these teeth were erupted at time of death.
2. *Lateral incisors* (I^2): Unerupted. Incisal edges within 1 mm of alveolar margin. Not shovel shaped. Left strongly rotated distolingually.
3. *Canines* (C^1): Unerupted.
4. *First premolars* (PM^1): Unerupted crown of right exposed due to loss of dm^1. It lay within 2 mm of alveolar margin and was fractured in its mesiodistal plane.
5. *Second premolars* (PM^2): Unerupted. Crown of right exposed owing to loss of dm^2. Occlusal surface of crown within 4 mm of alveolar margin.
6. *First molars* (M^1): Fully erupted bilaterally. Both displayed the normal 4-cusped crown pattern. On the left tooth was a weakly developed Carabelli's cusp; on the right, the Carabelli's trait was expressed as a slight groove.

Radiographic examination: Radiographs of the dentition allowed the visualization of the unerupted permanent teeth. From the x-rays, crown and root development was rated on Nolla's 1959 10-point scale (Moyers, 1958). These ratings, useful in estimating the individual's age, are given in a subsequent section of this chapter.

Vertebrae: Six cervical and four thoracic vertebrae were recovered. Although parts of some of them were missing, the cervical elements could be articulated to form a normal series from C1 (atlas) to C6. The seventh cervical (which has distinguishing features by which it can be recognized) was not recovered. The only completely intact thoracic vertebra was T1, which could be recognized by its reniform body and complete articu-

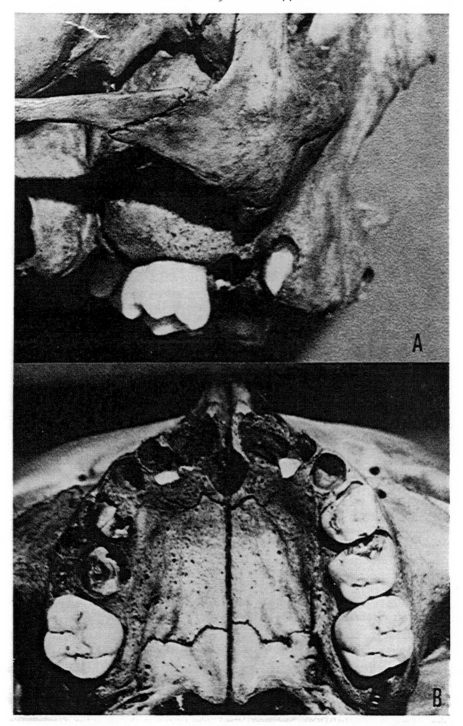

Figure 19-2. Dentition (A) right lateral view of maxilia showing defect of alveolar marginı (B) occlusal view of palate.

lar facet. The bodies of the other three thoracic vertebrae were missing, but judging from the size and other features of their arches, the fragments appeared to belong to the uppermost elements of the thoracic series. No sign of disease or anomaly was noted on any of the vertebrae. The ossification centers of the atlas and axis were completely united except for the odontoid epiphysis of the axis. The neurocentral joint of T1 was closed, but the line of union was still visible.

Ribs and clavicles: Ten right and nine left ribs were recovered. The assemblage included one lumbar rib from each side of the body; the remainder were thoracic. The first ribs were missing; the second ribs, which could be identified by well-developed scalene tubercles, were present. Six of the nineteen ribs had one or both ends missing. No anomalies were noted.

Both clavicles were found. The left, which was intact except for its missing epiphysis, was 9.4 cm long. The ends of the right clavicle were missing.

Left humerus: Both extremities of this bone were missing, leaving a midshaft of 15.8 cm.

Right radius: The proximal end of this bone was intact except for the missing epiphysis; the distal end was missing. The fragment was 12.8 cm long.

Right femur: A 25.3-cm femoral fragment was recovered. The proximal end was intact except for the three missing epiphyses; the distal end had been destroyed by animals.

Fibulae: The ends of both were missing. The right fragment was 19.0 cm long, the left 14.6 cm.

Phalanges: Two hand phalanges were recovered. They were not classifiable according to side of body. The proximal epiphyses of both were missing.

TABLE 19-II
MEASUREMENTS OF TEETH

Tooth	Buccolingual Diameter mm.	Mesiodistal Diameter mm.
Left dm^1	8.6	6.8
Left dm^2	9.9	8.5
Left M^1	11.2	11.2
Right M^1	11.8	11.7

Time of Death

None of the bones displayed the weathering cracks of the cortical surface that, in cold climates, appear during a single winter's exposure (Tappen, 1969). Although many bones had been damaged by carnivores, the delicate gnaw marks produced by wild rodents were not present. These latter animals, while occasionally feeding on carrion, are more apt to attack well-skeletonized remains, which serve them as a rich source of dietary mineral and protein. In our experience, it is rare to find bone exposed for a year or more that has not received their attention. Supporting these observations were other signs that the bones were recent. The cranium, for example, retained many of the more delicate structural details that are almost invariably lost with long exposure. The long bones had the "greasy" texture and splotchy brown discoloration indicative of fat retention. Taken together, the evidence indicated that the burial had occurred no earlier than the previous spring.

That several vertebrae and ribs, as well as the entire scalp, remained in the grave when the major portion of the skeleton was removed by scavengers suggested that decomposition was advanced when the grave was disturbed. From this a minimal time of burial of about two weeks was postulated. Once exposed, skeletonization can occur rapidly in Oklahoma's summer climate. For instance, Brues (1958) cites a local case in which a 300-lb. man was reduced to a skeleton and a few shreds of soft tissue during a month of warm weather. In the same year that the two girls disappeared, we examined the skeletonized bodies of two adult homicide victims. The first, a female, was strangled in late March and her body found 120 days later. The second was a male killed by gunshot in early July and discovered 47 days later. Both had lain exposed at sites similar in terrain and vegetation to that where the child's skeleton was found. Both retained about 12 lb. of soft tissue. Calculated from the known premortem body weights of the two victims, the overall rates of soft tissue disappearance were found to be 0.9 lb per day for the female and 2.9 lb per day for the male. The lower rate in the female can be attributed to slower decomposition during the cooler spring months. Applied to the 40-to-50-lb. body of a child, these rates would produce skeletonization within two to six weeks of summer exposure. The old spider webs and signs of insects within the otherwise empty cranium indicated that it was probably well skeletonized before the cold weather inhibited the activities of these animals. In sum, the findings suggested that the burial had occurred no later than early September. The evidence of summer burial, while of itself not finely drawn enough to determine which victim was involved, was consistent with the disappearance times of the two girls and thus helped rule out the possibility of the bones belonging to an unknown third child.

Four days after Barbara disappeared, police, in their search for her, visited the abandoned farm on which the grave was later located. One officer later recalled that he passed within 15 to 20 feet of the grave site and noticed nothing unusual. Had the grave been Anna's, who disappeared and was presumably buried about one month earlier, it is likely that it would have been opened and the remains scattered by the time of the police officer's inspection and he would have discovered them. If the grave was Barbara's it is probable that it was still undisturbed at this time and much easier to overlook. This finding gave further tenuous support to the hypothesis that the bones belonged to Barbara.

Manner of Death

The partial skeleton raised the possibility that the victim was dismembered and some of the parts deposited elsewhere. In such cases, the head and limbs are usually amputated and the torso left intact. Here such a pattern was not apparent: Parts of all the limbs, the head and upper torso were found and only the lower trunk was totally unrepresented. Carnivore activity offers a more likely explanation, since these animals are more apt to carry away the fleshy parts of a body and leave behind the more bony portions (Brues, 1958). These proclivities would account for the concentration of cranium, ribs, and vertebrae in and around the grave and the wider scattering or complete disappearance of the pelvic elements and many of the long bones.

In a child, a blow to the head often results in a separation of the cranial bones along the suture line instead of a fracture. In such cases, the impacted bone will be depressed and its outer table somewhat below the general plane of the cranial surface. While the cranium did display some vertical as well as horizontal separation of the coronal and sagittal sutures, the vertical component was due to an elevation of the left parietal rather than to a depression of the adjacent bones (Fig. 19-1A). The left side of the skull was considerably more bleached than the right—an indication that it had rested on its right side for a considerable period. In this position, the left parietal would be directly exposed to the sun. The heat and drying effects on the thin, fresh bone would cause it to warp and force open its sutural connections. Thus, postmortem warping rather than circummortem trauma accounts for the sutural separation observed in the cranium.

The loss of the lacrimal bone may also be ascribed to postmortem change. While this bone is delicate and easily broken, trauma to it almost invariably results in damage to the equally fragile surrounding bones of the orbital wall. On the other hand, it is often loosened and detached when a skull is cleaned and dried in laboratory preparations, and such losses are also frequently seen in otherwise well-preserved archaeological specimens. As in such cases, the margins of the surrounding bones were still intact.

Likewise, the loss of the anterior maxillary dentition (incisors and canines) could be attributed to postmortem change. These single-rooted teeth are easily lost with the decomposition of connective tissues binding them to their sockets, and it is rare to find an exposed skull in which at least some are not missing. In contrast, the loss of the multirooted right deciduous molars was more unusual and may have been associated with the bone damage to the alveolar ridge. The fractured crown (Fig. 19-2B) of the underlying permanent first premolar was also interesting, since, still deep in its socket and well protected by surrounding bone, considerable force would be required to cause such a fracture. While such trauma might be consistent with a facial blow delivered around the time of death, the possibility of postmortem damage by animals could not be ruled out. In summary, all damage observed in the recovered remains could be attributed to postmortem change— there was no bony evidence suggesting violence or other cause of death.

Commingling

Had there been duplications among the bones recovered, it would have been immediately evident that two skeletons were represented. However, it is possible that such an assemblage, through chance, might not include duplicate bones. If such were the case, commingling might pass undetected, since the two missing girls were similar enough in age and body size that their bones might not be distinguishable. For example, even if the cranium were proven to belong to Barbara, how could it be certain that one of the fibular fragments did not belong to Anna? This question was important, since the general similarity of the disappearances indicated that the two cases were connected.

To help rule out commingling, a mathematical approach was devised; the method has been treated in more detail in another paper (Snow and Folk, 1970). Essentially, it consists of making the null hypothesis that two skeletons are indeed involved and accepting or rejecting this hypothesis by determining the probability of not finding duplicate bones among the recovered remains. This probability can be calculated by the use of the following formula:

$$p = \frac{2^s \binom{S}{s}}{\binom{2S}{s}} \qquad \text{where}$$

S = the total number of bones that can, in isolation, be recognized and precisely classified as to their exact location in the skeleton.

s = number of bones in category S that are found in the recovered collection.

p = probability of commingling.

Of the 200-odd bones of the human skeleton, many are so small and delicate that they are often destroyed or lost during exposure. Others, such as most of the ribs, vertebrae, and phalanges, are serially homologous and can be precisely identified only if all (or nearly all) of their homologues are recovered. Others, e.g. the carpals, are not always distinguishable in their immature state. A review of the normal skeleton of a six year old reveals that there are only about forty-six elements both large and rugged enough to be recovered, and if recovered, precisely classifiable as to body location. Of these forty-six bones, twenty-two were represented in the assembled collection. In addition, a complete series of cervical vertebrae except C7 was found. Therefore, the four lower cervical vertebrae, C3, C4, C5, and C6, could be included, since the recovery of another midcervical vertebrae would indicate commingling. These additions raised S to 50 and s to 26. Substituting into the formula:

$$p = \frac{2^{26}\binom{50}{26}}{\binom{2.50}{26}}$$

$$p = .012$$

Because the odds were about 100 to one against it, the hypothesis of commingling was rejected.

Sex and Race

Since both missing children were white girls, any skeletal evidence of sex and race could only be used further to rule out an unreported third victim. Actually, the skeleton offered little positive evidence of either attribute. The most successful methods of sexing immature remains depend either on the recovery of a nearly complete skeleton and dentition (Hunt, 1955) or an intact pelvis (Reynolds, 1947)—neither condition being met in this case. Therefore, the assumption that the remains were female rested largely upon the long hair, dress, and girl's undergarment found with the bones.

Carabelli's cusp, an anomalous cuspule of the mesiolingual surface of the maxillary incisors, occurs in about 50 percent of Caucasians in the United States, 34 percent of Negroes, but only 5 to 20 percent of American Indians (Lasker, 1957; Kraus, 1959). Conversely, shovel-shaped incisors—so named because their lingual margins are raised, giving them the appearance of miniature scoops (Hrdlicka, 1920)—are found in 80 to 100 percent of American Indians (Lasker, 1950; Dahlberg, 1951) but usually in less than 10 percent of Caucasians and Negroes (Moorrees, 1957 and Carbonell, 1963).

The left first permanent molar of the specimen displayed a slightly developed Carabelli's cusp, and a dissection of the alveolar wall to expose the lingual surfaces of the unerupted lateral incisors revealed that they were not shovel shaped. Taken together, these findings tended to rule out American Indian ancestry—an important point in Oklahoma with its large Indian population. Again, however, the hair provided the best evidence of Caucasian racial affinity: It was slightly wavy, lightly pigmented, and of small diameter.

Age

While the skeleton was obviously that of a child, it was necessary to establish its age as precisely as possible to help rule out an unknown third individual and, it was hoped, to exclude one or another of the missing girls. Because of the many genetic and environmental variables influencing growth, estimates of developmental age, based on osseous and dental characters, seldom coincide with chronological age. For this reason, age assessments of unknown skeletons are best developed as age ranges rather than as point estimates of age (Stewart, 1954; Krogman, 1962).

In the cranium the occipital bone, which consists of four separate elements at birth, was solidly fused into a single unit with no persisting traces of union. Occipital union generally occurs at 4 to 5 years of age. Three long bone fragments—the proximal femur, proximal radius, and distal humerus—displayed open epiphyseal surfaces. Union of epiphyses at these sites generally occurs around the middle of the second decade. Thus occipital union and epiphyseal closure provided an immediate "outside" age range of about 4 to 15 years.

The anterior arch of the atlas vertebra (C1) had fused—an event usually occurring by 5 to 6 years (Girdany, 1952). The fusion of the neurocentral joint of the first thoracic vertebra also indicated an age of about the sixth year (Stewart, 1954). The apical epiphysis of the odontoid process of the axis (C1) had not fused to the main body, indicating an age of under 12 years (Todd, 1926). Taken in sum, the vertebral traits further narrowed the estimated age range to about 5 to 12 years.

Both first permanent molars (M^1) had erupted. In Caucasian girls in the United States this tooth erupts at a mean age of 6.22 years and a range, based on two standard deviations from the mean, extends from 4.65 to 7.79 years (Hurme, 1948, 1957). The latter statistics refer to "clinical" eruption—the age at which the crown pierces the gum. After clinical eruption, an additional 3 to 12 months is required for the teeth to reach the occlusal plane (Miles, 1963). Since the teeth of the specimen were fully erupted, a minimum of 3 months (0.25 year) was added to the above data to give a range of 4.90 to 8.04 years. While this agrees with the lower limit of the bone-based range, it reduced the 12-year upper limit substantially.

Although the permanent central incisors were missing, from their deep and well-formed sockets (Gron, 1962) it was obvious that they had erupted prior to death. The mean eruption age of I^1 in Caucasian girls in the United States is 7.20 years with a = 2 S.D. range of 5.61 to 8.79 years (Hurme, 1948, 1957). This allows an upward revision of the lower age limit to give a more constricted range of 5.61 to 8.04 years. Since both limits are based on = 2 S.D. values, we can be about 95 percent confident that the true age of the skeleton would fall within this range.

Another approach to the derivation of age from the dentition involves the maturation of the permanent teeth through the use of radiographs. From the time it first appears in a cystlike crypt of bone until it is fully formed, each tooth passes through a number of well-defined growth stages. Essentially, a tooth grows from the top down: First the crown appears and calcifies, then this is followed by the gradual elongation of the root. In age determination from children's skeletal remains, estimates based on tooth development have an advantage over those based on eruption because all of the teeth, erupted or unerupted, can be examined (Moorrees, 1963) and also because the maturation sequence displays somewhat less variability than that observed in dental eruption (Stewart, 1963; Garn, 1959; and Lewis & Garn, 1960).

In this case, the method devised by Nolla (1959) was used. This entails assigning each tooth a score of 0 to 10 based on crypt development, crown calcification, and root development as revealed by radiographs. These individual ratings are then compared to age standards based on Nolla's longitudinal study of Caucasian girls in the United States. The results are shown graphically in Figure 18-4. No crypt could be visualized for a third molar (M^3), giving it a score of 0. According to Nolla's tables, initial calcification of M^3 generally does not begin until the eighth year. Therefore, on the basis of this tooth alone an age less than eight years would be assigned. The ratings of the remaining teeth fell between 6.3 and 8.3 years on the chronological scale. The total of the average scores for the right and left teeth was 42.25, a little higher than Nolla's average of 41.2 for seven year olds. Interpolated into Nolla's tables, the specimen's score of 42.2 gave an age of 7.15 years.

Calculated to the dates of their disappearances, Anna was 5.77 years old and Barbara 6.71 years. Figure 19-4 shows the ranges of the skeletal and dental estimates compared to the chronological ages of the two girls. Both fell within the estimated ranges but with Barbara near the midpoint and Anna rather close to the lower limits. The weight of evidence, while not ruling out Anna entirely, favored the hypothesis that the bones belonged to Barbara.

Since eruption ages of the permanent teeth tend to be normally distributed (Hurme, 1948), calculation of the standardized deviate (z) affords more precise estimates of the probabilities of either Barbara or Anna displaying an eruption pattern similar to that of the specimen. This statistic is obtained

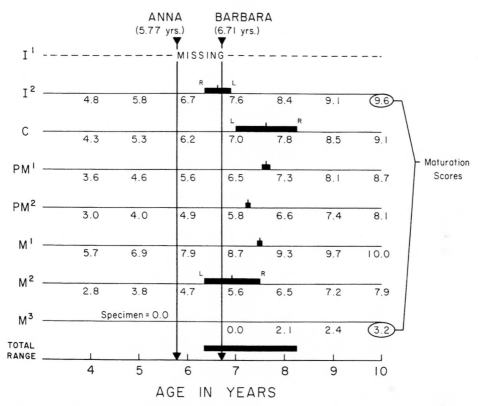

Figure 19-3. Age estimates based on tooth maturation (Nolla, 1959). Black bars indicate age span between right and left teeth of a given class.

by dividing the difference between the chronological age of the child and the mean eruption age of a given tooth by its standard deviation. From this value the probability of the child having erupted the tooth at a given age can be derived from normal curve-area tables. These relationships are shown in Figure 19-5, using the permanent central incisors as an example. Table 19-III gives the z score and their probabilities for M^1, I^1, and I^2 as calculated form the ages of the two girls at the time they disappeared. For the lateral incisors (I^2) the probabilities are remote that either girl would have erupted these teeth at the time they disappeared; had they been erupted on the specimen, serious consideration would have to be given to the possibility that it belonged to an older individual. The probabilities for the permanent molars indicate that these teeth have erupted in about 3 out of 10 girls as young as Anna. In contrast, eruption would have occurred in about 7 out of 10 girls by the time they reached Barbara's age. The most striking differences are noted in the central incisors (I^1) for which the data show that these

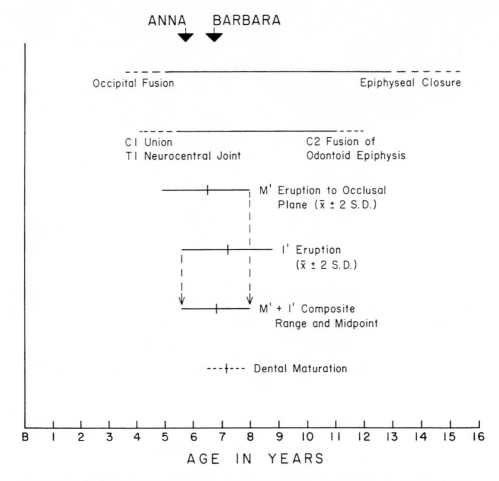

Figure 19-4. Estimated age ranges of the remains based on various osseous and dental traits.

teeth would be clinically erupted in only about four out of 100 girls of Anna's age. It will be noted that for Barbara also, this tooth would be somewhat premature (p=.27), but as will be seen below, this would not be unexpected, since she also seemed to be rather advanced for her age in general body growth.

Stature

Since long bone lengths are proportional to stature, they may be used to estimate an individual's height from his skeletal remains. Sex, race, and age influence this relationship, and many prediction formulae have been devised for males and females of various racial groups. These formulae are generally based on measurements of intact bones, and in this case the

TABLE 19-III
PROBABILITIES OF ERUPTION (*P*)
(BASED ON STANDARDIZED DEVIATES) OF THREE PERMANENT TEETH
PRIOR TO THE AGES OF ANNA (5.77 YEARS) AND BARBARA (6.77)
AT THE TIME OF THEIR DISAPPEARANCE

Teeth	Eruption Age (19) Mean	S.D.	Mean Age	−	Observed Age	Standardized Deviate (z)	p
	(Years)				(Years)		
M^1	6.22	0.80	Anna		0.45	0.562	.29
			Barbara		0.49	−0.612	.73
I^1	7.20	0.81	Anna		1.43	1.765	.04
			Barbara		0.49	0.605	.27
I^2	8.20	0.98	Anna		2.43	2.480	.01
			Barbara		1.49	1.520	.06

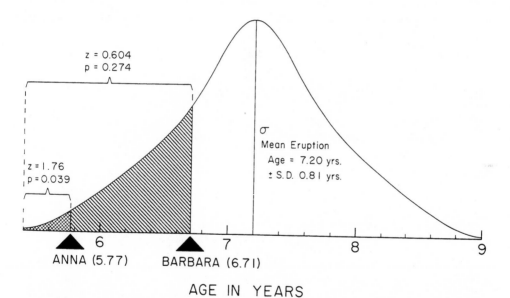

Figure 19-5. Distribution of eruption ages of permanent maxillary central incisors (Hurme, 1948) in Caucasian girls in U.S. with standardized deviates (z) and probabilities (p) of the two missing girls displaying I^2 eruption at their ages at the time of disappearance.

scavengers had left only two, the right femur and left humerus, reasonably undamaged.

Selecting these for study, the following steps were employed in deriving identification evidence based on stature:

1. Using the undamaged landmarks as reference points, estimates of the original lengths of the femur and humerus were derived.

2. Based on the above, statural estimates of the individual were calculated using several methods.

3. From various sources, statural estimates of the two missing girls were obtained and compared to those for the skeleton.

STATURE FROM DIAPHYSEAL LENGTH OF FEMUR: Using data from Stewart (1948), Olivier, (1969) relates the length of the femoral diaphysis to stature. In the recovered specimen, the proximal end of the femur was intact, except for the three missing epiphyses. The distal end had been destroyed, but its damaged margin lay well below the point where the femoral shaft flares out to form the broad distal condyles. It could then be inferred that the original diaphyseal margin was located only a centimeter or two beyond the broken edge of the specimen. Therefore, the total length of the fragment, 25.3 cm, could be considered a "short" approximation of true diaphyseal length. From Olivier's (1969) table, this estimate corresponds to a statural range of 49.2 to 51.3 inches.

STATURE FROM FEMORAL LENGTH: To estimate the maximal length of the femur with its epiphysis still intact, the following procedure was employed:

1. The femoral fragment was placed in a dioptograph, and a full-scale tracing was made with the bone oriented in its frontal plane.

2. The fragment was removed from the dioptograph and replaced with a femur of a normal adult white female selected randomly from a laboratory collection. The tracing of the fragment was kept in place.

3. With the adult femur oriented in the frontal plane, the platform of the dioptograph was lowered until its landmarks corresponded as closely as possible to those noted on the tracing of the specimen.

4. The adult femur was traced, superimposing its outline on that of the specimen.

Such a reconstruction is admittedly approximate, since it fails to take into account the individual variation in both the specimen and the reference femur and also ignores proportional changes that may occur during normal growth.

The maximal femur length (measured from the tracing) of 29.6 cm was substituted into the Trotter-Gleser formula for estimating stature of Caucasian females in the United States (Trotter & Gleser, 1952).

$$\text{Stature (cm)} = 2.47 \, (\text{femoral length, max.}) + 54.10$$
$$= 2.47 \, (29.6) + 54.10$$
$$= 127.2 \text{ cm} = 3.72 \text{ cm S.E. or}$$
$$\text{Stature (in.)} = 50.1 \text{ inches} = 1.46'' \text{ S.E.}$$

The regression formula used above was derived from data on adults, and the confidence with which it may be applied to children is not presently known (Trotter, 1969). As a partial check, a second estimate of stature from femur length was based on female data from the Brush Foundation growth study of American Caucasian children of North European ancestry (Simmons, 1944). Although femur length was not measured in the Brush study, it could indirectly be derived by taking the difference between two measurements, symphyseal height and knee height. Both were taken with the subject standing; the first is the vertical distance between the superior margin of the pubic symphysis (symphysion) to the floor and the second the distance between the mediosuperior margin of the tibia (tibiale) to the floor. The difference between the two is thus a measure of the upper segment of the limb, which we will refer to as "thigh length."

To relate thigh length to femur length, a standing AP radiograph was taken of the lower pelvis and femur of a normal 5.44-year-old girl. Two measurements were taken from this child's x-ray:

1. thigh length—symphysion to tibiale, 30.2 cm
2. maximum femur length—distance between femoral head and most distal point of the condyles, 31.3 cm

Assuming the relative difference between the two measurements to be constant, the mean thigh lengths of the Brush study girls were converted to estimates of femur length, as follows:

$$\text{femur length} = \frac{(31.3)}{(30.2)} = \text{thigh length}$$

The estimated femur length means were then plotted against the statural means for Brush study girls between 2 and 16 years of age. Since this relationship was highly linear, a least-square regression equation for estimating stature from femur length was calculated:

$$
\begin{aligned}
\text{Stature (cm.)} &= 3.113 \,(\text{femur length, cm}) + 35.11 \\
&= 3.113 \,(29.6) + 35.11 \\
&= 127.25 \text{ cm} \\
&= 50.1''
\end{aligned}
$$

Considering the many sources of error involved in each calculation, the exact agreement of the two estimates must be considered fortuitous. More important is that they both give a result in the neighborhood of 50 inches.

STATURAL ESTIMATE FROM HUMERUS: The left humerus of the recovered skeleton was missing its proximal end; distally, it was less damaged, and the upper portion of the olecranon fossa was intact. This latter finding was fortunate, since it provided the lower landmark that can be used to estimate the total length of the humerus from the incomplete bone. The upper landmark is taken as the apex of an inverted triangle of roughened bone formed by muscle attachments on the posterior surface of the bone (Krogman, 1962). On the intact humerus this point is located just inferior to the greater tubercle. In a series of 100 adult humeri, Müller (1935) found that the distance between this point and the upper margin of the olecranon fossa averaged 69.62 percent of the total length of the bone. On the specimen, the upper landmark could not be discerned, so it could be assumed that the level of the damaged margin occurred at some point below it. Measured from the lower landmark to the superiormost point of undamaged cortical bone on the posterior surface, the length of the fragment was found to be 13.8 cm. This distance therefore may be taken as a minimum measure of the distance between the two landmarks used by Müller if it is assumed that the break occurred at the tip of the apex of muscle attachment. Using the percentage relationship given by Müller, a length of 13.8 cm gives a total humeral length of 19.8 cm. Substituting this into Trotter and Gleser's formula (Trotter & Gleser, 1952) for statural estimate from humerus length of white females:

$$\text{Stature (cm.)} = 3.36 \, (\text{humerus length}) + 57.97$$
$$= 3.36 \, (19.8) + 57.97$$
$$= 124.50 \text{ cm} = 4.45 \text{ cm S.E.}$$

or 49.01 inches with a range based on $= 2$ standard errors of 45.51 to 52.52 inches.

Family members, teachers, and friends of the two girls generally described Barbara as tall for her age and Anna as short. In the description given to the police, Barbara's mother estimated her daughter's stature at 51 inches. Anna's mother gave her daughter's stature at 42 inches. The reliability of these estimates could be confirmed to some extent by comparing them with data on normal children to see if the girls fell within the expected statural ranges of their age groups. As a reference, the statural means and standard deviations for Caucasian females in the United States (Stoudt, Damon, & McFarland, 1960) were used. The estimates for both girls were found to fall within the limits of two standard deviations of the mean — a range that includes about 95 percent of normal girls. For Anna, a stature of 42 inches at her age (5.77 years) would be considered within normal limits, but she would still be noticeably shorter than her age peers. Barbara, on the other hand, at 51 inches would be considered tall, but not abnormally so, for her age of 6.71 years (Fig. 19-6).

From the time she was approximately six months old, Anna was routinely examined by her family pediatrician. On four such occasions her stature was recorded. The results further confirm the shorter-than-normal estimate of her stature, since throughout her life she had maintained a growth rate rather close to the lower limits of normal. In fact, the 42 inch estimate would lie remarkably close to the height predicted from her previous measurements.

In Figure 19-7 the statural estimates of the two girls and those based on the skeleton are shown. Barbara's stature of 51 inches falls within the range of all four skeletal estimates; Anna's stature of 42 inches, well below them. Only if her true height was underestimated by approximately 3.5 inches would

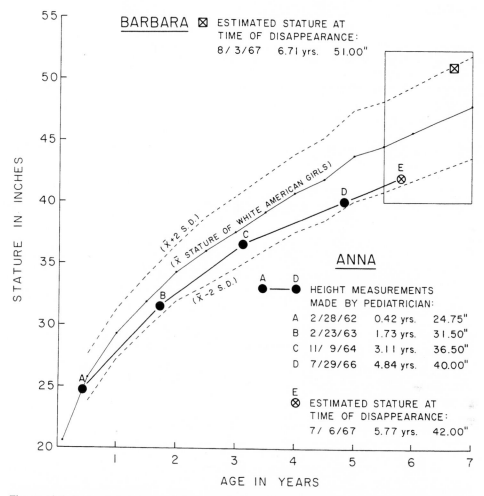

Figure 19-6. Estimated statures of the two missing girls compared to statural means of Caucasian females in the U.S. from birth to 7 years (Stoudt, Damon, and McFarland, 1960). Estimates for both girls fall within 2 standard deviations of the statural means of their respective ages, but Anna toward the lower limit and Barbara toward the upper.

Anna fall within the lower limits of the range of the humerus-based estimate, which, as noted above, may be considered minimal.

DISCUSSION AND CONCLUSIONS

This was an unusual case from two standpoints. First, it involved the skeletal identification of a young child. In most cases seen by the forensic anthropologist the bones are those of adults. Krogman (1962), one of the most experienced authorities in the field, states that among the hundreds of

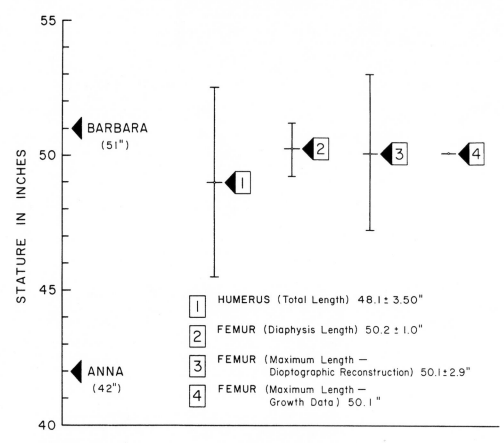

Figure 19-7. Statural estimates of the recovered skeleton compared to estimated statures of the missing girls.

skeletons brought to him for identification, only a "baker's half-dozen" have been those of children between 4 and 12 years of age. Second, identification problems are usually either of the "directed" or the "open" categories (Brues, 1958). In the former, the investigators already have a strong presumption of identity, and it is up to the physical anthropologist to test their hypothesis. In "open" cases, no a priori presumption of identification is available, and the physical anthropologist provides a general description of the remains, which the investigators attempt to match from their files of missing persons.

In review, the skeleton and contextual evidence surrounding the burial suggested the following conclusions:

1. From observational and statistical evidence, it was safe to assume that the remains were those of a single individual and not the commingled bones of two.

2. The bones were those of a child who had met his or her death through foul play as was evidenced by the attempt to hide the body.

3. The death occurred no earlier than a year before discovery and most probably during the summer of 1967.

4. Hair and clothing indicated sex was female.

5. Hair and dental evidence suggested that the victim was white.

6. Dental and osseous evidence suggested an age range of about 5 to 8 years with a likely age of about 7 years.

7. Four statural estimates, based on reconstructions of the fragmentary long bones, indicated that the victim's height was between 45 and 53 inches with a most likely estimate of about 50 inches.

Had this been an "open" case, the report submitted to the police would have been confined to the seven points listed above. In this instance, however, it appeared very probable that the remains were those of either Anna or Barbara.

The possibility that the bones belonged to a third child seemed remote, since there had been no other unsolved disappearances involving children of this age and sex in Oklahoma or surrounding states for several years. While it was possible that the bones were those of a child whose disappearance was not reported, experience has shown that such unreported cases far more frequently involve fetal remains or newborn infants than they do older children. If the latter disappear, and for some reason are not reported missing by the parents, the disappearance is very apt to be noticed by other relatives, neighbors, or school authorities, and sooner or later, police are informed. In short, it was most unlikely that a girl of the same age of the two missing children had been secretly buried during this period. Thus, the present case falls into the "directed" category. Yet it differs from the typical because there was not one but two presumptive subjects. Both were children of the same race and sex; they were less than a year apart in age. The assemblage of bones recovered represented less than one-third of a human skeleton.

Assuming the remains to belong to one of the two missing girls, the age estimate based primarily on the dentition would favor the victim being Barbara. Yet, as previously noted, Anna also tended to fall within or close to the lower limits of the various estimated age ranges. More convincing were the statural assessments, which clustered around the 51 inch estimate for Barbara and were well above that of 42 inches for Anna. Combined, the osteological evidence most strongly supported the identification made by Barbara's mother on the basis of the hair and clothing. As usual in such cases, chance played a role—had the two girls been a few months closer in age or a few inches closer in stature, their remains would probably have been indistinguishable. It is also of interest to note that statural estimates based on a single bone, the fragmented right femur, provided the most convincing evidence of identification, thus fully justifying the massive three day search for scattered remains.

Finally, a practical point might be emphasized to guide those involved in the investigation of similar cases. In the months and years that may elapse between the time of disappearance and the discovery of a skeleton, memories may dim and records may be lost or destroyed. Therefore, every available item of information useful in identification should be garnered from dental and medical histories, school health records, and interviews with the family and friends of the missing child as soon as possible after the disappearance.

REFERENCES

Brues, A. (1958). Identification of skeletal remains. *J Crim Law Criminol Police Sci, 48,* 551–563.

Carbonell, V. M. (1963). Variations in the frequency of shovel-shaped incisors in different populations. *Dental Anthropology.* D. R. Brothwell (Ed). Pergamon Press, Oxford, England.

Dahlberg, A. (1951). The dentition of the American Indian. Papers on the physical anthropology of the American Indian. The Viking Fund, Inc., New York City, NY.

Garn, S. M., A. B. Lewis, D. L. Polacheck (1959). Variability of tooth formation. *J Dent Res, 38,* 135–148.

Girdany, B. R., R. Golden (1952). Centers of ossification of the skeleton. *Am J Roentgenol, 68,* 922–924.

Gron, A. M. (1962). Prediction of tooth emergence. *J Dent Res, 41,* 573–585.

Hrdlicka, A. (1920). Shovel-shaped teeth. *Am J Phys Anthropol, 3,* 429–465.

Hunt, E. E., Jr., I. Gleiser (1955). The estimation of age and sex of preadolescent children from bones and teeth. *Am J Phys Anthropol, 13,* 479–487.

Hurme, V. O. (1948). Standards of variation in the eruption of the first six permanent teeth. *Child Develop, 19,* 213–231.

———— (1957). Time and sequence of tooth eruption. *J Forensic Sci, 2,* 377–388.

Kraus, B. S. (1959). Occurrence of the Carabelli trait in Southwest ethnic groups. *Am J Phys Anthropol, 17,* 117–124.

Krogman, W. M. (1962). *The Human Skeleton in Forensic Medicine.* Charles C Thomas, Springfield, Ill.

Lasker, G. W. (1950). Genetic analysis of racial traits of the teeth. *Cold Spring Harbor Symposia on Quantitative Biology, 15,* 191–204.

Lasker, G. W., M. M. Lee (1957). Racial traits in the human teeth. *J Forensic Sci, 2,* 401–413.

Lewis, A. B., S. M. Garn (1960). The relationship between tooth formation and other maturational factors. *Angle Orthod, 30,* 70–77.

Miles, A. E. W. (1963). Dentition in the assessment of individual age in skeletal material. *Dental Anthropology.* D. R. Brothwell (Ed). Pergamon Press, Oxford, England.

Moorrees, C. F. A. (1957). The Aleut dentition. A correlative study of dental characteristics of an Eskimoid people. Harvard University Press, Cambridge, Mass.

Moorrees, C. F. A., E. A., Fanning E. E. Hunt, Jr. (1963). Age variation of formation stages for the ten permanent teeth. *J Dent Res, 42,* 1490–1502.

Moyers, R. E. (1958). *Handbook of Orthodontics.* Year Book Publishers, Chicago, Ill., pp. 49–52.

Müller, G. (1935). Zur Bestimmung der Lange beschadigter Extremitatenknochen. *Anth Anzeig, 12,* 70–72.

Nolla, C. M. (1959). The development of the permanent teeth. *J Dent Child, 27,* 254–256.

Olivier, G. (1969). *Practical Anthropology.* Charles C Thomas, Springfield, Ill.

Reynolds, E. L. (1947). The bony pelvis in prepuberal childhood. *Am J Phys Anthropol,* (n.s.) *5,* 165–200.

Simmons, K. (1944). The Brush Foundation Study of Child Growth and Development. II. Physical growth and development. Monographs of the Society for Research in Child Development, Washington, DC 9, 1–87.

Snow, C. C., E. D. Folk (1970). Statistical assessment of commingled skeletal remains. *Am J Phys Anthropol, 32*:423–428.

Stewart, T. D. (1954). Evaluation of evidence from the skeleton. *Legal Medicine.* R. B. H. Gradwohl (Ed). C. V. Mosby, St. Louis, Mo., pp. 407–450.

———— (1948). Medico-legal aspects of the skeleton. I. sex, age, race, and stature. *Am J Phys Anthropol*, n.s. 6, 315–321.

———— (1963). New developments in evaluating evidence from the skeleton, *J Dent Res, 42*, 264–273.

Stoudt, H. W., A. Damon, R. A. McFarland (1960). Heights and weights of white Americans. *Hum Biol, 32*, 331–341.

Tappen, N. C. (1969). The relationship of weathering cracks to splitline orientation in bone. *Am J Phys Anthropol, 31*, 191–198.

Todd, T. W., J. D'Errico, Jr. (1926). The odontoid ossicle of the second cervical vertebra. *Ann Surg, 81*, 20–21.

Trotter, M. (1969) Personal communication.

Trotter, M., G. C. Gleser (1952). Estimation of stature from long bones of American whites and Negroes. *Am J Phys Anthropol, 10*, 468–514.

Chapter 20

SKELETAL AGING OF UNIDENTIFIED PERSONS

Judy Myers Suchey, Patricia A. Owings,
Dean V. Wiseley*, and Thomas T. Noguchi

Traditionally, forensic anthropologists deal with the identification of human remains that are skeletonized. In southern California, the role of the anthropologist has been expanded to include basic identification in soft tissue cases where the remains are decomposed, mutilated, burned, or mummified. Aging is accomplished by observations of epiphyseal union of the medial clavicle, anterior iliac crest, and pubic bone morphology. In addition, the same technique can be quite useful in young persons, from about 15 to 35 years of age, when the body is fresh and well preserved. Skeletal age identification in this range has been found to be more accurate than age estimation from soft tissue morphological features. For example, many females in their midteens present face and body morphology similar to physically mature females in their twenties. The true chronological immaturity of these females can readily be assessed from an examination of their skeletal features.

Forensic anthropologists generally use a variety of age indicators. However, with the present approach, attention is focused on the above three bones as a practical tool to assist in general age identification problems in a large autopsy room setting. The medial clavicle, anterior iliac crest, and pubic bone are generally well preserved even in burned remains. These bones can easily be removed at the time of autopsy using a stryker saw and can rapidly be defleshed by boiling them in tri-sodium phosphate until the morphological features of the bones become visible (usually less than one hour). In a majority of cases that fall from age 15 to 35, a relatively narrow age range may be determined from combined analysis of these three bones. The anterior iliac crest presents good age data for teenagers, whereas the medial clavicular epiphysis, being the last epiphysis to unite, is useful throughout

*Deceased

This publication is based on work supported by the National Science Foundation under Grant No. BNS78-13025.

The authors wish to thank Mr. James Njavro for the photography.

the twenties. The pubic bone is most reliable in individuals under 40.

The purpose of this chapter is twofold: (1) to discuss aging methodology using the iliac crest, medial clavicle, and pubic bone, and (2) to present actual forensic cases in which this technique has been employed. Five cases are selected that represent bodies in various states of preservation. Both sexes and a variety of ages are represented.

CHOICE OF TECHNIQUE

Prior studies on epiphyseal union essential to the development of this technique include Stevenson (1924), Todd and D'Errico (1928), and McKern and Stewart (1957). The research done in the 1920s was based on the Western Reserve Collection, the 1950s research on the American males killed during the Korean War. These two samples do not adequately cover young individuals under 18, lack Mongoloid individuals, and have limited data on females. The current technique was developed on a modern sample of 859 Americans autopsied at the Department of the Chief Medical Examiner-Coroner, Los Angeles. This sample is racially diverse, has a significant number of females, and includes a significant number of individuals from age 11 to 17. In addition, the autopsy sample is more representative of the general American population than were the former studies. Furthermore, it should be noted that age data are reliable, being based on death certificates and, in some cases, birth certificates.

The currently employed technique uses four stages for epiphyseal union: (1) nonunion without epiphysis, (2) nonunion with epiphysis, (3) partial union, (4) complete union. Figure 20-1 illustrates these stages on the anterior iliac crest; Figure 20-2 illustrates these stages on the medial clavicle. Table 20-I presents the data for the left anterior iliac crest for males and females. As can be seen from Table 20-I, crests with no union (stages 1 and 2) can be seen in males 19 years and younger and in females 15 years and younger. Partial union occurs in both males and females from age 14 to 23. Complete union occurs as early as age 17 in males and 18 in females. Table 20-II presents the data for the left medial clavicular epiphysis for males and females. Clavicles with no union (stage 1 and 2) can be seen in males 25 or younger and in females 21 or younger. Partial union can be seen in males 17 to 30 and in females 16 to 33. Complete union is seen as early as age 21 in males and 20 in females.

Prior studies in pubic symphyseal aging essential to the development of this technique include Todd (1920, 1921), Brooks (1955), McKern and Stewart (1957), and Gilbert and McKern (1973). Todd's studies done on an Ohio dissection room sample (the Western Reserve Collection) were the first attempt to develop a systematic method for pubic symphyseal aging. Limita-

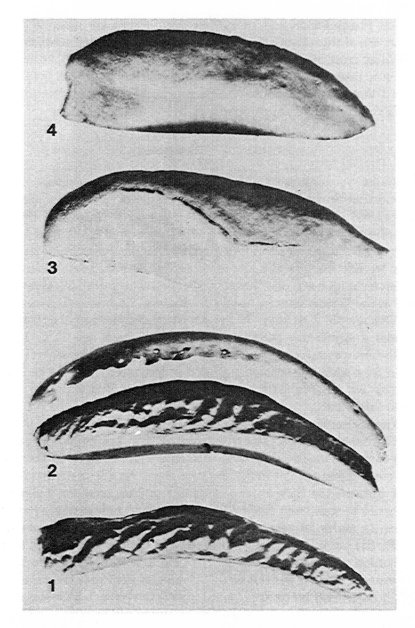

Figure 20-1. Stages for epiphyseal union on the iliac crest (from bottom to top): (1) nonunion without epiphysis; (2) nonunion with separate epiphysis; (3) partial union; (4) complete union.

tions to the sample include poor representation of males under 35 and females of all ages. In addition, reliability of the age data is in question, and parturition data are not considered in the study of female symphyses (Todd 1921, III). Todd describes 10 typical phases in symphyseal development,

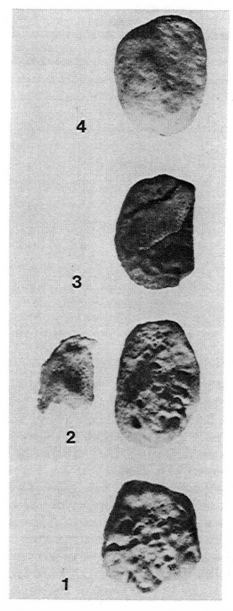

Figure 20-2. Stages for epiphyseal union of the medial clavicle (from bottom to top): (1) nonunion without epiphysis; (2) nonunion with separate epiphysis; (3) partial union; (4) complete union.

though it should be noted that sample sizes in the younger years were not sufficient to determine the statistical distribution of the relevant features. In 1955, Brooks reanalyzed Todd's Western Reserve sample. She modified certain of Todd's phases to correct for an error of underaging and described

TABLE 20-I

EPIPHYSEAL UNION OF THE LEFT ANTERIOR ILIAC CREST
IN A MODERN MULTIRACIAL SAMPLE OF PERSONS AUTOPSIED
AT THE DEPARTMENT OF CHIEF MEDICAL EXAMINER-CORONER, LOS ANGELES (IN %)[1]

| Age | No. | Males (n = 522) | | | | Age | No. | Females (n = 198) | | | |
| | | Stage of Union[2] | | | | | | Stage of Union | | | |
		1	2	3	4			1	2	3	4
11	2	100	—	—	—	11	1	100	—	—	—
13	3	67	33	—	—						
14	7	43	43	14	—	14	3	—	—	100	—
15	12	25	67	8	—	15	9	—	44	56	—
16	24	4	33	63	—	16	4	—	—	100	—
17	22	—	9	82	9	17	6	—	—	100	—
18	30	—	7	53	40	18	16	—	—	69	31
19	34	—	9	47	44	19	9	—	—	56	44
20	28	—	—	25	75	20	14	—	—	14	86
21	29	—	—	10	90	21	8	—	—	—	100
22	38	—	—	—	100	22	13	—	—	8	92
23	30	—	—	3	97	23	10	—	—	10	90
24–40	263	—	—	—	100	24–39	105	—	—	—	100

[1]For additional information on epiphyseal union of this sample, consult Owings (1981).

[2]Stages of union: (1) nonunion without epiphysis, (2) nonunion with epiphysis, (3) partial union, (4) complete union

alternative morphological patterns of the symphyseal face that varied from Todd's typical 10 phases. McKern and Stewart's 1957 study of American males killed in the Korean War included a large number (349) of young individuals with reliable age data. McKern and Stewart are to be commended for their concern with variability. They divided the symphyseal face into three major components (The Dorsal Plateau, The Ventral Rampart, and The Symphyseal Rim) and developed a six-stage system for each component. This system allows individuals falling outside the typical developmental scheme to be aged. Gilbert and McKern (1973) extended this system to females using a sample of 120 females. Age data were reliable for this sample, and parturition data were available on over half the sample. The major limitation to this sample was the scarcity of young females under 35.

At present, a large sample (400 females, 739 males) of pubic bones from modern Americans autopsied at the Department of the Chief Medical Examiner-Coroner, Los Angeles is being studied in an effort to develop improved pubic aging systems. The male sample has been studied (Suchey et al., 1980) using both the McKern-Stewart system and the Todd system. Analysis of the individuals was done with the age unknown to the investigator. The results are presented in Tables 20-III and 20-IV. When Todd's system is applied to the male sample, it can be seen that the mean of the Los Angeles

TABLE 20-II

**EPIPHYSEAL UNION OF THE LEFT MEDIAL CLAVICLE
IN A MODERN MULTIRACIAL SAMPLE OF PERSONS AUTOPSIED
AT THE DEPARTMENT OF CHIEF MEDICAL EXAMINER-CORONER, LOS ANGELES (IN %)**

Age	No.	*Males (n = 597)* Stage of Union[1]				Age	No.	*Females (n = 247)* Stage of Union			
		1	2	3	4			1	2	3	4
11	2	100	—	—	—	11	1	100	—	—	—
13	3	100	—	—	—	13	1	100	—	—	—
14	7	100	—	—	—	14	2	100	—	—	—
15	12	100	—	—	—	15	9	100	—	—	—
16	25	92	8	—	—	16	6	66	17	17	—
17	23	83	—	17	—	17	7	43	14	43	—
18	33	52	18	30	—	18	16	19	31	50	—
19	33	55	21	24	—	19	11	18	18	64	—
20	27	30	15	55	—	20	15	7	—	86	7
21	33	9	3	85	3	21	9	11	11	78	—
22	40	12	10	70	8	22	15	—	—	80	20
23	32	6	—	78	16	23	12	—	—	83	17
24	29	3	—	62	35	24	16	—	—	50	50
25	38	3	—	45	52	25	7	—	—	43	57
26	21	—	—	38	62	26	16	—	—	37	63
27	35	—	—	37	63	27	9	—	—	33	67
28	22	—	—	23	77	28	19	—	—	5	95
29	22	—	—	5	95	29	11	—	—	—	100
30	30	—	—	7	93	30	11	—	—	9	91
31–40	130	—	—	—	100	31	10	—	—	—	100
						32	10	—	—	10	90
						33	12	—	—	17	83
						34–39	22	—	—	—	100

[1]Stages of union: (1) nonunion without epiphysis, (2) nonunion with epiphysis, (3) partial union, (4) complete union.

sample is lower than the age range suggested by Todd. Standard deviations are fairly small for Todd's younger phases, substantiating the utility of the system. The age ranges are fairly broad, especially in the older phases; thus caution must be used, as certain individuals may fall far from the mean. In southern California, the technique currently being used for forensic cases is that of McKern and Stewart. This system is selected due to the flexibility it presents for younger age patterns. The Todd system is found to be too static and not applicable to some cases. Table 20-IV compares the Los Angeles sample statistics to the statistics on the Korean War dead sample. The Los Angeles sample produced broader age ranges—as might be expected because the Los Angeles sample was larger than the one used for the McKern-Stewart system (739 compared to 349). The mean ages correspond fairly well. In the younger ages, mean ages are slightly less in the Los Angeles sample. In the

TABLE 20-III
AGING THE MODERN MULTIRACIAL SAMPLE OF MALES AUTOPSIED
AT THE DEPARTMENT OF CHIEF MEDICAL EXAMINER-CORONER, LOS ANGELES
WITH THE TODD PUBIC SYMPHYSIS SYSTEM

Todd's Phases	Todd's Age Range	Los Angeles Sample Size	Los Angeles Range	Los Angeles Mean	Los Angeles Standard Deviation
I	18–19	19	14–19	16.68	1.46
II	20–21	50	14–23	18.12	1.74
III	22–24	52	17–24	20.38	1.90
IV	25–26	30	20–36	24.83	3.72
V	27–30	51	19–45	24.57	4.58
VI	30–35	43	22–51	28.81	5.89
VII	35–39	56	20–64	34.04	9.47
VIII	39–44	97	23–71	38.33	9.43
IX	45–50	241	21–87	51.00	13.64
X	50+	100	26–92	62.74	12.40

TABLE 20-IV
STATISTICS ON THE MCKERN-STEWART SYSTEM OF AGING THE MALE OS PUBIS
COMPARED TO THE STATISTICS WHEN THE SYSTEM IS APPLIED
TO THE LOS ANGELES SAMPLE OF MALES

McKern-Stewart Sample (n = 349)					Los Angeles Sample (n = 739)				
Total Score	No.	Age Range	Mean Age	S.D.	Total Score	No.	Age Range	Mean Age	S.D.
0	7	–17	17.29	.49	0	2	14–19	16.50	3.54
1–2	76	17–20	19.04	.79	1	14	14–23	17.50	2.14
					2	3	16–17	16.33	.58
3	43	18–21	19.79	.85	3	26	15–23	18.08	1.98
4–5	51	18–23	20.84	1.13	4	7	16–18	17.00	.82
					5	23	16–23	18.83	1.95
6–7	26	20–24	22.42	.99	6	35	17–25	20.46	2.13
					7	5	21–26	22.60	2.30
8–9	36	22–28	24.14	1.93	8	48	18–37	23.73	4.56
					9	0	—	—	—
10	19	23–28	26.05	1.87	10	54	19–49	27.30	6.52
11, 12, 13	56	23–39	29.18	3.33	11	45	20–78	35.91	12.48
					12	26	20–59	33.27	9.94
					13	93	21–71	36.26	9.96
14	31	29+	35.84	3.89	14	201	24–80	47.00	12.16
15	4	36+	41.00	6.22	15	157	25–92	61.27	13.89

older ages, mean ages are greater, especially for the final two categories (total scores 14 and 15) where the Los Angeles sample is noticably larger.

The female sample collected at Los Angeles has been extensively studied using a variety of techniques. The Gilbert-McKern (1973) system, the female counterpart to the McKern-Stewart system, has been found to be difficult to use (Suchey, 1979). Suchey et al. (1981) modified the Gilbert-McKern system and analyzed the Los Angeles sample. The females were found to exhibit extreme variability, which apparently makes the formulation of a reliable aging system almost impossible. Brooks (1981) studied the same sample using a modified Todd system; this approach also failed to verify the existence of a reliable standard. The variability in females was again found to be great, and the pregnancy data do not help to explain the extreme variations observed. It should be noted that the complete female sample used here has the ages verified by birth certificates; the accuracy of the chronological ages cannot be questioned.

Currently the technique used for aging female pubic bones in southern California forensic cases is limited to the use of a few general rules (Suchey et al., 1979b). The youngest pattern in the female pubic bone is characterized by deep, distinct ridges on both the dorsal and ventral demifaces. At this stage the ventral rampart has not yet begun formation. Females showing these traits are almost always 24 years or younger. Ossific nodules (Fig. 20-3) generally occur in females 28 or younger (Brooks, 1981).

APPLICATIONS

John Doe 1

John Doe 1 was a mummified and skeletonized individual in an advanced state of decomposition (Fig. 20-4). The body was devoid of internal viscera. The coroner's investigator originally described the individual as a Negro male of 40 or more years. Cause of death was determined by the pathologist to be a gunshot wound to the base of the skull.

Anthropological examination provided a confirmation of the sex and race. Sex was determined to be male from traits of the os pubis (Phenice, 1969). This determination was consistent with the maximum diameter of the head of the left femur (50 mm). The individual was determined to be Negro from morphological features of the cranium: fairly heavy maxillary prognathism, long and narrow cranial vault, wide nasal aperture, broad and low nasal bridge, and slight nasal sill. Stature was estimated to be from 5 feet 7½ inches to 5 feet 10½ inches. This estimate was based on the maximum length of the left femur (49.7 cm). Measurement was made with an osteometric board, and Trotter and Gleser's (1958) formula for Negro males was used.

Age determination was made by observations of the pubic bone and medial clavicle (Fig. 20-5). The pubic bone exhibited a 4-2-0 pattern using the McKern-Stewart system. The dorsal plateau, exhibiting vestiges of billowing, extended over most of the dorsal demiface. Ventral beveling extended inferiorly along the ventral border, but the ventral rampart had

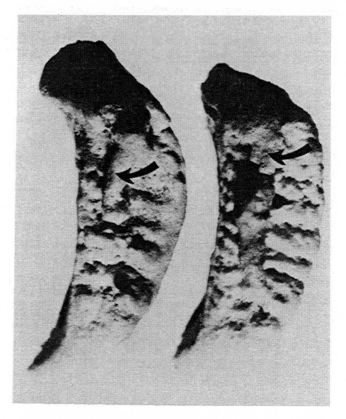

Figure 20-3. Ossific nodules (arrow) on ventral aspect of right pubic bones. Left from black female age 18; right from white female age 21.

not yet begun formation. The symphyseal rim was absent. These observations yielded an age range of 20 to 24 years based on the McKern-Stewart system. The clavicle exhibited partial epiphyseal union, suggesting an age range of 17 to 30. Thus, observation of the clavicle provided estimates consistent with the pubic age estimate but did not help to narrow it further.

Identification of John Doe 1 was made by dental records; he was a Negro male 20 years of age.

John Doe 2

John Doe 2, a badly decomposed body, was subjected to anthropological examination because attempts at identification had remained futile for almost a month (Fig. 20-6). The original pathologist's report indicated John Doe 2 to be a Caucasoid male 40 to 60 years of age. Examination of the pubic bone and skull supported the initial sex and race diagnosis. Sex was determined to be male by pubic traits (Phenice, 1969). Race was based on features

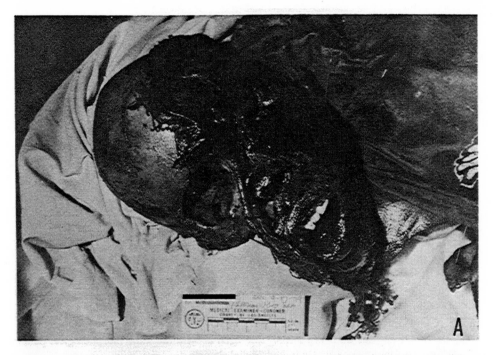

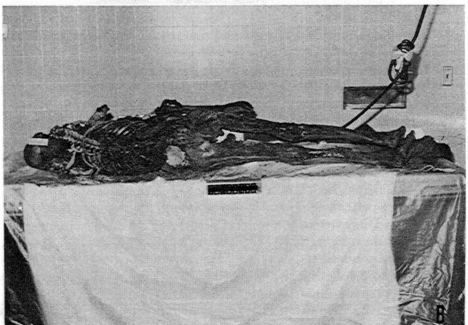

Figure 20-4 A & B. John Doe 1, a mummified and skeletonized individual in an advanced state of decomposition.

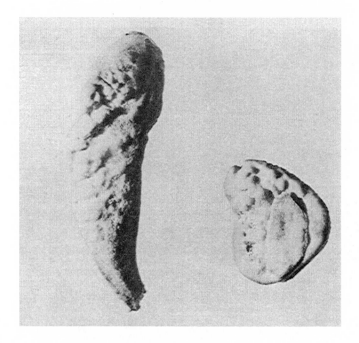

Figure 20-5. Left pubic bone of a white male aged 21 with the same morphological pattern (4-2-0) as John Doe 1 and partially united medial clavicle.

of the cranium (projecting nasal bones, sharp nasal sill, orthognathism) as well as examination of the remaining soft tissues.

The general appearance of the body was suggestive of an older individual. All teeth were missing antemortem. Examination of the pubic bone provided a younger assessment (Fig. 20-7). A pattern of 4-4-2 was observed. The dorsal plateau extended over most of the dorsal demiface; the ventral rampart was extensive, but gaps were still evident. The dorsal aspect of the symphyseal rim was complete, and the ventral part was beginning to form. This pattern yielded an age range of 23 to 28 when the McKern-Stewart system was strictly used. Given the morphological appearance of the body, the range was extended to 25 to 35 years. Due to the disparity between the pubic age and the external features of the body, arrangements were made for an age assessment by microscopic examination of a fibula midshaft (Kerley, 1979). Kerley provided an age range of 28 to 39 for John Doe 2. This estimate was similar to the skeletal age provided by the pubic bone and was clearly younger than the original estimate by the pathologist.

John Doe 2 was identified nearly one and a half years later by radiographic comparisons of the cervical vertebrae. He was 27½ years of age. Following the identification of John Doe 2, two midwestern men were brought to trial for his murder. Anthropological testimony was needed to clear up the

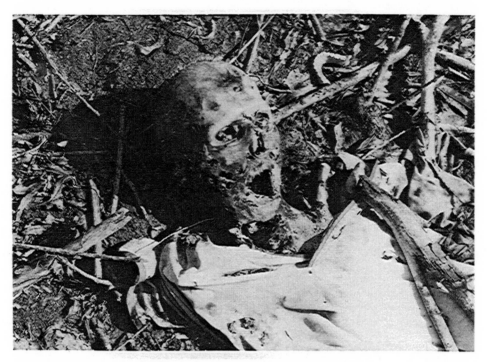

Figure 20-6. John Doe 2, a badly decomposed body.

confusion of the age. Principles of pubic aging were explained to the jury, whose interest was greatest when diagrams were roughly sketched on a paper board. The identity of John Doe 2 was accepted by the jury, and the defendants were subsequently found guilty. From discussions with law enforcement personnel after the trial, it became evident that the reevaluation of the age of John Doe 2 was the breakthrough in discovering his true identity. Prior attempts at identification were futile because an older man was being sought.

Jane Doe 1

Jane Doe 1 consisted of the body of a young Negro female with the head, hands, and feet removed (Fig. 20-8). The body appeared clean and relatively fresh when found. The head, hands, and feet were never recovered. The original age estimate, by the coroner investigators and police, was age 20. At the time of autopsy the pathologist placed an upper age estimate of 25 by the external appearance of the body.

Anthropological examination focused on age and stature; since the torso was in excellent condition, sex and race were immediately evident. At the time of autopsy, the anterior iliac crest, medial clavicle, and pubic bones

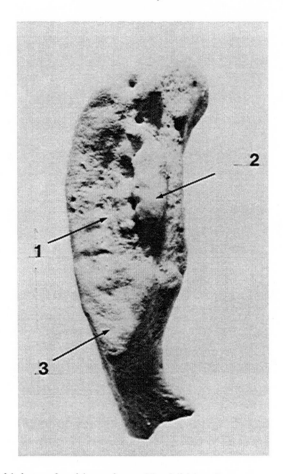

Figure 20-7. Left pubic bone of a white male age 27 exhibiting the same morphological pattern as John Doe 2. (1) dorsal plateau (stage 4); (2) ventral rampart (stage 4); (3) symphyseal rim (stage 2).

were removed for aging (Fig. 20-9); the femur was removed for a stature estimate. After defleshing, the iliac crest was found to have partial union of the epiphysis (14–23 years), the medial clavicle was found to have no union (21 or younger), and the pubic bones exhibited distinct ridges (24 or younger). Using these three criteria, the age range of 14 to 21 was obtained.

Jane Doe 1 was identified within a week by information supplied by the family. Identification was made by certain distinct traumatic marks on the right knee and on the thighs as well as comparisons of chest x-rays. Jane Doe 1 had just reached her fifteenth birthday; thus she was noticeably younger than the original soft tissue age estimates. The anthropological age assessment, making use of the anterior iliac crest, introduced the possibility that she was in her mid teens. This was a crucial step in establishing individual identity.

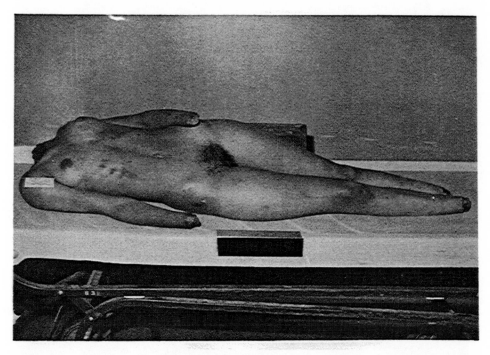

Figure 20-8. Jane Doe 1, a young Negro female with the head, hands, and feet removed by assailant.

The case of Jane Doe 1 illustrates the importance of age estimates through evaluation of multiple indicators.

Jane Doe 2

Jane Doe 2 consisted of a complete body in good condition (Fig. 20-10). She was found soon after death. Cause of death was strangulation, which left only minor trauma to the neck area. In the autopsy report, she was described as a well-nourished young Negro female about 18 years old.

Sex, race, and stature were clearly evident from external observations of the body. Anthropological examination was made for the age factor; it is important to note that females 15 to 30 can be aged more accurately from the skeletal structures than from soft tissue morphological observations alone. At the time of autopsy, the anterior iliac crest, medial clavicle, and pubic bones were removed and defleshed (Fig. 20-11). The iliac crest showed complete epiphyseal union (18 or older); the medial clavicle showed no union (21 or younger). Based on these two features alone, an age range of 18 to 21 is indicated. The pubic bones showed distinct ridges and no ventral rampart. These data (24 or younger) are consistent with the above age range but do not help to narrow it further.

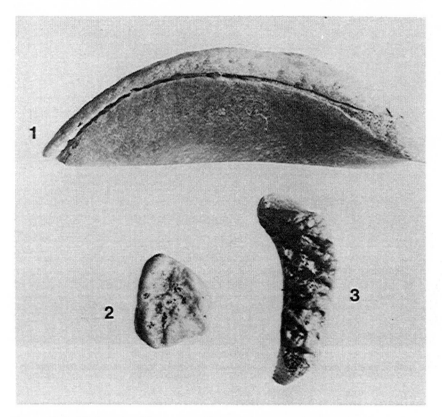

Figure 20-9. (1) Anterior iliac crest with partial union; (2) medial clavicle with no union; (3) right pubic bone with deep, distinct ridges indicating age of Jane Doe 1.

Jane Doe 2 was identified by dental x-rays. She was found to be 20 years of age. The original coroner investigator's age estimate, the anthropological skeletal age estimate, and the exact chronological age of the young Negro female were all in agreement.

Jane Doe 3

A female body, badly burned in a hotel fire, required identification (Fig. 20-12). Anthropological estimates for age and stature were requested. Stature was estimated by removing the femur to obtain the maximum length, and the pubic bones were removed for age analysis. The pubic bone exhibited a complete ventral rampart and symphyseal rim (Fig. 20-13A). An estimate of 30 + was given, based entirely on the pubic bone. Jane Doe 3 exhibited extremely large dorsal pits on the pubic bones (see Fig. 19-13B). Once believed to be evidence for childbirth, it is now known that nulliparous females, and in rare cases even males, can exhibit these changes. Further,

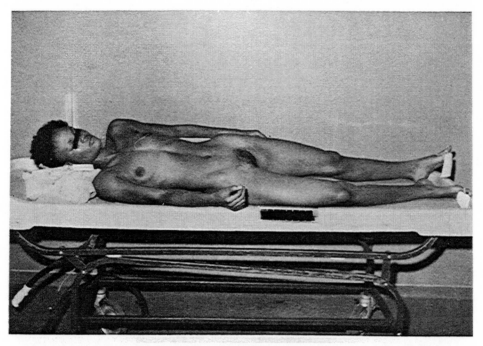

Figure 20-10. Jane Doe 2, a complete body of young black female in good condition.

there are multiparous females who show no dorsal changes. Additional information on the relationship between dorsal pitting, number of full-term pregnancies, interval since last pregnancy, and age of decedent can be found in Suchey et al. (1979a).

Jane Doe 3 was identified by physical evidence in her possession and the description of unusual teeth. She was a 48-year-old Mexican-American female who was known to have had at least one child. The pubic age proved to be correct in this particular case; however, it is now known that many females in their twenties show a completed ventral rampart and/or symphyseal rim (Suchey et al., 1979b).

SUMMARY

Obtaining a good age estimate is vital to the analysis of unidentified bodies. Age determination of individuals from age 15 to 35 can rapidly be achieved by examining the medial clavicular epiphysis, anterior iliac crest, and pubic bone. These bones can easily be removed at the time of autopsy and rapidly defleshed for observation on the spot. Although forensic anthropologists are traditionally called for skeletonized or badly decomposed remains,

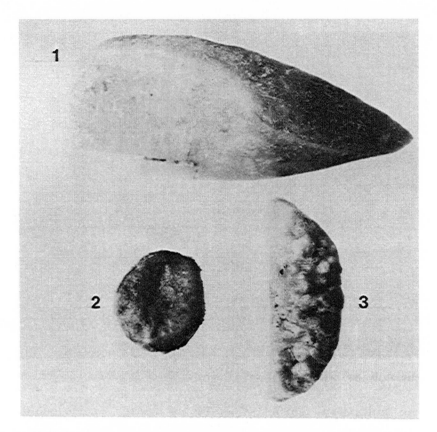

Figure 20-11. (1) Anterior iliac crest with complete union; (2) medial clavicle with no union; (3) right pubic bone with distinct ridges indicating age of Jane Doe 2.

this technique can also be profitably applied to well-preserved bodies. Cases and research in southern California have shown that the data from the skeletal structures provide a more accurate age assessment than external morphological features.

The strategy employed here has been elaborated from prior standards, using data from an extensive multiracial sample of modern Americans, of known identity, autopsied at the Department of Chief Medical Examiner-Coroner, Los Angeles. This article presents standards for epiphyseal union of the iliac crest and medial clavicle as well as pubic symphyseal changes. Five case studies are included to illustrate the application of the technique. These cases illustrate bodies in various states of preservation. Cases are both male and female and of various ages.

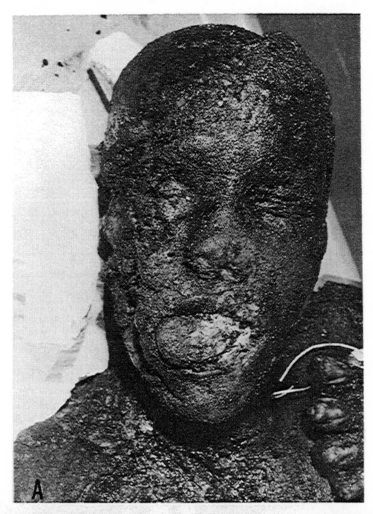

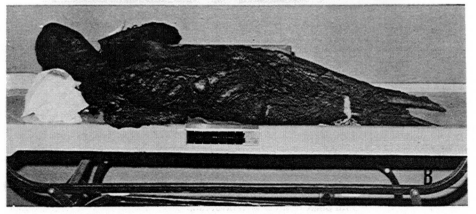

Figure 20-12 A & B. Jane Doe 3, a female body, badly burned in a hotel fire.

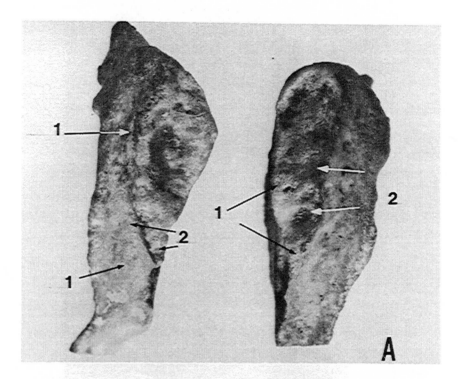

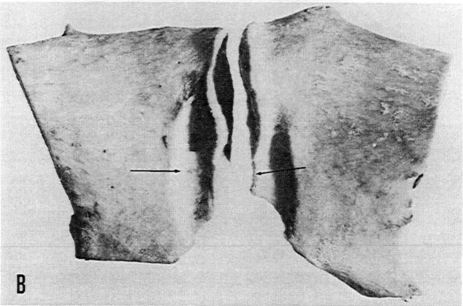

Figure 20-13 A & B. A. Both pubic bones with ventral rampart (1) and symphyseal rim (2) complete from Jane Doe 3. B. Large pits (arrow) on dorsal aspects.

REFERENCES

Brooks, S. T. (1955). Skeletal age at death: the reliability of cranial and pubic indicators. *Am J Phys Anthropol, 13*:367–597.

—— (1981) Personal communication.

Gilbert, B. M., and McKern, T. W. (1973). A method for aging the female os pubis. *Am J Phys Anthropol, 38*:31–38.

Kerley, F. R. (1979). Personal communication.

McKern T. W., and Stewart, T. D. (1957). *Skeletal Age Changes in Young American Males, Analyzed from the Standpoint of Identification.* Natick, Massachusetts: Headquarters Quartermaster Res. and Dev. Command, Tech. Rep. EP-45.

Owings, P. A. (1981). "Epiphyseal Union of the Anterior Iliac Crest and Medial Clavicle in a Modern Multi-racial Sample of Males and Females." Master's Thesis, California State University, Fullerton.

Phenice, T. W. (1969). A newly developed visual method of sexing the os pubis. *Am J Phys Anthropol, 30*:297–301.

Stevenson, P. H. (1924). Age order of epiphyseal union in man. *Am J Phys Anthropol, 7*:53–93.

Suchey, J. M. (1979). Problems in the aging of females using the os pubis. *Am J Phys Anthropol, 51*:467–470.

Suchey, J. M., Wiseley, D. V., Green, R. F., and Noguchi, T. T. (1979a). Analysis of dorsal pitting in the os pubis in an extensive sample of modern American females. *Am J Phys Anthropol, 51*:517–540.

Suchey, J. M., Wiseley, D. V., and Noguchi, T. T. (1979b). Age changes in the female os pubis. American Academy of Forensic Science, Annual Meeting, Atlanta, Georgia, February, 1979. (Typescript copy)

—— (1980). Aging the male os pubis. American Academy of Forensic Sciences, Annual Meeting, New Orleans, Louisiana, February, 1980. (Typescript copy)

—— (1981). Age changes in the female os pubis in an extensive sample of modern American females. American Academy of Forensic Science, Annual Meeting, Los Angeles, California, February, 1981. (Typescript copy)

Todd, T. W. (1920). Age changes in the pubic bone. I: The male white pubis. *Am J Phys Anthropol, 3*:285–334.

—— (1921). Age changes in the pubic bone. II. The pubis of the male Negro-white hybrid. III. The pubis of the white female. IV. The pubis of the female Negro-white hybrid. *Am J Phys Anthropol, 4*:1–70.

Todd, T. W., and D'Errico, J. (1928). The clavicular epiphyses. *Am J Anat, 41*:25–50.

Trotter, M. and Gleser, G. C. (1958). A re-evaluation of estimation of stature based on measurements of stature taken during life and of long bones after death. *Am J Phys Anthropol, 16*:79–123.

Chapter 21

MICROSCOPIC AGING OF HUMAN BONE

Ellis R. Kerley

The microscopic method of age estimation has been described in detail elsewhere (Kerley, 1965, 1970). Basically, it involves making ground sections of the midshaft of human femur, tibia, and/or fibula and counting microscopic structures in four 100-power fields in the outer third of the cortex using a standard laboratory binocular microscope with polarizers. The numbers of osteons, fragments of old osteons, and nonhaversian canals are added for all four fields to provide a representative count for the outer third of the cortex for each bone examined. A visual estimate of the percentage of the field that is composed of circumferential lamellar bone is made for each field also, and the results are averaged for all four fields. Anyone who plans to use this method should read either of the above references describing the technique in detail. The original research involved 126 specimens and demonstrated that osteons and fragments increase with age as they replace decreasing amounts of circumferential lamellar bone and nonhaversian canals. Although four factors are measured by this method, what is actually being examined is the rate of osteon turnover, or replacement.

Some of the advantages of this method include its simplicity, its application to the midshaft areas of long bones, where thick cortical bone is preserved best under most postmortem conditions, and its ability to cover the entire age range from birth through 95 years of age with particular utility in dealing with older age specimens. Also, its accuracy and reliability have been statistically determined, whether one uses the regression formulae for osteons and fragments or the age profile method of age estimation. The latter method provides a reliability of 87 percent when a range of accuracy of ± 5 years is used. Disadvantages include the need to make ground sections of bone and consequent alteration of the specimen and the inherent difficulty of deciding whether borderline structures should be considered osteons or fragments for purposes of counting.

Although modifications of this method have been suggested (Ahlqvist and Damsten, 1969; Singh and Gunberg, 1970), they have not improved the accuracy or reliability of the original method, which has proved to be rather useful in forensic applications (Kerley, 1969). Recently, however, the original regression formulae were revised and a method presented for compensating for variations in actual field size in different microscopes at 100 power (Kerley and Ubelaker, 1978). These should improve the reliability with which this method can be applied in different laboratories. The following cases are from actual forensic files and illustrate some of the unusual circumstances in which the microscopic method can provide important evidence for identification of human remains.

CASE 1

A forensic pathologist from the Armed Forces Institute of Pathology brought several fragments of bone to the Forensic Anthropology Laboratory of the University of Maryland and requested an opinion as to what they might represent. He stated that there was reason to believe they might be human. The largest fragment was about the size of a half-dollar piece and included some cortical surface. The other fragments were rather small and irregular in shape, having been fractured on several borders.

Examination

The fragments appeared to be part of a massive comminuted fracture and were compatible with human bone in terms of their texture and cortical thickness. If human, they were most likely from the femoral diaphysis. The largest fragment had cut marks in several different planes, and there was what appeared to be dried soft tissue impacted in the marrow spaces of the medullary, or endosteal, surface of the bone. A fine network of root tendrils had invaded the dried mass and the vascular spaces of the bone in some areas. A histological ground section representing about one-third of the cortical circumference of an intact bone was made from the largest of the fragments and examined microscopically to estimate the age at the time of death. Little else could be determined from the fragments available.

Findings

Microscopic examination for age estimation was undertaken (Kerley, 1965), although the specimen was surely marginal for such estimation. The report emphasized the tentative nature of such an estimate from less than half the normal circumference of the femur, if indeed it was human femur. Since the specimen was only sufficient for one ground section, the resulting slide was examined and osteons counted on four separate occasions spaced several days apart. Both the Age Profile Method and the original regression formulae were used in estimating age. The results are shown in Tables 21-I and 21-II. Using the regression formulae, the most probable age was between 26 and 51 when the counts obtained on four separate trials were used and their age ranges averaged. The age ranges obtained by the Age Profile Method excluded all but the years between 19 and 47, when the results of all four trials were used. The median year and most probable age at death was 33 years, with a probability of 87.3% that the actual age at death was between 28 and 38. The formulae and probabilities used were originally derived from anatomically selected fields in complete cross sections of bone, however, and that was pointed out to the forensic pathologist. The bone appeared human.

TABLE 21-I
AGE PROFILE CHART

Histology					*Averaged Measurements*							*Age Range*
FEMUR:	0	10	20	30	40	50	60	70	80	90	100	
Osteons	.	.				.	.	.	.	.	.	19–47
Fragments	.	.				.	.	.	.	.	.	18–47
Lamellar	.	.				.	.	.	.	.	.	13–50
Nonosteon	.	.				.	.	.	.	.	.	13–47
TIBIA:	0	10	20	30	40	50	60	70	80	90	100	
Osteons	.	.		.	.	.	.	.	.	.	.	
Fragments	.	.		.	.	.	.	.	.	.	.	
Lamellar	.	.		.	.	.	.	.	.	.	.	
Nonosteon	.	.		.	.	.	.	.	.	.	.	
FIBULA:	0	10	20	30	40	50	60	70	80	90	100	
Osteons	.	.		.	.	.	.	.	.	.	.	
Fragments	.	.		.	.	.	.	.	.	.	.	
Lamellar	.	.		.	.	.	.	.	.	.	.	
Nonosteon	.	.		.	.	.	.	.	.	.	.	

					RESORPTION							
	0	10	20	30	40	50	60	70	80	90	100	
Outer	.	. +++		.	.	.	.	.	.	.	.	+++
Middle	.	++		.	.	.	.+++.++++.+++.+					++
Inner	.+	.		.	+++++++++++++++++++++							++

Profile range	19–47 (33)	Number	Case 1
Visual Estimate	Young Adult	Sex	M Race
Other		Section	1/4 cross decal H&E
Microscopic Age	28–38 [33]	Date	October 23, 1972

TABLE 21-II
AGE ESTIMATION

Feature	Trial #1	Trial #2	Trial #3	Trial #4	Average
Osteons	81	81	84	96	85.5
Age Range	18–43	18–43	19–45	23–52	19–47
Fragments	24	23	30	36	28.2
Age Range	17–44	16–43	20–48	23–52	18–47
Lamellar	30	32.5	26.2	22.5	27.8
Age Range	13–47	12–47	17–51	19–56	13–50
Non-Osteon	8	10	6	7	7.75
Age Range	13–46	12–43	15–48	14–47	13–47
					19–47
TOTAL RANGE	18–43	18–43	20–45	23–47	23–43
		REGRESSION FORMULAE			
Osteons Age	34.8	34.8	36.7	44.9	37.7
Age Range	16–54	16–54	18–56	26–64	18–57
Fragments Age	28.8	28.0	33.8	38.8	32.3
Age Range	4–53	3–53	9–58	14–63	7–57
Lamellar Age	27.3	24.9	31.6	36.5	30.1
Age Range	3–51	1–49	8–55	12–60	6–54
Non-Osteon Age	44.8	41.8	47.9	46.3	45.2
Age Range	17–72	14–70	20–76	18–74	17–73
REGRESSION RANGE	17–51	16–53	20–55	26–60	26–51

There appeared to be remnants of soft tissue with well-preserved cells with clearly defined nuclei. The remaining portion of the largest fragment was decalcified, and stained sections were made from it. The cell nuclei stained normally, and cell walls were visible in most areas. Although the tissue was not readily identifiable itself, the cells appeared to be compatible with bone marrow cells. There was an extensive network of small root tendrils permeating the tissue mass and invading larger vascular spaces of the bone. The most reasonable explanation for this paradox of a tissue mass being so well preserved for a sufficient length of time for roots to grow through it and into the bone was that it had been kept at a continuously cold temperature, possibly at a high altitude just below the tree line, or at least lichen line, or in an arctic area where lichens grew. The possibility was mentioned in the report of examination. The time since death under such circumstances was estimated as somewhere between one and two years, with the usual qualification that such estimates are quite tenuous.

Grossly the fragments of bone, and particularly the largest one, showed signs of high-speed impact damage. There were both cut and fractured edges present, and the cuts were oriented in several planes. Those on the largest fragment were on the external, or periosteal, surface and showed signs of deflection. Air crash or other high-speed impact was suggested in this case.

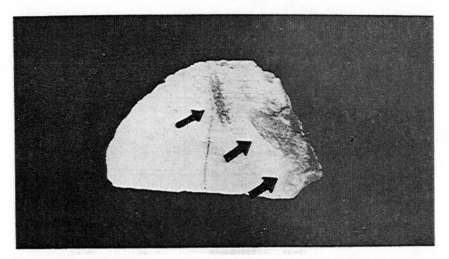

Figure 21-1. Largest fragment of bone found in Case 1. The arrows point to multiple cuts in different directions made when metal fragments were driven through the body by high-speed impact.

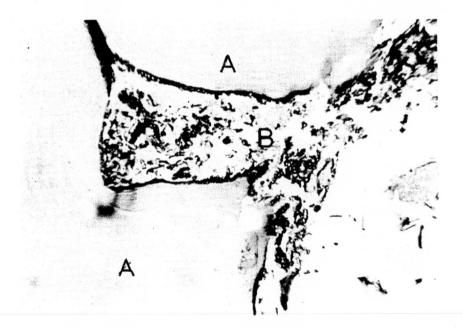

Figure 21-2. Photomicrograph of the endosteal surface of the bone fragment showing bone (A) with preserved marrow cells (B) filling spaces in the bone. The dark areas in the cellular mass are root tendrils.

Follow-Up

When the report of examination was submitted, follow-up information was made available. The fragments of bone had been recovered by digging under the point of impact where a U.S. Navy jet aircraft had crashed one-and-a-half years previously. They were recovered by the civilian climber who had initially discovered the crash site seven months after the crash occurred. Those bone fragments were all that had ever been recovered of the pilot, as the disintegration of the aircraft had been extensive. The crash occurred above 8,000 feet in the Sierra Nevada Mountains. The question was whether the recovered bone fragments were from the pilot or were at least consistent with his description. He was 28 years old at the time of the crash, 75 inches tall and weighed 190 pounds. Ironically, a set of anthropometric measurements was available for this pilot, but could not be compared to the small fragments that had been recovered. He was identified on the basis of agreement of all available data, including age, and the lack of any conflicting evidence.

CASE 2

Several specimens wrapped in blue plastic dry cleaner's bags individually were brought to the laboratory by agents of the Federal Bureau of Investigation for possible identification. Each had been found in a different jurisdiction around a major midwestern city at about the same time. The questions were: Are all of the parts from the same individual? and Who was it? The specimens consisted of a heart, thorax that had been skinned, flesh-covered right thigh, legs, and feet.

Examination

All submitted specimens were examined together grossly. The thorax had been skinned, and all superficial muscles had been removed. The intercostal muscles were intact, as were portions of the serratus and deep dorsal muscles. The attachments of the pectoral muscles had been dissected in a knowledgeable manner. The heart was of an appropriate size for the thorax. No cause of death could be determined from the heart or thorax. The right thigh and both lower legs were smooth and had been shaved. There were thicker than average deposits of subcutaneous fat on the anterior and medial aspects of the thigh and over the peroneal region of the lower legs. The feet appeared fairly small, short, and broad for the size of the legs. The skin of the legs was light in color and Caucasoid in appearance. There was fine, slightly dark terminal hair over the upper unshaved portion of the thigh.

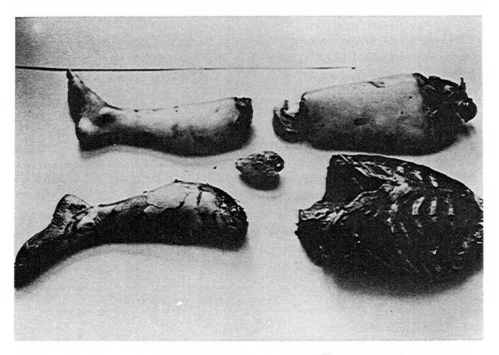

Figure 21-3. Human remains that were recovered and examined in Case 2.

Radiographs were made in anterior-posterior and lateral planes. They revealed that the rib sternal ends were rounded and that all epiphyses were fused in the rib cage, vertebrae, and legs. The leg bones were all similar in terms of size, cortical thickness, and trabecular pattern. The left and right lower leg long bones matched radiographically. No discrepancies were found.

Measurements were made of the vertical diameter of the femoral head and the lengths of the major long bones. The femoral head diameter was 42 mm, which is well in the female range (Washburn; Thieme & Schull). The gross appearance and shaved lower legs were consistent with female sex also, although the possibility of shaving the legs of a male victim was mentioned in the report. In this case, all indications were of female sex, however. The femoral length was 420 mm. That and the femur+tibia measurements suggested a stature of 61 to 62 inches using the Trotter & Gleser (1952, 1958) tables for female Caucasoids.

Histologic sections of the femur were prepared as ground bone sections about 100 microns thick and examined under polarized light at 100 power using a standard binocular microscope with 10X oculars and a 10X objective lens. The number of osteons, fragments of old osteons, nonhaversian canals, and percentage of lamellar bone were recorded for four selected fields and added together to estimate the age at death (Kerley, 1965). The age was estimated to have been between 15 and 25 years at death, with 20 being the median and most probable actual year.

TABLE 21-III
CROSS SECTION HISTOLOGY AGE ESTIMATE PROFILE

Histology	Averaged Measurements											Age Range
	0	10	20	30	40	50	60	70	80	90	100	
Femur Osteons	.				.	.	.	.	.	.	.	8–28
Femur Fragments	.	.			.	.	.	.	.	.	.	12–38
Femur Lamellar	.	.			.	.	.	.	.	.	.	12–35
Femur Pseudo-haver	.	.			.	.	.	.	.	.	.	7–31
	0	10	20	30	40	50	60	70	80	90	100	
Tibia Osteons	.	.	.	.	.	.	.	.	.	.	.	
Tibia Fragments	.	.	.	.	.	.	.	.	.	.	.	
Tibia Lamellar	.	.	.	.	.	.	.	.	.	.	.	
Tibia Pseudo-haver	.	.	.	.	.	.	.	.	.	.	.	
	0	10	20	30	40	50	60	70	80	90	100	
Fibula Osteons	.	.	.	.	.	.	.	.	.	.	.	
Fibula Fragments	.	.	.	.	.	.	.	.	.	.	.	
Fibula Lamellar	.	.	.	.	.	.	.	.	.	.	.	
Fibula Pseudo-haver	.	.	.	.	.	.	.	.	.	.	.	

RESORPTION

	0	10	20	30	40	50	60	70	80	90	100	
Outer	.	+++	+	.	.	.	.	.	.	.	.	15–25
Middle	. ++ .	+	.	+++++++++++++++					.	.	.	
Inner	+	.	.	+++++++++++++++++++++								

Age Profile	12–28 (20)	Number	Case 2
Visual Estimate	15–20	Sex (Female)	Race Caucasoid
Other	Microradiograph also	Section	Ground
Microscopic Age	15–25 (20)	Date	31 May 1963

Remarks   No medullary resorption or osteone enlargement.

Summary: It was concluded that all of the remains examined could have belonged to the same individual and that all three segments of legs did belong to one individual. It was suggested that the individual was slightly overweight, as evidenced by the thick subcutaneous fat.

Sex: female
Age: 15 to 25 years, probably 20
Race: Caucasoid
Stature: around 61 to 63 inches

Injuries: postmortem dismemberment and reflection of the pectoral muscles suggest some knowledge of anatomy. No other evidence of injury or cause of death.

Time since death: For the area and time of year, about one week to a week and a half.

Follow-up: Victim was a Caucasoid female age 24 at the time of death, 63 inches tall and somewhat overweight. She was married, and her husband (who was a first-year medical student) admitted to killing her and dismembering her body, when he was confronted with the identification.

REFERENCES

Ahlqvist, J., and Damsten, O. (1969). A modification of Kerley's method for the microscopic determination of age in human bone. *Forensic Sci, 14*:205–212.

Kerley, E. R. (1965). The microscopic determination of age in human bone. *Am J Phys Anthropol, 23*:149–163.

———— (1969). Age determination of bone fragments. *J Forensic Sci, 14*:59–67.

———— (1970). Estimation of skeletal age: after about age 30. In T. D. Stewart (Ed): *Personal Identification in Mass Disasters*. Washington, D.C.: Smithsonian Institution, pp. 57–70.

Kerley, E. R., and Ubelaker, D. (1978). Revisions in the microscopic method of estimating age at death in human cortical bone. *Am J Phys Anthropol, 49*:545–546.

Singh, I., and Gunberg, D. (1970). Estimation of age at death in human males from quantitative histology of bone fragments. *Am J Phys Anthropol, 33*:373–381.

Thieme, F., and Schull, W. (1957). Sex determination from the skeleton. *Hum Biol, 29*:242–273.

Trotter, M., and Gleser, G. (1952). Estimation of stature from long bones of American whites and Negroes. *Am J Phys Anthropol, 10*:463–514.

———— (1958). A re-evaluation of estimation of stature taken during life and of long bones after death. *Am J Phys Anthropol, 16*:79–123.

Washburn, S. L. (1948). Sex differences in the pubic bone. *Am J Phys Anthropol, 6*:199–207.

Chapter 22

ADULT AGE DETERMINATION FROM THE DENTITION

DELLA COLLINS COOK

INTRODUCTION

The teeth are perhaps the single most durable and informative body part that forensic anthropologists analyze. Dental age is widely accepted as the most reliable source of age information in juveniles, and dental morphology is commonly used for both race assessment and individuation. While crown wear and degenerative changes in the alveolar bone are routinely consulted when other skeletal elements are missing or when other age indicators are discordant, teeth are less commonly a primary source of information about age in adults. This point can be illustrated by examining four recent summaries of forensic anthropology as practiced in the United States. Two (Krogman, 1962; El-Najjar and McWilliams, 1978) do not discuss adult age changes in the teeth, while two (Kerley, 1978; Stewart, 1979) cite Gustafson's (1950) system for age assessment on tooth sections. Stewart's discussion is the most complete (1979) and includes a brief review of related methods.

Forensic odontology receives more attention in Europe than in the United States, and it is not surprising that age changes in the teeth of adults are discussed more extensively in the literature of this specialty (Gustafson, 1966; Cameron and Sims, 1974). In the 30 years since Gustafson published his six-feature scoring system for determining age from tooth sections, several independent tests of his system have appeared, and modifications of his procedure as well as other techniques for evaluating age-related changes in dental histology have been proposed. The application of several of these techniques to the case presented here illustrates the problems and advantages posed by age determination from adult teeth.

The author would like to thank Jane E. Buikstra for making the teeth described here available for study as well as for sharing her observations on the case. This study was supported in part by the National Science Foundation, Contract BNS 77-2310.

307

SL 0976-80

The case, SL 0976-80, is the essentially complete, articulated skeleton of an adult male found sitting in a chair in an abandoned building in a poorer section of St. Louis, Missouri in April, 1980. Some extremely decomposed soft tissue was still present, as were several articles of clothing and other personal effects that may have been associated with the remains. In a preliminary report, the St. Louis medical examiner suggested that the individual was black and extremely old, basing this opinion on a diagnosis of osteoarthritis and osteophytosis. A radiologist consulted by the medical examiner's office found the individual to be white and suggested an age range of 55 to 75 with a best estimate of 60, citing trabecular bone loss in the long bones, vertebral spurring, and degenerative changes in the spine as evidence. Degenerative disc disease and Forestier's disease were considered as appropriate diagnoses.* The remains were sent to Jane Buikstra for a resolution of these issues.

Buikstra reached a much younger age estimate, suggesting a range of 40 to 55 and a best estimate of 45 to 50. She assessed the pubic symphysis age as Todd phase IX (45–50), and the author agreed with her findings (Buikstra, 1980). There is extensive ossification of intervertebral ligaments, predominantly lateral to the anterior intervertebral ligament. Free body and osteophytic ossification of the annulus fibrosus at all levels have resulted in complete fusion of C2–3, C5–6, C7–T1, T3–6, and T8–L1; there is limited motion throughout the spine. The capsular ligaments of most joints of the appendicular skeleton are ossified. There is extensive ossification of muscle attachments. Intervertebral disc space is preserved except in the cervical spine, Schmorl's nodes and other disc herniations are absent, and there is little or no evidence for degenerative change in any of the synovial joints. The right sacroiliac joint is fused by bony bridging on the superior margin with no loss of joint space, and several ribs are fused to the sternum. These characteristics suggest ankylosing spondylitis, as argued in Buikstra's report, rather than osteoarthritis as the most probable diagnosis (Masi and Medsger, 1979; Bluestone, 1979). Forestier's disease can be excluded because sacroiliac fusion is absent in this syndrome (Bluestone, 1979; Moskowitz, 1979; Sokoloff, 1979). Since ankylosing spondylitis generally appears in young adulthood or adolescence and can be quite advanced before middle age, joint disease in SL 0976-80 has no significance for age determination.

Buikstra found that most skeletal criteria suggested that the individual was black. There are two lingual cusps on the mandibular P1 as well,

---

*Post Mortem Examination Report Case No. 0976-80, 4/19/80 Radiologic Consultation Report OME No. 0976-80, 4/23/80

a condition that Kraus (1957) considered as racially diagnostic. While ankylosing spondylitis is less common in American blacks than in whites, it is not so rare as to make the diagnosis of the condition useful in race determination.

The dentition of SL 0976-80 poses several interesting problems related to the application of dental age standards. Extensive recession of alveolar bone has resulted in the antemortem loss of nine of the posterior teeth, as indicated in Table 22-I. As a result of severe periodontosis, the distance between the cementoenamel junction and the buccal alveolar bone is roughly equivalent to crown height. There are heavy calculus deposits throughout, especially on the left maxillary molars. (Fig. 22-1) These teeth lack opponents, and there is calculus several millimeters thick on their buccal and occlusal surfaces. Among the posterior teeth, only the right M2/2 and P2/2 are in functional occlusion, and the lack of occlusal wear facets on the remaining molars suggests that the tooth loss was long-standing. In contrast to the relatively light wear on the posterior teeth, the anterior teeth are quite worn. Dentin is exposed and deeply cupped, a pattern more suggestive of bruxism than of functional wear. Only the mesiobuccal root of the right maxillary M1 remains, and this root is carious. The right maxillary P1 is missing antemortem, and there is an extensive periodontal abscess surrounding the alveolus. The right maxillary P2 is fractured and carious. The anterior teeth present severe linear enamel hypoplasia.

Because most of the age changes seen in adult teeth are related to tooth function and because the relationship of pathology to the rate at which these changes occur is largely unknown, SL 0976-80 provides an interesting context for evaluating the various techniques for age estimation that are available from the literature. We can ask as well whether any of these techniques provide conclusive support for one or the other of the general age estimates that have been made for this individual.

AGE ASSESSMENT TECHNIQUES

Techniques of age determination based on gross evaluation of dental wear (Miles, 1963a, 1963b; Murphy, 1959) are predicated on a model for abrasion and attrition that presumes normal functional occlusion and a relatively complete dentition. They are widely recognized as population-specific (Miles, 1963a; Dahlberg, 1960). For these reasons such techniques are not appropriate in this case. The wear on the anterior teeth of SL 0976-80 is quite pronounced. The degree of exposure of dentin can be matched only in the oldest of specimens from archaeological populations in which wear was rapid and would certainly suggest advanced age in a modern American.

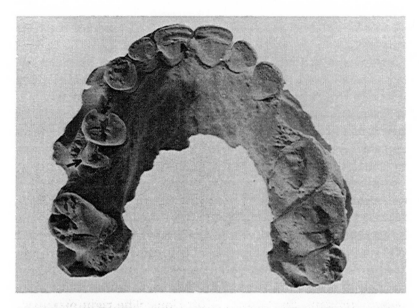

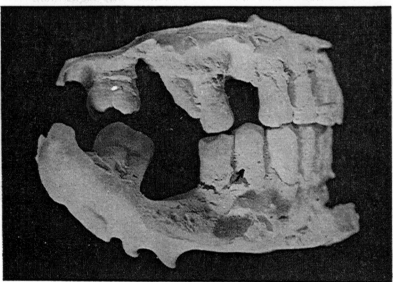

Figure 22-1 A & B. A. Occlusal view of the cast of the maxillary dentition. Arrows indicate severe linear enamel hypoplasia on the lingual surface at the central incisors, caries of the right P2, and remaining carious root of the right M1. Note the heavy calculus deposits on the occlusal surfaces of the left M1 through M3 and cupping wear of the dentin on the right C. B. Right lateral view of the casts of the teeth of SL 0976-80 in occlusion. Note the mesial drift of the maxillary P2 and M1 root and mandibular M2, hypereruption of the mandibular P1, loss of alveolar bone, and heavy calculus deposits (arrow).

TABLE 22-I
TEETH PRESENT IN SL 0976-80[1]

right	x	M2	M1	P2	x	C	12	11	11	12	C	x	x	M1	M2	M3	left
	x	M2	x	P2	P1	C	12	11	11	12	C	P1	P1	x	x	x	

[1]Buikstra suggests that the missing third molars may have been congenitally absent.

However, the wear pattern is quite unusual. The plane of the wear facets on the incisors is consistent with translation movements in normal centric occlusion. The jaw must be retracted several millimeters to bring the remaining wear facets into contact. In this position the left maxillary canine fits a deep groove on the labial and interproximal surfaces of the mandibular canine and anterior premolar, and the distal surface of the second mandibular premolar has an extensive contact facet corresponding to a facet on the mesial surface of the maxillary M1. On the right the canines and premolars form a similar set of wear planes that have resulted in pulp exposure in both canines. The facets that are in contact when the jaw is retracted are arranged in a pattern that is consistent with limited lateral movements of the lower jaw, and they suggest that the extreme wear seen in SL 0976-80 is a product of bruxism rather than normal functional occlusion. In contrast, wear in the functional right upper and lower second molars does not penetrate the dentin, but it is difficult to assign a meaning to this relatively slight degree of wear in a dentition as incomplete as this one.

Histological techniques for age assessment are more promising. However, the effects of function, pathology, and population-specific rates of age change are important, just as they are in gross evaluation of wear. I would like to discuss each of the histological aging techniques in the light of these issues.

The Gustafson technique is a summed score of point scores assigned to six variables: attrition, secondary dentin deposition, paradontosis, cementum deposition, root resorption, and root transparency. All variables are scored on a scalar 0-to-3-point basis, and all are weighted equally. Buccolingual longitudinal sections are used. Tooth position is not taken into account. Scores for single teeth are interpreted against a linear regression of score against age. Gustafson claims an average error of about 3.6 years in a sample of 41 teeth or a 95 percent confidence interval of about seven years. The nature of the sample is not described, but he does suggest that poor dental care may result in higher than usual scores (Gustafson, 1950). Because this technique weighs attrition equally with other age changes, the attrition component of the score may underestimate age for SL 0976-80 when posterior teeth are considered and overestimate it when anterior teeth are considered. On the other hand, the advanced periodontal disease in this specimen will result in a high age estimate.

Several tests and modifications of Gustafson's technique have appeared since 1950. Johanson (1971) applied Gustafson's technique to a sample of 162 teeth from 46 individuals. Gustafson derives from Johanson's work the following technical recommendations (Gustafson 1966): that anterior teeth are more reliable than premolars and molars, that the six variables together are more reliable than any single variable, that scores from several teeth should be averaged where possible, that paradontosis must be scored on the alveolus rather than on the isolated tooth, and that the optimal section thickness for scoring transparency is 0.25 mm. Because these recommendations are somewhat more accessible to workers in the United States than is Johanson's original article, they require some comment. First, 98 percent of Johanson's sample consisted of single-rooted teeth, and position-specific formulae are not given. For this reason, it is best to consider the question of choice of tooth for sectioning as not answered in this study. Second, Johanson's discussion indicates that he used gross rather than microscopic evaluation of root transparency. His discussion of section thickness relates to photography rather than to the observation of transparency per se.

Johanson made several modifications of Gustafson's technique. He refined the scale by introducing half point values between the four whole point values proposed by Gustafson. Since the Gustafson values are attained stages and the interpolated values include the whole point value, this will have the effect of increasing the summed score for a given tooth. For this reason, the resulting regression lines are not strictly comparable. Johanson presents regression analyses for each variable and for the summed score, as well as multiple regression analysis of combinations of the variables. Correlations between age and score for the individual variables range from .24 for resorption to .86 for transparency. The correlation coefficient between age and the sum of all six variables was .92. Johanson's study yielded a 95 percent confidence limit of 14 years for the summed score and 10 years for a weighted score on the same sample.

Other investigators have tested Gustafson's technique on independent samples with mixed results. DeChaume (1960) reached age estimates within five years of actual age in 80 percent of a sample of 100 individuals, but excluded some showing pathological changes before evaluating the results. Errors larger than five years were systematically distributed, young adults being assigned older ages because of periodontal disease or abrasion accompanied by secondary dentin formation, and certain older adults being under aged because they lacked age changes in these three variables. All other investigators who have replicated Gustafson's study have, like Johanson, found the technique to be less accurate than Gustafson claimed (Miles, 1963; Naldabian and Soggnaes, 1960; Burns and Maples, 1976). Maples and Rice have pointed out that Gustafson's original error analysis was incorrect. They reanalyze his data, finding a standard error of about seven years (Maples and Rice 1979), a figure that is consistent with the other replication studies.

Apart from this statistical problem, several other issues cloud the interpretation of the Gustafson study and the various replication studies. In none of the five studies is the nature of the sample described in any detail. All appear to be based on samples of clinically extracted teeth. One would expect such samples to include carious teeth, teeth from prospective denture patients with advanced periodontal disease, and healthy teeth from orthodontic patients, the mixture depending on the nature of the clinic population. Maples and Rice (1979) have argued that this factor explains many discrepancies in the published estimates and that more heterogenous, less selected samples can be expected to give more precise results. There has yet been no systematic attempt to evaluate the effects of caries and periodontal disease on the Gustafson technique or to construct standards that take dental pathology into account.

A second issue concerns the definition of the sample. Most authors report the number of teeth studied. Both Gustafson and Johanson discuss determinations based on averages of scores from several teeth, but neither reports the number of individuals included in his sample. The number of ties in true age figures in Gustafson's table of raw data suggests that his study may be based on teeth from as few as 25 individuals; Nalbandian's plot also contains many ties. Johanson's regression analysis is based on 46 individual estimates using a variable number of teeth per individual. Both of these procedures are statistically suspect and may artificially reduce the error of estimate.

In addition to this series of studies replicating Gustafson's method, there are several studies that have proposed modifications reducing the number of variables. Vlček and Mrklas (1975) were unable to score root transparency or paradontosis in archeological specimens. They present a reanalysis of Gustafson's data omitting these variables. Nalbandian and Soggnaes (1960) suggest that two of Gustafson's variables—attrition and root resorption—provide little useful information in their sample, and they propose a reevaluation of the technique using only the four remaining variables. Fanning (1962) reports increased root resorption in carious teeth, a result that supports Nalbandian and Soggnaes's proposal.

These studies raise the issue of the relative reliability of the variables included in Gustafson's summed score. Burns and Maples (1976) have investigated the relationship between age, tooth position, and Gustafson's variables considered independently and in combination. They found that root transparency is the most reliable age indicator and that root resorption is least correlated with age, a result similar to Johanson's. Maples (1978) has presented position-specific regression formulae for calculating age from the five variables excluding root resorption and from secondary dentin and root transparency alone. Standard errors for these formulae range from 9 to 13 years. Half point values were used as a refinement of the original 0 to 3 scale proposed by Gustafson. Burns and Maples (1976) report that tooth position, sex, and race as well as presence of diagnosed periodontal disease made significant contributions to the multiple regression determination of age and that weightings of variables derived from multiple regression analysis allowed more accurate age determination than did Gustafson's unweighted technique. While improvements over the accuracy obtained in the various tests of Gustafson's method are modest in Maples's studies, there is some improvement, and the formulae he presents for calculating age from root transparency and secondary dentin formation alone are least likely to be influenced by pathological conditions, functional considerations, abrasiveness of the diet, and related factors that alter the relationship between age and Gustafson score in interpopulation comparisons (Cook and Rusch-Behrend, n. d.).

In addition to these tests and modifications of Gustafson's technique, several age determination systems based on single histological indicators have been proposed. Zander and Hurzeler (1958) present an elaborate technique for calculating cementum thickness on serial transverse sections. Cementum thickness is calculated from the area of cementum in the transverse section, the length of the internal boundary of the cementum, and the length of the external boundary of the cementum. These values are evaluated at the apex, midroot, and cervical regions of the root as well as extrapolated to the root as a whole. A sample of 233 single-rooted teeth showing no periodontal disease was used in their study. No analysis of accuracy of age assessment is given, but regression curves for their data are plotted with 95 percent confidence intervals. Tooth position was found to be unimportant. Decreased cementum formation was found in a second sample of diseased teeth (Hurzeler and Zander 1959).

Philippas and Applebaum have considered secondary dentin formation in the anterior teeth (1966, 1967, 1968). Their data are presented as age-typical stages for each tooth position without statistical analysis. Secondary dentin formation is evaluated in longitudinal buccolingual sections, as in the Gustafson technique. Their sample consisted of 273 teeth obtained at autopsy. Specimens were selected for absence of severe attrition, caries, or erosion. An interesting perspective on this study is provided by Lantelme et al. (1976). They evaluated secondary dentin formation in healthy and periodontally diseased teeth in Zander and Hurzeler's serial transverse sections by measuring average pulp canal diameter following the methods of Zander and Hurzeler (1958). Diseased teeth showed narrowing of the canal at all levels. While pulp canal size decreased with age in both samples, age changes are quite small with respect to the difference between the diseased and healthy teeth. Contributions of both age and disease to analysis of variance were significant, except that age made no significant contribution to apical pulp canal diameter.

Transparent dentin formation has been evaluated in univariate studies by Miles and by Johnson. Miles published regression data on the length of the transparent or sclerotic portion of the root (1963a, 197). Scatter in these data is pronounced, but Miles found the technique as accurate as Gustafson's for the same sample. This technique assumes some regularity in the progression of transparency from apex to crown. While this is commonly the case, cementum to pulp patterns also occur (Nalbandian and Soggnaes, 1960). Nalbandian and Soggnaes (1960) report that these changes are generally symmetrical and consistent from tooth to tooth in an individual, but the effects of caries and periodontal disease on this indicator have not been systematically evaluated. Johnson (1968) measured the area of transparent and opaque dentin in both the crown and root dentin of a sample of 27 individuals. He calculated ratios of transparent to opaque dentin for the crown, root, and secondary dentin as well as for the total dentin from longitudinal sections. None of these data showed significant correlation with age.

ANALYSIS

Undecalcified buccolingual longitudinal sections of six teeth from SL 0976-80 were prepared. Teeth were cast in dental stone to provide a permanent record of crown features, embedded in epoxy, cut in the desired plane using a Buehler Isomet® low-speed saw, mounted on slides, sectioned to 150 microns, and polished using a Buehler Minimet® polisher. The Gustafson variables and other required observations were then made using a 10x hand lens and a 40x polarizing microscope equipped with a measuring reticle. Observations appear in Table 22-II, as do evaluations following the various standards discussed in the text.

Examining first the raw scores, we note that the paradontosis, cementum, and transparency scores are high for all teeth, while the attrition and secondary dentin scores are low. The anomalies of dental wear in this individual are reflected in the anteroposterior gradient in attrition scores, and differences in eruption age are mirrored in the differences in the left M1, M2, and M3. Despite the absence of functional occlusion on the left, the left and right M2 are quite similar. The right M2 was assigned a 2.5 cementum score because there is a thick mass of interradicular cementum on this tooth. Cementum on the lingual root of the right M2 is actually somewhat

TABLE 22-II
EVALUATION OF GUSTAFSON VARIABLES AND AGE ESTIMATES

Variable	L11	LC	LM1	LM2	LM3	RM2		
Attrition	2	2	0	0.5	0	1		
Paradontosis	3	3	3	3	3	3		
Secondary dentin	1	1	1	1	0	1.5		
Cementum	2.5	2.5	2.5	2.5	2.5	2.5		
Transparency	2.5	2.5	2.5	2.5	2.5	2.5		
Root resorption	0	0	0	0	0	0		
TOTAL[a], whole points	10	10	9	8	8	9		
TOTAL[b], half points	11	11	9.5	9.5	8.5	10.5		
Standards							*Range*	*Mean*
Gustafson[a]	53	53	51	44	44	51	44–53	49
Nalbandian[a]	54	54	50	43	43	50	43–54	49
Johanson[b]	68	68	60	60	54	65	54–68	62
Johanson ST[c]	58	58	58	58	52	61	52–61	58
Johanson APSCTR	65	65	60	60	52	64	52–65	61
Maples ST[c]	55	70	35	53	60	59	35–70	55
Maples APSCT	63	70	41	49	55	58	41–70	56

[a]Based on sum of points rounded down to whole values
[b]Based on sum of points including fractional values
[c]Letter abbreviations refer to variables included in the summed score for a standard

less thick than on the left. On the other hand, there is somewhat less sclerosis of the dentin in the functional M2 than in the nonfunctional one (Fig. 22-2), but this does not result in a different score. None of these teeth show root resorption, and the irregular area at the apex of the canine represents a section through the root wall rather than the Howship's lacunae characteristic of this lesion (Nalbandian and Soggnaes, 1960).

Age estimates for SL 0976-80 obtained from the various standards published for the Gustafson technique and its modifications vary widely. Age estimates for the canine are highest for the techniques that ignore position, and not surprisingly, estimates for the M3 are generally lowest. The nonfunctional left molars are somewhat "younger" than the remaining teeth. Ranges for the six teeth vary from 9 to 35 years, depending on the standards applied. Given this broad range, the means for the various techniques are fairly consistent. Appropriate confidence intervals are difficult to assign because they are sample-specific, and samples on which the published intervals are calculated are unlikely to be representative for this individual. A confidence interval of plus or minus 15 years is an appropriately conservative estimate, however. It is interesting to note that Maples's and Johanson's ST[c] techniques do not give results that differ greatly from the remainder, although these formulae exclude variables that one would expect to be most sensitive to pathological changes.

Results of the univariate techniques are less extensive because standards are published only for the anterior teeth (Table 22-III). Miles's technique for metric evaluation gives a lower best estimate than do the various applications of the Gustafson technique or its modifications, but the published confidence interval is broad enough to include all of the latter means. The Phillippas stage technique for secondary dentin formation suggests a markedly low age for the incisor, but this technique produces an age that is consistent with the Gustafson ages for the canine.

TABLE 22-III
UNIVARIATE OBSERVATIONS AND AGE ESTIMATES

Technique	Observation		Estimate	Confidence Interval
Miles root transparency	LI1	5mm	44	20–65
Philippas secondary dentin stage	LI1	VI	31–35	—
	LC	VI–VII	46–60	—
Zander cementum thickness	LI1 Apex	.113	56	±40
	Mid-root	.194	50	±40
	Cervical	.788	82	±48
	LC Apex	.068	32	±40
	Mid-root	.369	90	±40
	Cervical	1.15	113	±48

Application of the Zander and Herzeler technique can only be approximated because a tooth that has been longitudinally sectioned cannot be sectioned transversely for their procedure. To approximate their observation, I measured cementum thickness perpendicular to the occlusoapical axis of the tooth using a reticle. Buccal and lingual measurements were averaged at each of three levels: .75 mm cervical to the apex of the dentin, midroot and .75 mm apical to the cementoenamel junction. These average thicknesses are evaluated according to the standards published by Zander and Herzeler. The resulting estimates illustrate erratic behavior of this indicator in periodontal disease. The apical estimate is the only one to include tissue still in the alveolus in this specimen. These results are roughly consistent with the Gustafson results, although the confidence limits for this technique are so broad as to limit its usefulness.

Estimates from the Gustafson, Nalbandian, Miles, and Philippas standards support the osteological age assessment of 40 to 55. Estimates from the Johanson and Zander techniques largely support the medical examiner's assessment, while the Maples standards produce an age estimate that lies in the range of overlap between the two. In summary, although this group of techniques produces a rather wide range of estimates, it does suggest a best age estimate of approximately 55. The wide range of estimates may reflect uncontrolled population differences in the rate of accumulation of age changes or the effect of pathological conditions on aging, small sample size in the original studies, statistical problems arising from the conversion of

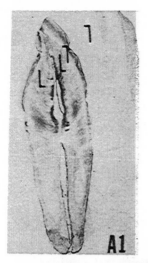

A1

Figure 22-2 A–F. These tooth sections range from 75 to 100 microns in thickness. Views of whole teeth are photographed in transmitted light, and all are photographed at the same scale. Micrographs are taken at 13×. The camera field is approximately 2.5 by 3.5 millimeters. Markers indicate locations of the micrographs on the tooth sections. Letters indicate enamel (e), dentin (d), opaque dentin (o), transparent dentin (t), cementum (c), calculus (k), secondary dentin (s), and pulp (p). A1. Upper left central incisor, buccal side to the right. A2 (upper markers). Occlusal extreme of the pulp cavity, showing moderate secondary dentin formation. A3 (lower markers). Buccal enamel showing linear enamel hypoplasia and prounced striae of Retzius. There is early caries in the deepest part of the hypoplastic depression. Dentin of pulpal margins is opaque.

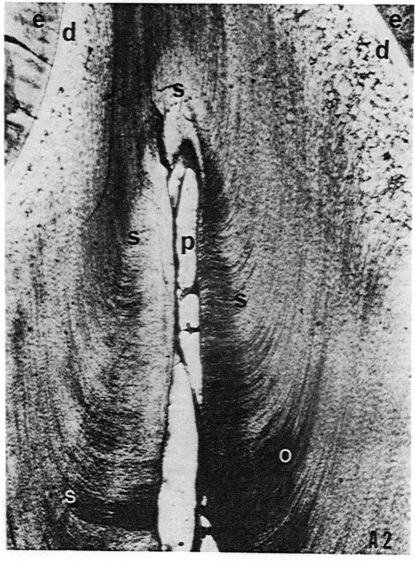

A2

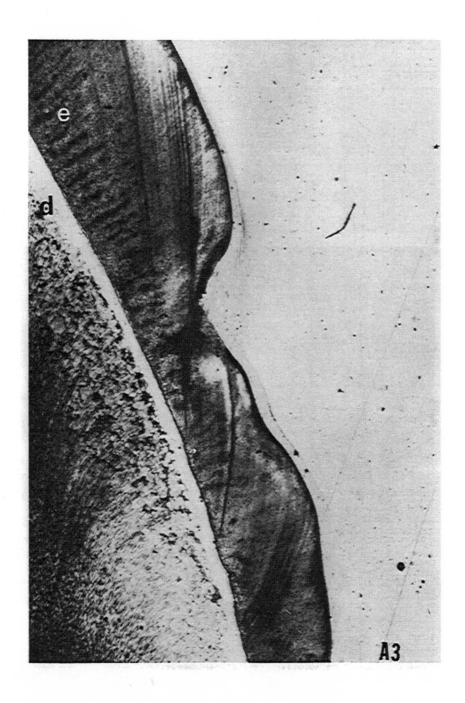

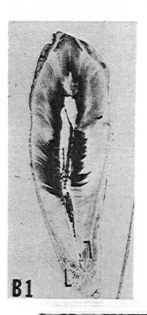

B1. Upper left canine, buccal side to the left. Note the wear and heavy cementum formation B2. The micrograph shows irregular form of the apex of the root. Howslip's lacunae are not present; hence this appearance is not evidence for root resorption as coded by Gustafson. Most of the dentin is opaque.

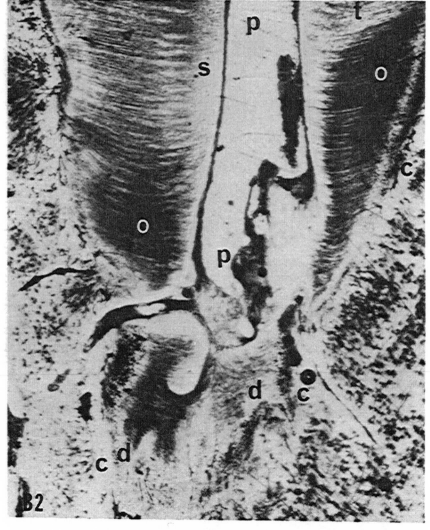

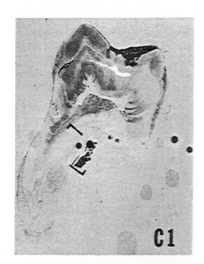

C1. Upper left M1, buccal side to the left. Note the lack of wear and calculus deposition in the occlusal caries and in the interradicular space. Secondary dentin formation is relatively slight. C2. The micrograph, taken in polarized light, shows calculus, cementum, and transparent dentin.

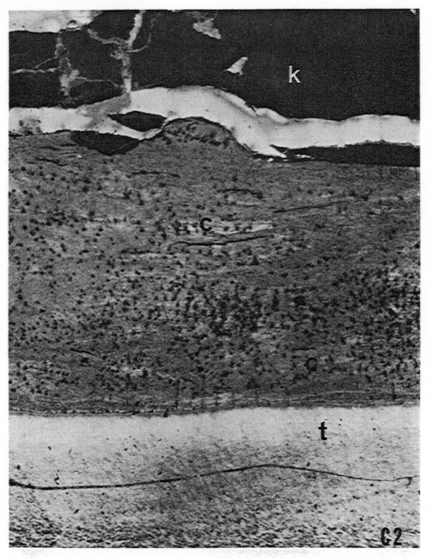

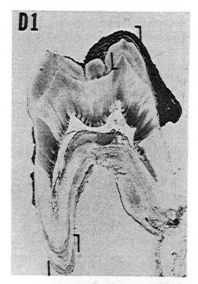

D1. Upper left M2, buccal side to the right. Calculus deposits on the occlusal surface are quite thick. D2 (upper markers). Micrograph of the buccal cusp, showing layered calculus covering a chip in the enamel of the cusp tip. Apart from this fracture, this cusp shows no wear, indicating that the opponent was lost very early in life. D3 (lower markers). Micrograph of the cementum at the apex of the lingual root. There is no root resorption.

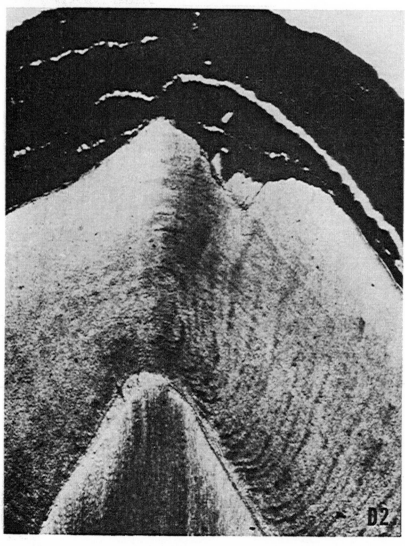

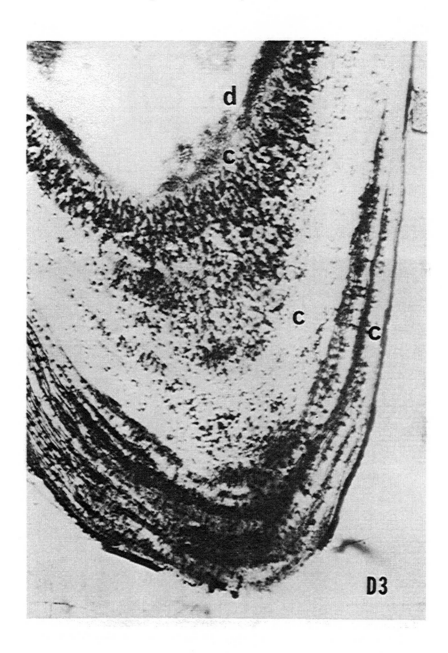

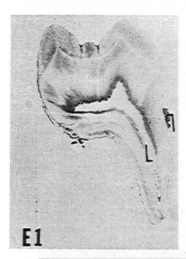

E1. Upper right M2, buccal side to the left. E2. The micrograph shows opaque and transparent dentin and cementum. Compare this with D.

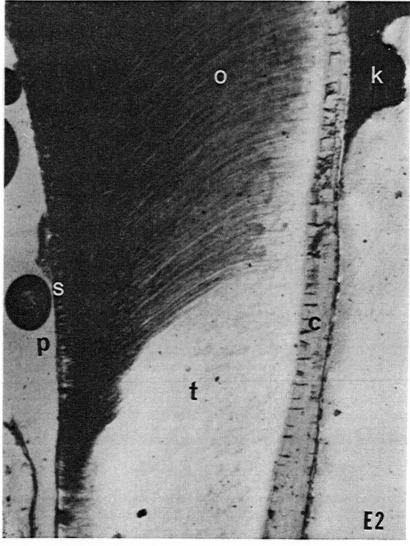

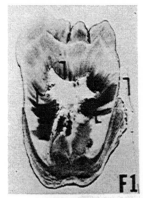

F1. Upper left M3, buccal side to the left. Note the relatively slight formation of secondary dentin, extensive opaque dentin, and heavy cementum deposition. F2 (upper markers). Micrograph of the pulp cavity, showing minimal secondary dentin formation. The structure marked X and the circular structures in the dentin are bubbles in mounting medium. F3 (lower markers). Cementum at the periodontal margin, 2 millimeters removed from the cementoenamel junction. Note the opaque and transparent dentin.

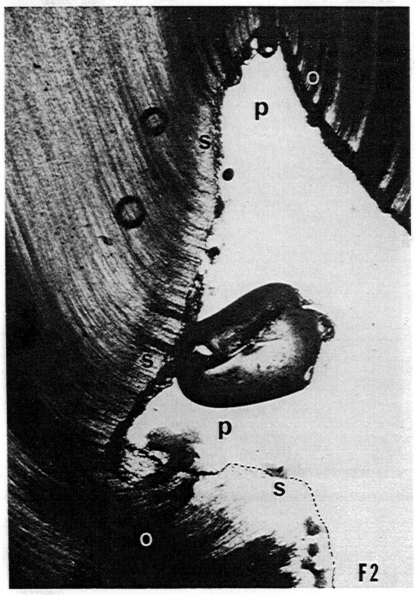

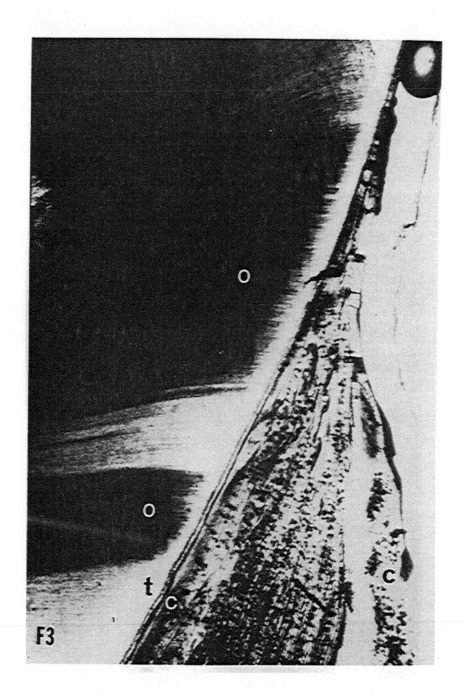

scalar variables to continuous ones for the purposes of regression analysis, or some combination of these factors. The techniques are promising, however, and more attention to their standardization and application to known ages cases is certainly desirable. Until such studies are available, it seems wisest to use more than one standard, to evaluate as many teeth from each case as is feasible, and to approach the published error estimates with some caution.

DISPOSITION

SL 0976-80 remains unidentified.

REFERENCES

Bluestone, R. (1979). Ankylosing spondylitis. In D. J. McCarty (Ed.): *Arthritis and Allied Conditions*. Philadelphia: Lea and Febiger.

Buikstra (1980). Osteologist's report on #976-80.

Burns, K. R., and Maples, W. R. (1976). Estimation of age from individual adult teeth. *J Forensic Sci*, 21:343–356.

Cameron, J. M., and Sims, B. G. (1974). *Forensic Dentistry*. Edinburgh: Churchill, Livingstone.

Cook, D. C., and Rusch-Behrend, G. (n.d.). Calibration of the Gustafson dental age estimation method in a prehistoric Amerindian sample: A perspective on the need for population-specific standards. In preparation.

Dahlberg, A. A. (1960). Clinical aging patterns in teeth of different population groups. In N. W. Shock (Ed.): *Aging: Some Social and Biological Aspects*. American Association for the Advancement of Science Publications No. 65.

DeChaume, M., DeRobert, L., and Payen, J. (1960). De la valeur de la détermination de lââge par l'examen des dentes coupes minces. *Annales de Médicine Légale, de Criminologie, et de Police Scientifique*, 40:165–167.

El-Najjar, M. Y., and McWilliams, K. R. (1978). *Forensic Anthropology*. Springfield: Charles C Thomas.

Fanning, E. (1962). The relationship of dental caries and root resorption of deciduous molars. *Arch Oral Biol*, 7:595–601.

Gustafson, G. (1950). Age determinations of teeth. *J Am Dent Assoc*, 41:45–54.

Gustafson, G. (1966). *Forensic Odontology*. New York: American Elsevier.

Hurzeler, B., and Zander, H. A. (1959). Cementum apposition in periodontally diseased teeth. *Helv Odontol Acta*, 3:1–3.

Johanson, G. (1971). Age determinations in human teeth. *Odontologisk Revy, 22 (supplement 21)*:1–126.

Johnson, C. C. (1968). Transparent dentine in age estimation. *Oral Surg*, 25:834–848.

Kerley, E. R. (1978). Recent developments in forensic anthropology. *Yearbook of Physical Anthropology*, 21:160–173.

Kraus, B. S. (1957). The genetics of human dentition. *J Forensic Sci*, 32:420–428.

Krogman, W. M. (1962). *The Human Skeleton in Forensic Medicine*. Springfield: Charles C Thomas.

Lantelme, R. L., Handelman, S. L., and Herbison, R. J. (1976). Dentin formation in periodontally diseased teeth. *J Dent Res*, 55:48–51.

Maples, W. R. (1978). An improved technique using dental histology for estimation of adult age. *J Forensic Sci, 23:*747–770.

Maples, W. R., and Rice, P. M. (1979). Some difficulties in the Gustafson dental age estimations. *J Forensic Sci, 24:*168–172.

Masi, A. T., and Medsger, A. T. (1979). Epidemiology of the rheumatic diseases. In D. J. McCarty (Ed.): *Arthritis and Allied Conditions.* Philadelphia: Lea and Febiger.

Miles, A. E. W. (1963a). Dentition in the estimation of age. *J Dent Res, 42:*255.

——— (1963b). The dentition in the assessment of individual age in skeletal material. In D. R. Brothwell (Ed.): *Dental Anthropology.* Oxford: Pergamon.

Moskowitz, R. W. (1979). Clinical and laboratory findings in osteoarthritis. In D. J. McCarty (Ed.): *Arthritis and Allied Conditions.* Philadelphia: Lea and Febiger.

Murphy, T. (1959). Gradients of dentine exposure in human molar tooth attrition. *Am J Phys Anthropol, 17:*179–186.

Nalbandian, J., and Sognnaes, R. F. (1960). Structural changes in human teeth. In N. W. Shock (Ed.): *Aging: Some Social and Biological Aspects.* American Association for the Advancement of Sciences Publication No. 65.

Philippas, G. C., and Applebaum, E. (1966). Age factor in secondary dentin formation. *J Dent Res, 45:*778–789.

——— (1967). Age changes in permanent upper lateral incisors. *J Dent Res, 46:*1002–1009.

——— (1968). Age changes in the permanent upper canine teeth. *J Dent Res, 47:*411–417.

Sokoloff, L. (1979). Pathology and pathogenesis of osteoarthritis. In D. J. McCarty (Ed.): *Arthritis and Allied Conditions.* Philadelphia: Lea and Febiger.

Stewart, T. D. (1979). *Essentials of Forensic Anthropology: Especially as Developed in the United States.* Springfield: Charles C Thomas.

Vlček, E., and Mrklas, L. (1975). Modifications of the Gustafson method of determination of age according to teeth on prehistorical and historical osteological material. *Scripta Medica, 48:*203–208.

Zander, H. A., and Hurzeler, B., (1958). Continuous cementum apposition. *J Dent Res, 37:*1035–1044.

Chapter 23

A FORENSIC TEST CASE
FOR A NEW METHOD OF
GEOGRAPHICAL RACE DETERMINATION

GEORGE W. GILL

INTRODUCTION

For years a human identification problem has existed in the northwestern Great Plains of North America in distinguishing the skeletal remains of whites from those of native American Indians. This is true in both archaeological and forensic contexts, since both major geographical races have inhabited the region for over a century and a half.

When a cranium possesses anterior dentition, race determination problems are lessened due to the much higher incidence of shovel-shaped incisors among the American Indians (and related Mongoloids). Race differences for this trait are far from absolute, however (Carbonell 1963), and incisors are often missing from skulls postmortem. The Giles and Elliot (1962) craniometric discriminant function method for differentiating the three main geographical races of North America (black, white, American Indian) works well in many regions, but often misclassifies American Indian crania of the northwestern plains (Gill and Lanum, n.d.). Many of the American Indian crania from Wyoming and Montana are classed by the method as "Negroid."

Due to these region-specific problems I began nearly a decade ago to develop a visual method of assessing crania based upon interorbital shape of the frontal process of the maxilla, in conjunction with other features of midfacial projection. Alice Brues (1980), University of Colorado, has apparently faced similar challanges of race determination in an adjacent

I wish to extend a special thanks to Dr. William M. Bass, University of Tennessee, for assisting me with the first interorbital study beyond the initial student class project and for helping me get to the 31st Annual Meeting of the American Academy of Forensic Sciences in Atlanta in 1979 to announce the results. I also want to thank Mr. Norman Newlon and Mr. Ronald Sargent of the Wyoming State Crime Laboratory for their encouragement and assistance in tracing the ancestry of the subject. Important assistance was also provided by Alonzo T. Spang, Superintendent of the Wind River Indian Agency, and the family of the decedant in obtaining the precise geneological details for this study. — George W. Gill region of the West and has developed somewhat similar visual methods. The Brues method is concerned more with differences in slope of the nasal bones and less with the adjacent maxilla but focuses on precisely the same area of the face.

After a few years of successful use of the visual method, metric quantification and further testing of the technique were done by Susan S. Hughes as part of a graduate seminar class at the University of Wyoming in 1978. The success of the Hughes pilot study on the small University of Wyoming skeletal sample stimulated three subsequent projects and reports designed primarily to expand sample sizes (Gill and Hughes, 1979; Bennett, 1979; Gill, Gilbert, Bennett, and Hughes, n.d.) and also resulted in preliminary publication of the 1978 pilot study (Hughes, 1980).

In the fall of 1979, at a point in the investigation when the sample size of whites and American Indians surpassed 195 and the technique was well tested, the University of Wyoming Physical Anthropology Laboratory received Forensic Case 17 (Wyoming State Crime Lab Case 79392). The case consisted of a fully clothed, completely skeletonized young male of unknown racial affinity found by duck hunters near Glenrock, Wyoming. The details of this case illustrate two points: (1) the problems of race determination from specimens exhibiting mixed ancestry and (2) the possible utility of our new metric method in solving difficult race identification cases like the one discussed here.

MATERIALS AND METHODS

Background details of the new interorbital technique are available from the author in a number of preliminary reports (Gill and Hughes, 1979; Bennett, 1979; Gill, 1980; Hughes, 1980), and further considerations are soon to be presented elsewhere (Gill, Gilbert, Bennett, and Hughes, n.d.). So, only a few historical comments and theoretical issues will be addressed here.

The Hughes (1980) project uncovered four measurements useful for the estimation of American Indian–white differences in midface projection (Appendix 1, definition sections 1 and 2). These and the two indices derived from them, maxillofrontal index and zygoorbital index, are defined in the available literature (Bass, 1971; Howells, 1973). One of these measurements requires specialized coordinate calipers (simometer), which are illustrated by Howells (1973). These calipers were constructed at the University of Wyoming according to the Howells plan. Hughes then developed two additional important measurements with the same instrument (Appendix 1, definition section 3), which result in what we have termed the *alpha index*.

Sample sizes were still small at the conclusion of the Hughes project, but through the cooperation of colleagues at the University of Tennessee, I was able to begin expanding numbers of both white and American Indian racial groups (Gill and Hughes, 1979). Bennett (1979) later increased the total sample size to 195 individuals and used American Indian collections from various regions of North America. This allowed the establishment of the cutoff points of 40, 40, and 60 for each of the three indices (see Appendix 1, page 1). Even though none of the three indices by itself produces more than about 80 percent accuracy in separating American Indians from whites, by using all three in conjunction (a simple two-out-of-three notation), Bennett (1979) was able correctly to classify slightly over 90 percent of her sample. This compares quite favorably with the craniometric method of Giles and Elliot (1962), which is capable of producing 82.6 percent accuracy for males in some instances and 88.1 percent for females. The Giles and Elliot method, however, has been found lacking when applied to American Indian samples of the Southwest (Birkby, 1966) and the northwestern plains (Gill and Lanum, n.d.). This probably has to do with the limited geographical distribution of the Giles and Elliot (1962) American Indian sample (from Indian Knoll only). It is hoped that the broadly selected samples of both American Indians and whites in the present study will assist in avoiding the problems encountered through wide application of the Giles and Elliot method.

B. Miles Gilbert, Anthropology Museum, University of Wyoming, provided additional data from 103 whites and 101 blacks from the Smithsonian Terry Collection. He also collected simometer measurements from a small sample of Eskimos. Later Gilbert conducted a discriminant function analysis using not only the metric variables defined here but also some midfacial measurements. Some of these eventually proved to be poor discriminators, and thus the total was reduced to the six variables defined here. The discriminant function analysis has provided useful information on the ways in which blacks and Eskimos pattern for these same traits, but does not suggest any better way for separating American Indians from whites. As Eugene Giles, University of Illinois, predicted in 1979 when reviewing a preliminary report of this study, the three indices in combination have turned out to be a simpler, more accurate, and more efficient way of making the American Indian–White separations than the use of discriminant function formulae.

Preliminary results of Gilbert's work indicate that both Eskimos and blacks pattern similarly to the American Indian with regard to the three indices. Therefore our separations seem to be defining more than merely American Indian–white differences. The indices are possibly quantifying a part of white midface projection that will allow separation of them from all nonwhites. This is certainly a possibility being explored at present, but since the existing cutoff figures have been developed for whites and American Indians only, the present method should not be extended beyond these two geographical racial groups.

FORENSIC CASE 17

The Office of the Attorney General, State of Wyoming, has a Forensic Human Identification Team as an adjunct to the Wyoming State Crime Laboratory. The team consists of a coordinator from the Crime Laboratory and three additional certified forensic scientists: a forensic pathologist, forensic anthropologist, and forensic odontologist. As forensic anthropologist, I am normally summoned for autopsies in cases involving unidentified human remains, especially when the remains are partially or wholly skeletonized. Such a case arrived at the Ivinson Memorial Hospital morgue, Laramie, Wyoming, in mid-October 1979 (U.W. Forensic Case 17; Wyoming State Crime Lab Case 79392). The specimen was a completely skeletonized young adult male, fully clothed in trousers, a jacket, and laced boots. He had several coins in one pocket but no identification. The remains had been found by duck hunters along the banks of the North Platte River near Glenrock, Wyoming. Small saplings had grown through the clothing, so the skeletal deposit was known to have been at least a few years old.

Due to the condition of the remains, the pathology examination was brief, and after radiographic analysis the entire specimen was turned over to the Physical Anthropology Laboratory. An inventory of remains showed the skeleton to be nearly complete except for a missing right radius, the left patella, cervical vertebrae 4 & 5, three coccygeal segments, a portion of the hyoid, three right carpals, and 24 phalanges. Three teeth were also missing postmortem, but the central incisors were present and in good condition.

The corroded coins from the trousers pocket were cleaned and the inventoried bones examined for skeletal pathology. No pathological conditions were found other than a divided right occipital condyle, which probably did not affect neck movement or carriage of the head.

Examination of the coins showed that all were dated 1972 or before, and most of the one cent pieces were nearly uncirculated 1972 Denver mint coins. These were then returned to the Crime Laboratory with the suggestion that 1972–73 records of missing persons be given priority.

The basic skeletal identification results were then obtained and were listed as follows in the October 19, 1979 report to the Wyoming State Crime Laboratory:

Sex: Male. Twelve of the 15 criteria utilized in sex determination point clearly to maleness and some of them (limb dimensions and shoulder breadth) should be conclusive.

Race: Caucasian. Nearly all key features of the skull, face and palate, as well as the

Giles-Elliot discriminant function metric analysis all indicate this racial affinity.

Age: 20 years. An age range of 18–21 years with a most probable age of 20 is suggested by eight cranial and post-cranial criteria. All criteria point to this same age bracket.

Stature: 5' 10 ¾". This adult living stature estimate of 179.64 ± 3.62 cm is based upon calculations from well preserved long bones of the legs (the most reliable indicators).

General comments: No indication of cause of death was found on the skeleton and no unusual anomalies other than a double right occipital condyle. This probably did not affect neck movement or carriage of the head, however. Numerous filled cavities of the teeth were observed on molars and premolars. The Part II report will list these in detail.

Of the above determinations only racial affinity appeared somewhat troublesome. All visual criteria pointed clearly to white ancestry except for a set of distinctly shovel-shaped central incisor teeth. Results of the study of Carbonell (1963), however, have shown that this trait alone cannot be relied upon as a definite indicator of Mongoloid affinities.

Even though the Giles-Elliot (1962) discriminant function analysis often misclassifies northwestern plains Indians (as Negroid), it appears to sort out whites with good reliability. In this case the Giles-Elliot results indicated white affinities (white-black 32.4 and white-Indian 19.3).

Two other forensic anthropologists in the region were consulted on race determination because of the apparent conflict between the incisor teeth and all other criteria. One concurred strongly in the white determination and the other was less certain because of the teeth. Some of the traits reviewed by us are listed in the case file as follows:

Cranial height and contour: Caucasoid
Sharp nasal spine and sill: Caucasoid
Mid-line prominence and retreat of the malars: Caucasoid
Limb proportions and femoral characteristics: Caucasoid
Shovel-shaped incisor teeth: American Indian or Mongoloid
Visually assessed shape of ascending ramus of maxilla and nasal bones: Caucasoid
Parabolic palate form: Caucasoid

At this point it seemed important to examine the precise amount of midface projection. Given, however, that the simometer was in use halfway across the country (for the Gilbert study of the Terry Collection) it was decided that a cast of the cranium should be made in case the remains were recalled before the simometer was returned. In this way the interorbital features test could at least be applied to a high quality cast of the decedent's cranium, if not the actual skull itself. With the help of Michael Charney, Center for Human Identification, Ft. Collins, Colorado, the cast was made.

Not long thereafter, in early December (the simometer still on loan), the team coordinator at the Wyoming State Crime Laboratory reported that a possible match had been made between a missing persons file and the decedent and that the individual had disappeared in 1972. However, he went on to say, if the match is correct then the person was an American Indian, not a white. "Could the specimen possibly represent an American Indian?" A response was made by letter on December 4, 1979 (see Appendix 2) with full confidence in the white racial assessment. Previously, difficult cases for racial identity had been analyzed for the Crime Laboratory and none had been missed before. So, as exemplified by the tone of the December 4 letter, little reason was seen to question the results, based upon traditional, previously established procedures (and especially in conjunction with the time-tested visual method). Not having the simometer was somewhat irritating but certainly not considered critical to the case.

Not long after this final communication of December 4, however, a positive identification of Victim 17 was made. Notification came from the Wyoming State Crime Laboratory that the forensic anthropology examination had been completely correct in all evaluations of the skeleton, except one — racial identity. The victim had been American Indian and not white. What had happened? A few law enforcement people were mildly amused. The forensic anthropologist was mildly irritated but, perhaps more important, deeply curious about just what had happened. Photographs of the victim were obtained and a complete geneological record requested from the Bureau of Indian Affairs, Wind River Indian Agency, Ft. Washakie, Wyoming. The photograph revealed very little white appearance to the young man's face, but the family history chart (281-U07044) produced the information that was strongly suspected by this time — significant American white ancestry. In fact, white ancestry was traced back through both paternal and maternal lines. The young man's father is recorded at the Wind River Bureau of Indian Affairs Office as unmixed Arapahoe, but thanks to follow-up investigation by the office superintendent, it was later learned that he was 1/2 white. The mother is fully documented as 17/32 Shoshone and 15/32 white. In other words, the decedent was approximately 1/2 white, 1/4 Shoshone and 1/4 Arapahoe.

The leading question then at this point was whether a person slightly more than 1/2 American Indian, showing largely native features externally, and obviously classed by all agencies as a Native American, could slip by as an unmixed white skeletally? The simometer was recovered and measurements of the skull cast taken to see if the interorbital features could add anything not previously revealed by the other metric and anthroposcopic techniques. The following measurements and indices were obtained:

Measurements			*Indices*	
1.	Nasomaxillofrontal subtense	8	Maxillofrontal	38.10
	Maxillofrontal breadth	21		
2.	Nasozygoorbital subtense	21	Zygoorbital	35.00
	Zygoorbital breadth	60		
3.	Nasoalpha subtense	18	Alpha	50.00
	Alpha chord	36		

As may be seen from the Appendix 1 charts and cutoff numbers, the cranium is classified American Indian by all three indices, even though figures are close to those for whites on maxillofrontal index.

CONCLUSIONS

A new osteometric method for distinguishing American Indian crania from those of whites has been developed based upon a sample of 298 (the 101 blacks are not included here), and the results so far indicate a very high percentage of accuracy in the placement of individuals of unmixed ancestry. This surpasses the results obtained by the more widely used Giles and Elliot (1962) discriminant function method, especially in areas of the American West where the Giles and Elliot system quite often misclassifies Native Americans. The new method would likewise seem to be more effective than previously used visual techniques and certainly in this latter instance has the advantage of objectivity for use in court testimony.

Since its use with Case 17 the method has also been used successfully during autopsy with cases where all soft tissue still remained (within 4 days after death in one case). This merely requires dissection of thin tissue over the nose and below the eyes to reveal the craniometric points. This, of course, constitutes another advantage of this method over the traditional Giles and Elliot system. In a recent Wyoming State Crime Laboratory case where I correctly classified an American Indian homicide victim on the autopsy table, using the interorbital feature method, the cranium was later skeletonized for casting and facial reconstruction. This allowed an opportunity to repeat the simometer measurements on the dry cranium. One of the six measurements varied by 1 millimeter, but no variation was exhibited among the other five, and all results were the same as previously obtained during autopsy. Apparently, then, very little, if any, distortion occurs when taking the measurements on recently deceased individuals where small amounts of fascia still adhere to the interorbital skeleton.

The forensic identification of Case 17 presented here suggests that American Indian midfacial features as revealed by use of the simometer may be more entrenched genetically than some other commonly studied skeletal features and therefore more likely to be of value in modern forensic examinations where varying amounts of white admixture are often present in the native populations. Certainly a single case does not prove this assertion, but it does stand as a single example suggesting intriguing possibilities that should be tested further. Certainly in the instance of Forensic Case 17 the mistaken conclusion of unmixed white ancestry would *not* have been reached had it been possible to apply the new interorbital method during preparation of the report.

REFERENCES

Bass, William M.: *Human Osteology: A Laboratory and Field Manual of the Human Skeleton.* Columbia, Missouri Archaeological Society, 1971.

Bennett, Suzanne M.: "The Use of Discriminant Function Analysis in the Assessment of Race." Laramie, Senior Honors Paper, Department of Anthropology, University of Wyoming, 1979.

Birkby, Walter: An evaluation of race and sex identification from cranial measurements. *Am J Phys Anthropol, 24*: 21–28, 1966.

Brues, A. M.: Discussant comments of the Forensic Anthropology Symposium. Denver, 40th Annual Meeting of the Society for Applied Anthropology, 1980.

Carbonell, Virginia M.: Variations in the frequency of shovel-shaped incisors in different populations. In Symposia of the Society for the Study of Human Biology: vol. V, *Dental Anthropology*, D. R. Brothwell (Ed.). Oxford, Pergamon, 1963.

Giles, Eugene, and Elliot, Orville: Race identification from cranial measurements. *J Forensic Sci, 7*:147–157, 1962).

Gill, George W.: Interorbital Skeletal Features in Race Identification: Additional Findings. Denver, paper presented at the 40th Annual Meeting of the Society for Applied Anthropology, 1980.

Gill, George W., Gilbert, B. Miles, Bennett, Suzanne M., and Hughes, Susan S.: Race Determination from Projection of the Mid-facial Skeleton (unpublished manuscript).

Gill, George W., and Hughes, Susan S.: Race Determination from Interorbital Skeletal Features. Atlanta, paper presented at the 31st Annual Meeting of the American Academy of Forensic Sciences, 1979.

Gill, George W., and Lanum, Philip: A Test of the Giles-Elliott Discriminant Function Approach on Northwestern Plains Skeletal Populations (unpublished manuscript).

Howells, W. W.: Cranial variation in man. A study by multivariate analysis of patterns of difference among recent human populations. *Papers of the Peabody Museum of Archaeology and Ethnology*, Harvard University, 67(xvi): 259pp., 1973.

Hughes, Susan S.: Differences in nasal projection between American Indian and Caucasian crania. Laramie, *Wyoming Contributions to Anthropology, 2*: 96–113, 1980.

APPENDIX 1

University of Wyoming Physical Anthropology Laboratory checklist for the interorbital features method or race determination.

2 *Mid-orbital breadth*--the breadth between zygoorbitale left and right.

Zygoorbitale is defined by Howells as "the intersection of the orbital margin and the zygomaxillary suture" (Howells 1973:170). Occasionally the suture meanders along the orbital border; then its most mesial location is chosen as zygoorbitale.

Naso-zygoorbital subtense--subtense from the zygoorbital points to the deepest point along the nasal bridge.

3 *Alpha cord*

The point alpha is the deepest point on the maxilla, left and right, on a tangent run between the naso-maxillary suture where it meets the nasal aperture, and zygoorbitale.
To determine alpha, a straight line is pencilled connecting the above two points, then a straight edge is placed across the two points, and the skull is turned upwards until the profile of the straight edge and pencilled line are visible. The deepest point is easy to find and it is marked on the pencilled line. The deepest point usually coincides with the slight concavity from which the maxilla rises anteriorly to the nasal aperture. When the concavity forms a long shallow depression in profile and the deepest point is difficult to determine, then the mid-point along the pencilled line is chosen.

Naso-alpha subtense--subtense from the alpha points to the deepest point on the nasal bridge.

Definitions adapted from Hughes (1980)

Bennett, S.M. (1979) The Use of Discriminant Function Analysis in the Assessment of Race. Senior Honors Paper, University of Wyoming, Laramie.

Gill, George W. (1980), see page 1 reference.

Gill, George W. and Susan S. Hughes (1979) Race Determination from Interorbital Skeletal Features. Paper presented at the 31st Annual Meeting of the Am. Academy of Forensic Science, Atlanta.

Hughes, Susan S. (1980) Differences in Nasal Projection Between American Indian and Caucasoid Crania. <u>Wyo. Contributions to Anthropology</u>, Vol. 2. pp. 96-113.

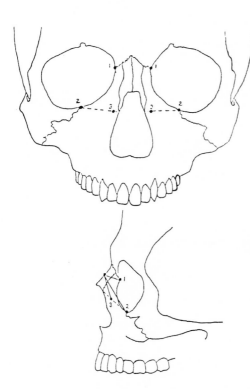

1 *Maxillofrontal breadth*--breadth between maxillofrontale left and right.

Maxillofrontale is defined by Bass (1971:60) as the intersection of the fronto-maxillary suture and "anterior lacrimal crest, or the crest extended (medial edge of the eye orbit)".

Naso-maxillofrontal subtense--subtense from the maxillofrontal points to the deepest point on the nasal bridge.

INDIAN–WHITE RACIAL DIFFERENTIATION

Interorbital Features Method

(Gill 1980)

Specimen:_____ Sex:_____

Location:_____ Age:_____

| Measurements | Indices | ■ Amer/Indian | □ White |

1. Naso-maxillo frontal subtense ____

   ÷ = _____ _____ 40 _____
   (maxillofrontal)

   Maxillofrontal breadth ____

2. Naso-zygoorbital subtense ____

   ÷ = _____ _____ 40 _____
   (zygoorbital)

   Zygoorbital breadth ____

3. Naso-alpha subtense ____

   ÷ = _____ _____ 60 _____
   (alpha)

   Alpha cord ____

   Race:_____

Maxillofrontal Index

15 20 25 30 35 40 45 50 55 60 65

Zygoorbital Index

15 20 25 30 35 40 45 50 55 60 65

Alpha Index

35 40 45 50 55 60 65 70 75 80

Gill, George W.
   1980 Interorbital Skeletal Features in Race Identification: Additional Findings. Paper
       Presented at the 40th Annual Meeting of the Society for Applied Anthropology, Denver.

APPENDIX 2

Letter to the coordinator of the Human Identification Team, Wyoming State Crime Laboratory, December 4, 1979.

December 4, 1979

Mr. Ron Sargent
Latent Fingerprint Examiner
State Crime Laboratory
591 Hathaway Bldg.
Cheyenne, WY 82002

Dear Ron:

I assume that you received my telephone message from Howard last week, regarding the recent skeletal I.D. (case #79392), but I thought a written follow-up for the file couldn't hurt. After discussing the question about racial affinities with you on the phone I did go back to my analysis sheets and take another look. Certainly the skeleton is basically Caucasian as I mentioned earlier in the full report; however, two more things are of interest here. Firstly, the upper central inciser teeth are clearly shovel-shaped to an extent that occurs with only about 10% of Whites, but most Indians. Secondly, the Giles-Elliot discriminant function analysis (based on cranial metrics) even though it classifies the skull as Caucasion does place it in a zone of overlap with American Indians.

So, the above information, even though it does not change my conclusion, does open up the possibility that the individual could have possessed some American Indian ancestry - perhaps even enough to live on the reservation as an American Indian, culturally. As I told Howard, though, the chances that the individual was unmixed American Indian are next to zero, but the possibility that he was mixed American-White racially (as many of our reservation Indians are) would be about 15-20%. Still, the vast majority of traits point squarely at Caucasian ancestry and the best over all conclusion from the skeletal evidence remains Caucasian.

I hope that this follow-up letter is of some value to you. When the I.D. of this individual is pretty well confirmed please let me know. Each one of these identified ones helps us "calibrate" our techniques.

Sincerely,

George W. Gill
Associate Professor

Section IV
INDIVIDUAL IDENTIFICATION

Besides the significance of establishing identity when criminal activity is suggested, specific identification of human remains may have legal ramifications in marital, economic, insurance, and historical realms. The forensic physical anthropologist can initially contribute in attempts to establish identity by identifying general biological categories of skeletal remains. Once these general features such as age and sex of the remains have been established, subsequent identification of unique skeletal or dental characters may be matched with existing information to develop a positive or a circumstantial identification.

Specific identity is usually established by a medical examiner, coroner, or law enforcement identification officer. In some instances, the level of evidence to establish identity may have to be evaluated by the court or an inquest. Decisions on specific identity often rest on the expert opinions of a number of consultants. Identification consultants contributing to the process usually include forensic odontologists for the teeth and surrounding structures, physical anthropologists for osteological data, clinical radiologists for cellular structure and internal bony characteristics, and crime lab personnel for identification of available hair or fingerprints. Collaboration among these specialists may also lead to productive new lines of investigation.

Biological data that allow positive identification include visual comparisons, fingerprints, dental records, and medical x-rays. In many jurisdictions, positive identification rests on congruous matches of fingerprints or dental characters with existing records. Circumstantial identification may sometimes be established and accepted from associated materials and the general compatibility of demographic aspects of a decedant with the skeletal remains.

The steps in identification in a given case depend upon the records available for comparison as well as the completeness and degree of preservation of the remains. Most standard reference texts for legal medicine and identification outline general procedures. Reviews that include procedures with reference to skeletonized remains and forensic anthropology are those by Stahl (1980), Snyder (1977), and Charney (1974, 1978). Svensson et al. (1981) document the importance of physical evidence and associated materials at the scene of discovery of remains for subsequent identification. Stewart (1979) provides anthropological examples of specific unique features that may lead to personal identification through comparisons with dental and medical records.

Although the case presentations in Sections II and III emphasize various categories for the identification process, individual identification is an element in most of them. The cases presented by Brooks and Brooks and by Bass in Section II illustrate the application of historical information as part of the battery of information sometimes necessary to document identity. The use of all available indicators in cases like these is exemplified by the analysis of Snow and Reyman and by Finnegan in this section. As with many of the examples in this volume, collaboration among specialists was important for final resolution of the cases.

Although fingerprints allow for positive identification if the tissues are preserved and records exist (see Chapter 24 for an example), skeletalized remains are frequently identified through comparison of dental and skeletal features with existing records. The importance of collaboration between anthropologists and odontologists is documented by Gladfelter (1975) and Snow (1982). Dental features such as rotated teeth, restorations, extractions, pathologies, and development are important considerations. In his discussion of burned remains, Heglar illustrates the importance of collaboration by an odontologist, radiologist, and anthropologist. Dental characters were also important in determining age and identity of the adolescent female in the example given by Perzigian and Jolly in Section III. Dental comparisons are often critical for positive identification, but frequently the teeth are lost after death, dental work is absent, or no records can be found. Even when medical or dental records exist, a lead or tentative identification is necessary to know which records to request and examine. Ubelaker (Chap. 29) documents frontal sinus comparisons.

For skeletonized materials without teeth, the most likely characters that would appear in medical records or x-rays are old fractures, evidence of surgical procedures, and in some instances, skeletal anomalies. The importance of such indicators is documented in the case presented by Rhine. In his case even after a tentative identification had been established through leads developed from a facial reproduction, positive identification depended upon congruent factors seen in the skeleton and the medical records of the decedent after the correct ones were obtained.

When traditional means of identification cannot be applied, leads can often be generated through less standard channels. Facial reproductions cannot yet be used to establish positive identity, but as both Rhine and Rathbun show, the publication of the results may stimulate investigative leads. The publicity factor is important in these instances. Both cases also suggest that improvements in the technique depend upon further research and testing of results. The availability of new tissue thickness standards for North American groups is an important step. Caldwell

(1981) has generated a useful bibliography on the technique and has compared the various guides to modeling facial features with death masks and skulls of known individuals. Further research and testing of the validity and replicability of results of facial reproductions should strengthen the acceptability of the approach.

Although facial reproduction techniques have experienced a revival of interest, other similar techniques such as the use of photo overlays with skulls and comparisons of skulls with portraits or photographs have considerable historical depth. Stewart (1979) and Krogman (1962) provide a number of examples. Direct comparisons of skulls with photographs, although apparently relatively simple, frequently require complex adjustments for correct alignment and leave considerable room for interpretation. Janssens et al. (1979) have documented some aspects of this type of superimposition. Snow and Reyman illustrate the creative use of new technology as it becomes available by superimposing television images of a skull and a photograph, as in the McGurdy case. This technique can be used also by forensic odontologists to compare smiling photographs with tooth size and anomalies in a particular skull. Dr. Tadao Furue, a physical anthropologist at Hawaii's Central Identification Laboratory, demonstrated a superimposition system with cameras and mirrors for comparisons of both skulls and teeth with photographs and dental x-rays at the 1981 annual meeting of the American Academy of Forensic Sciences.

Skeletal indicators of pathology can help establish identity. In the case presented by Maples, the analysis of the standard classes of information from the skeleton coupled with the diagnosis and interpretation of a specific pathology led to identification. Since many forensic anthropologists have developed expertise in the recognition and interpretation of skeletal pathologies, collaboration with pathologists is an important step in the medical interpretation. Maples makes the important point that description and identification of a particular condition alone frequently are not sufficient. Interpretation of the pathological features and the implications of the symptoms in the living are important aspects of the forensic analysis. Not only must the condition be recognized, it must be understandable to the nonspecialist. Snow and Reyman, as well as Finnegan, provide examples of how other pathologies during life such as trauma, scars, dental pathologies, and additional disease factors can provide direct and indirect evidence for identifying historical personages. It may also be important to relate skeletal features to activities of the decedent. In Section II Angel suggested sports and music hobbies from anatomical variation of the victim's skeleton. Documentation of other habitual activities and morphological changes, however, needs to be developed. Pathologies, life conditions, and skeletal indicators are important features in all the cases in this section.

Chemical analysis of the bone and surrounding tissue can be used to develop supportive evidence in the identification process. Trace elements incorporated in the bone during life, or in the mummified tissue from embalming as in the case presented by Snow and Reyman, have potential in documenting events surrounding death. For both trace element analysis as well as the chemical analysis of hair and blood factors, Finnegan correctly stresses the importance of collecting soil samples at the site of recovery. Although this information by itself cannot be used to establish positive identity, it forms part of the battery of physical evidence that can be used to develop a specific identity from circumstantial evidence.

The process of establishing specific identity will vary with individual circumstances, as do the necessary techniques with the completeness of the remains. The forensic physical anthropologist, as part of the identification team, can contribute expertise with bone and suggest lines of investigation for colleagues with different specialties that can corroborate some findings. Success in developing positive identifications frequently depends upon collaboration among a number of consultants and the availability of anatomical records. Cooperative research in this area will likely remain important in future developments in the forensic field.

REFERENCES

Caldwell, M. C. (1981). "The Relationship of the Details of the Human Face to the Skull and its Application in Forensic Anthropology." Master's thesis, Arizona State University.

Charney, M. (1974). Individual identification from human skeletal Material. In C. W. Wilber, *Forensic Biology for the Law Enforcement Officer*. Springfield: Charles C Thomas, pp. 288–332.

_____ (1978). Forensic anthropology. In D. J. Nash: *Individual Identification and the Law Enforcement Officer*. Springfield: Charles C Thomas, pp. 67–91.

Gladfelter, I. A. (1975). *Dental Evidence: A Handbook for Police*. Springfield: Charles C Thomas, pp. 24–47.

Janssens, P. A., Hansch, C. F., and Voorhamme, L. L. (1978). Identity determination by superimposition with anthropological cranium adjustment. *Ossa*, vol. 5, pp. 109–122.

Krogman, W. M. (1962). *The Human Skeleton in Forensic Medicine*. Springfield: Charles C Thomas.

Snow, C. C. (1982). Forensic anthropology. In J. A. Cottone and S. M. Standish (Eds.), *Outline of Forensic Dentistry*. Chicago: Yearbook Medical Publishers, pp. 34–53.

Snyder, L. (1977). Identification of dead bodies, In L. Snyder (Ed.), *Homicide Investigation*, 3rd ed. Springfield: Charles C Thomas, pp. 61–85.

Stahl, C. J. (1980). Identification of human remains. In W. U. Spitz and R. S. Fisher (Eds.), *Medicolegal Investigation of Death*. Springfield: Charles C Thomas, pp. 32–65.

Stewart, T. D. (1979). *Essentials of Forensic Anthropology*. Springfield: Charles C Thomas.

Svensson, A., Wendel, O., and Fisher, B. A. (1981). *Techniques of Crime Scene Investigation*, 3rd ed. New York: Elsevier, pp. 87–113.

Chapter 24

PERSONAL IDENTIFICATION
Facial Reproductions

TED A. RATHBUN

Recent media coverage has stimulated public interest in facial reproductions on unidentified skulls. Although the historical development and the application of the process have been well summarized (Krogman, 1962; Stewart, 1979), the technique has not been without criticism (Brues, 1958; Montagu, 1947; Stewart, 1954; Suk, 1935, Rathbun, 1966). Even after some testing of the results of reproductions (Krogman, 1946; Snow et al., 1970) and reports of the utility of reproductions in developing leads in a forensic setting (Rhine, 1977; Charney et al., 1978; Rhine and Campbell, 1980a; Ilan, 1964; Gerasimov, 1971; Rhine, this volume), the professional anthropological response has still been somewhat less than enthusiastic. Besides the questions of needed skills and time to complete a facial reproduction, reservations are often expressed about the applicability of tissue thickness standards from older European data and skepticism about average proportions of distinctive individual features such as the lips, nose tips, and eyes. New standards for American blacks have been published (Rhine and Campbell, 1980b), and data collected for American whites (Moore, 1980) are now available (Rhine and Moore, 1982).

The following case documents the utility of facial reproductions in developing potential leads through public response to published likenesses when traditional means of personal identification have been unsuccessful. Technical suggestions for the process are considered, and the case illustrates the effectiveness of the newly developed facial tissue thickness standards for American black females.

Appreciation is extended to Stanley Rhine and Homer Campbell for sharing prepublication data on facial thickness, Michael Charney for the cast and photo, Betty Pat Gatliff for advice on materials and procedures in reproduction, Coroner Frank Barron III for the opportunity to try the procedure on a forensic case, Sgt. R. E. McGee for making the positive identification through dermatoglyphics, Lieutenant Connie W. Lewis for the investigative work, and the Stokes Eye Clinic for providing prosthetic eyes. Kay West and Laura McGuire were responsible for most of the reproduction work on the cast and the case.

CASE REPORT

An extensively decomposed body was discovered in a wooded area outside the city limits by two men who smelled and then saw the body on Labor Day, September 2, 1979. They reported the finding to the County Sheriff's Department, and the Forensic Science Squad collected the remains and conducted the scene investigation. They determined two separate locations for the body from foliage decay and stains and noted that the feet were missing bilaterally, the central maxillary incisors were absent, and no clothing or jewelry was present. A bra was later found tangled with the ribs and vertebrae. The fingers, which were covered with leathery, dehydrated skin, were amputated by the investigators, secured in formalin, and taken to the Sheriff's Office laboratory. The skull, found near the legs, and the mandible, found 7 feet away in the brush, were almost totally void of soft tissue.

The consulting pathologist viewed the scene, and the remains were taken to the county hospital morgue for x-ray and further examination. When I was called to the morgue late in the afternoon, I found that connective tissue still united most of the postcranial skeleton, although the degree of articulation had been disturbed in transit. The thorax and distal extremities showed extensive animal chewing marks. The pathologist and I were in general agreement in our provisional assessment that the remains were of an adult black female of medium height and muscular build. The final pathologist's report indicated that the cause, manner, and time of death could not be determined because of the advanced state of decomposition.

I removed the skull, mandible, right innominate, and right femur to my osteology laboratory for further analysis. Since cartilage still adhered to certain areas of these bones, the innominate and femur were soaked in tap water overnight and then alternately immersed in solutions of enzyme detergents and sodium hypochlorite. As much tissue as possible was removed manually as it loosened. Snyder et al. (1975) and Stephens (1979) discuss this and other methods of preparing specimens for analysis.

Morphological characters of the innominate and the skull were characteristically female. The Giles and Elliot (1962) discriminate function score of the metric dimensions for the skull was 838.63, which is well below the female range cut point of 891. Racially definitive morphological characters included alveolar prognathism, nasal gutter, wide nasal aperture, low nasal bridge, and femora with little torsion and straight diaphyses. The sex-specific racial discriminate function score of the skull was 96.21 and in the black range of the black/white dichotomy. The white/Indian score was 13.89, which is just into the Indian range, which starts at 13.01 in the Giles and

Elliot (1962) matrices. Some possible Indian heritage was also suggested by slight shoveling on the lateral mandibular incisors and flat zygomatic bones.

Gross anatomical and radiographic examination indicated adult status. All of the epiphyses, including the medial clavicle, had completely united. No indications of degenerative joint changes or osteophytosis were noted by the radiologist. Pubic symphysis metamorphosis was assessed as a 6 with the Gilbert and McKern standards (1973), which indicated a mean age of 29 and a range of 25 to 36 years. (See Chapter 20 for discussions of methods and accuracy of age estimates using pubic symphyseal remodeling.) The completely obliterated sagittal suture and the extensive loss and alveolar resorption of the mandibular molars led me to suggest the upper portion of the range as the probable age at death.

The dentition exhibited no restorations even though large caries were noted and some periodontoclasia (alveolar resorption) around the roots was evident. Postmortem loss of the central maxillary incisors, which were never recovered, was indicated by the sharply defined root sockets with no signs of remodelling. Individualized features of the skull included depressed zygotemporal sutures, multiple mental foramina, and an old healed trauma on the left frontal. Maximum femur length yielded a calculated stature of 167 to 174 centimeters, 5 feet 5¾ inches to 5 feet 8½ inches (Trotter, 1970).

The results of the analysis were made available to law enforcement agencies and were released for publication in the local newspapers by the coroner. After a year, there were still no leads to identification.

FACIAL REPRODUCTION

The decision to attempt a facial reproduction on the unidentified skull developed informally from the confluence of academic, forensic, political, and public interests. Two undergraduate students in my forensic physical anthropology class requested the opportunity to learn the process and test the reliability of the reproductions by comparisons with premortem photographs. A skull cast and premortem photograph of a 26-year-old white female were obtained from Michael Charney of the Colorado State University Casting Laboratory. By working with a cast of a known individual not only could the final results be compared, but also individual inaccuracies in the process might be illuminated. I knew from my previous experience with facial reproductions of archaeological specimens (Rathbun, 1966) that some areas of the face were easier to model than others. Technical and logistical problems could also be solved before attempting a reproduction on a forensic case.

The procedures and older tissue thickness standards are clearly documented by Krogman (1962) and Gatliff and Snow (1979). After sex, age, and race have been determined, the mandible is attached and the skull is mounted in the Frankfort plane. Depth markers for the appropriate average tissue thickness are attached at 18 to 32 landmarks. Prosthetic eyes are inserted in the orbits, and then facial contours are built up by filling in the spaces between the markers with modeling clay. Individual features such as nose length and projection, mouth width, and ears are modeled by using standard proportions and anatomical features as reference points. Hair and skin coloration may be added. The demonstration videotape by Gatliff (1979) is especially useful for the neophyte. Rhine and Campbell (1980b) supplied a prepublication draft of the new tissue thickness standards for American populations.

Some unanticipated technical complications arose with the trial reproduction. Skull mounts were very expensive to purchase, so wooden stands with a large dowel that could be inserted into the foramen magnum were made locally. Although the stand was serviceable, there was a tendency for the skull to skip forward as work progressed. Gatliff recommends electric eraser material for markers at the tissue thickness landmarks, but it is sometimes difficult to cut the material straight and to glue the erasers on points that fall on crests around the nose and teeth. Splitting the erasers to make narrower markers helped; others have suggested the use of balsa wood. Prosthetic eyes can sometimes be difficult to obtain. We also found some types of modelling clay to be a frustrating factor. Although clay with a high oil content is easier to work with, the high summer heat and humidity caused the clay to slump overnight. This was partially solved by keeping the partial reproduction in a refrigerator when not under construction. Plaster casts absorb some of the excess oils, but skulls sometimes contribute additional oils and make the slumping problem worse. Approximating skin tones is another problem with most commercially available clays, which are usually green or grey. Some workers in the field recommend photographs in black and white with variations in exposure times to indicate skin darkness variation, but we wanted to attempt the closest likeness to living conditions possible. We tried a number of preparations but finally found that a cream base, totally opaque line of stage makeup worked best. The combined oil content of the clay and cosmetics made application a bit messy and smudging a continual problem, but hair spray and artists' fixative helped stabilize the application.

Although the skull gives no clues as to hair length, style, or color, a variety of wigs, purchased from a local thrift store, were used to produce a range of possible likenesses for comparison. When the premortem photograph was revealed, there was a reasonable likeness. Major inconsistencies included hollow cheeks, too much bilateral symmetry, and too much glamor in the fine details such as eyelashes and cosmetic styles. Comparisons with other independently executed reproductions done on the same cast (Charney et al., 1978) revealed a general resemblance among the four reproductions. This similarity of results provides some credence to the procedures, since all of the reproductions were done independently, but with variations in land-marks and tissue standards.

As part of an exploratory project to determine critical factors in the recognition aspect, slides of a variety of likenesses with different hair colors, styles, lengths, and glasses and the premortem photograph were shown to introductory anthropology classes. The students were asked to match the closest approximations with the photograph. Females were generally more astute than males in their observations and recognized that all the slides were of the same person. Snow et al. (1970) also found that civilian females were better at matching premortem and reproduction photographs. Race, age, or regional origin of the students did not significantly influence the results. When asked about the details considered to be most significant in recognition, the eyes and lips were most important, but nasal form and hairstyle were influencing factors. These results are consistent with findings in experimental work on eye movements and gaze. Subjects staring at a photograph spend the majority of time on the eyes and mouth, less on nose and hair, and least on lateral contours (Yarbus, 1967; Morris, 1977). In addition, intensities of expression have been reported to be more pro-nounced on the left side (Ekman et al., 1980), so we might pay more attention to subtleties in that area when attempting subsequent reproductions.

CASE SPECIMEN FACIAL REPRODUCTION

During the summer of 1980 the local coroner learned of our work with facial reproductions. Since the case reported earlier had not been identified after a year and no further leads were forthcoming, he requested that a facial reproduction be attempted on the skull, which he had retained as evidence when the remainder of the body had been buried. This was the only unidentified case remaining during his tenure in office, so he was especially interested in a resolution.

After the skull was mounted and secured on a wooden stand, the tissue thickness standards for American black females provided by Rhine and Campbell (1980b) were applied at 32 points. Intervening spaces and the individual features were modeled from the techniques by Gatliff and Snow (1979), and the videotape by Gatliff (1979) was repeatedly viewed as the reproduction progressed.

Special problems arose as the work continued. Attempts to form lips and ears were complicated by the consistency of the clay, which was thinned by the heat and additional oils from the skull. Since the maxillary central incisors were missing, the mouth had to be depicted closed. The inferior nasal spine, which is critical for the determination of nose projection, was unbroken but very short, and the projections from the nasal bones did not seem to coincide. The final product was a compromise of the two indications. Since there are no published recommendations for the depiction of scars or healed trauma, the depressed area on the frontal bone was contoured, slightly roughened for contrast, and depressed in the clay. The final touches included application of cosmetics and a wig. No attempt was made to provide individual expression or fine details such as eyelashes.

CASE RESOLUTION

When the coroner viewed the results, he arranged for a newspaper reporter to do a story on the process and publish photos of the reproduction with the background information. The story appeared in the morning paper, and that very afternoon a local grocer called the sheriff to report a likeness to a customer's daughter who had been missing for about a year. Subsequent investigation revealed that besides the general demographic congruity and facial resemblance seen in the photos, the missing woman had sustained a forehead injury when hit with a pocket watch during childhood.

Another agency provided fingerprints and official photos of the missing woman. The premortem photo was compared to the photograph of the reproduction as well as the original depiction, and a close resemblance was noted. The preserved fingers, which had been retained by the sheriff's office, had been printed and were then compared with those on file from the police report. A 10 point match conclusively established the identity. Police reports indicated that the decedent was a black female, 24 years old, 5 feet 6 inches to 5 feet 8 inches tall, weight 110 to 130 pounds, with an open face gold crown in the upper front teeth. She had a nine-year-old son, and her great-grandmother was an Indian. The missing mandibular molars were extracted after her sister had hit her with a board two to three years previously. No dental records or the missing incisors with the crown were ever found. The case is still pending with no determination of cause, manner, or mode of death.

DISCUSSION

The successful identification of the decedent in this case was gratifying in itself, but the project illustrates the potential of attempting facial reproductions to develop investigative leads. Although the fingers had been preserved, there were no suspects to attempt to match. It was fortunate that both a

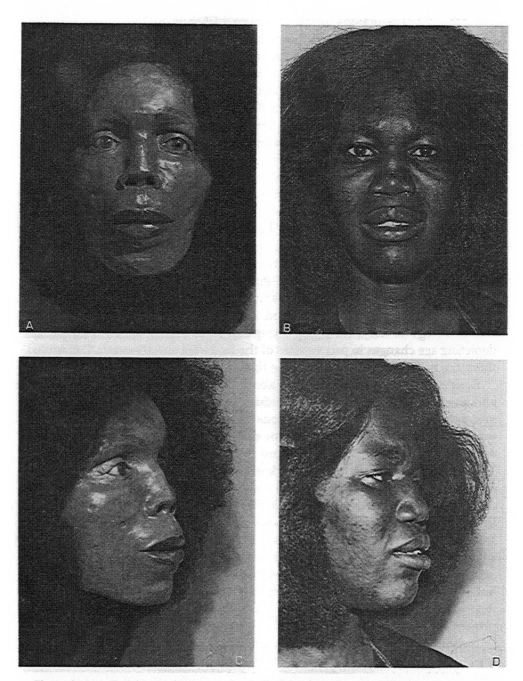

Figure 24-1. A. Facial reproduction on the skull of the decedent. B. Official law enforcement premortem photo of the decedent. C. Facial reproduction on the skull of the decedent, lateral view. D. Official law enforcement premortem photo of the decedent, lateral view.

recent official photograph and the fingerprints of the decedent were available. Since facial reproductions usually produce a likeness rather than a portrait of a decedent, recent, relatively large photographs are important. The forehead scar also illustrates the importance of attention to individual anomalies and anatomical asymmetries. The relatively short time between the disappearance of the decedent and the recognition in the paper may have played a role. The grocer and his wife reported in a later interview that the general depiction was good, but the eyes, cheeks, and general expression of the mouth were especially important in their decision to call the sheriff. They also knew that the woman was missing.

The new facial tissue thickness standards (Rhine and Campbell, 1980b) worked well in this instance, but refinement of the methods and additional data around the nose, lips, and eyes need to be documented. Not only are these areas critical for recognition, but they are also the hardest to depict correctly. A larger sample, including regional variations, should further the reliability. Although some reproductions for black males have been reported with older tissue data (Krogman, 1946; Wilder, 1912), I could find no published accounts for black females. Variations of tissue thickness with age at specific points also need to be verified. In this case, the decedent was close to the mean age of the Rhine and Campbell sample (1980b), so attempts at depicting age changes in proportions of the face were not necessary. Currently there are no published data on tissue thickness for children either.

Besides the reservations of some about the reliability of tissue thickness and average proportions of individual features, replicability has been questioned on the basis of variations in the artistic skills of individual workers. For the case in question, none of us had artistic training in sculpting or drawing, and the available discussions provided good guides to the neophyte. The initial work with the cast of a known individual was important, since experience improved our use of the techniques and reduced the amount of time involved. The first attempt took about 40 hours, but the case reproduction took considerably less. More experienced workers report time spent from a few hours to two days. When identification results, the investment appears worthwhile. The materials are relatively inexpensive, and fees depend upon individual circumstances. No fee schedules have been established, but reports from others range from free to $500 per reproduction. The reproduction in this case was done gratis since it was part of an academic project. Charges for future work will depend upon circumstances.

It should be noted that facial reproductions, as such, are not yet considered to be proof of identity, but Rhine (Chapter 25) reports the admission of one as evidence in court. The utility of facial reproductions depends upon expert, thorough osteological analysis of the remains, and then when traditional identification techniques do not quickly produce an identification or are inapplicable, the reproduction may develop alternative leads. A strong case can be made for routinely producing facial reproductions in the early stages of investigation and before the potential trails of evidence grow even colder.

As more data become available, techniques and materials refined, reproductions attempted, and factors in recognition tested, progress should be made in validating facial reproduction as another useful technique in the forensic application of physical anthropology.

REFERENCES

Brues, A. M. (1958). Identification of skeletal remains. *Journal of Criminal Law, Criminology and Police Science, 48*:551–563.

Charney, M., Snow, C. C., and Rhine, J. S. (1978). The Three Faces of Cindy M. Presented at 30th Annual Meeting of the American Academy of Forensic Sciences, St. Louis, Missouri.

Ekman, P., et al. (1980). Asymmetry in facial expression, *Science, 209*:833–836.

Gatliff, B. P. (1979). Facial Reconstruction in Forensic Medicine. Videotape, Department of Biomedical Communications, University of Texas Health Science Center at Dallas.

Gatliff, B. P., Snow, C. C. (1979). From skull to visage. *Journal of Biocommunication, 6(2)*:27–30.

Gerasimov, M. M. (1971). *The Face Finder.* Philadelphia, J. B. Lippincott Co.

Gilbert, B. M., and McKern, T. W. (1973). A method for aging the female *os pubis. Am J Phys Anthropol, 38*:31–38.

Giles, E., and Elliot, O. (1962). Race identification from cranial measurements. *J Forensic Sci, 7*:147–157.

Ilan, E. (1964). Identifying skeletal remains, *International Criminal Police Review, 175*:42–45.

Krogman, W. M. (1946). The reconstruction of the living head from the skull. *FBI Law Enforcement Bulletin,* July, pp. 11–18.

———— (1962). *The Human Skeleton in Forensic Medicine,* Springfield, Charles C Thomas.

Montagu, M. F. A. (1947). A study of man embracing error. *Technological Review, 49*:345–362.

Moore, C. E. (1980). Facial Tissue Depths in American Whites. 32nd Annual Meeting of the American Academy of Forensic Sciences, New Orleans.

Morris, D. (1977). *Manwatching.* New York: Harry N Abrams, Inc., pp. 71–76.

Rathbun, T. A. (1966). An attempt at facial restoration, Appendix A in "An Analysis of the Skeletal Material Excavated at Hasanly, Iran." MA thesis, University of Kansas, Lawrence, pp. 66–70.

Rhine, J. S. (1977). A Comparison of Methods of Restoring Living Facial Features to the Skull. Presented at Pan American Conference of the International Reference Organization in Forensic Medicine and Sciences, Mexico City.

Rhine, J. S., and Campbell, H. R. (1980a). The Body in the Plain Brown Wrapper. 32nd Annual Meeting of the American Academy of Forensic Sciences, New Orleans.

———— (1980b). Thickness of facial tissues in American blacks. *J Forensic Sci, 25(4)*:847–858.

Rhine, J. S., and Moore, C. E. (1982). Facial reproduction tables of facial tissue thicknesses of American Caucasoids in Forensic Anthropology. *Maxwell Museum Technical Series,* #1. Albuquerque.

Snow, C. C., Gatliff, B. P., and McWilliams, K. R. (1970). Reconstruction of facial features from the skull: an evaluation of its usefulness in forensic anthropology. *Am J Phys Anthropol, 33*:221–227.

Snyder, R. G., Burdi, A. R., and Gaul, G. (1975). A rapid technique for preparation of human fetal and adult skeletal material. *J Forensic Sci, 20(3)*:576–580.

Stephens, B. G. (1979). A simple method for preparing human skeletal material for forensic examination. *J Forensic Sci, 24(3)*:660–662.

Stewart, T D (1954). Evaluation of evidence from the skeleton. In R. H. B. Gradwohl (Ed.), *Legal Medicine*. St. Louis, Mosby, pp. 407–450.

———— (1979). *Essentials of Forensic Anthropology*. Springfield, Charles C Thomas, pp. 255–274.

Suk, V. (1935). Fallacies of anthropological identification and reconstructions, a critique based on anatomical dissections. *Publications of the Faculty of Science, Universita Masaryk, Brno, 207*:1–18.

Trotter, M. (1970). Estimation of stature from intact long limb bones. In T. D. Stewart (Ed.), *Personal Identification in Mass Disasters*, Washington, National Museum of Natural History, pp. 71–83.

Wilder, H. H. (1912). The Physiognomy of the Indians of southern New England. *American Anthropologist, 14*:415–436.

Yarbus, A. L. (1967). *Eye Movement and Vision*. New York, Plenum.

Chapter 25

FACIAL REPRODUCTION IN COURT

J. STANLEY RHINE

Facial reproduction, the process of modelling a face directly onto a human skull, is being used with increasing frequency in forensic anthropology. Such three-dimensional reproductions serve as a means of stimulating investigative leads, with identity being firmly established through the application of other forensic techniques such as those described in Section III.

The process of building a face on a skull for identification was first employed by Welcker (1883, 1888) to reproduce the faces of Schiller and Kant, and later by His (1895) on the skull of J. S. Bach. Kollmann and Büchly (1898) collected additional data on facial tissue thicknesses and compiled tables that have continued in use to the present day in most laboratories working on facial reproductions. The method used by these investigators was to place depth markers on the skull at the 18 measurement points and to build up the face in clay to those levels. After the turn of the century, the method was occasionally applied to skulls of archaeological origin (Wilder, 1912).

Criticized as unreliable and more art than science (Suk, 1935; Brues, 1958), the method languished until Ilan (1964) applied it to a forensic case, and Snow, Gatliff, and McWilliams (1970) tested its efficacy. Publication of these results stimulated new interest in the process in the United States, and considerable subsequent effort by a number of investigators has gone into exploring its application. Much of this effort has been directed toward an attempt to stimulate leads for investigation (Snow, 1977; Charney, Snow and Rhine, 1978; Heglar, 1978; Birkby, 1981). This average tissue thickness method of facial reproduction has recently been refined by increasing the measurement points to 32 and collecting data on blacks (Rhine and Campbell, 1980). A new and larger white sample, replacing the outdated standards of Kollmann and Büchly, has also been collected (Moore, 1980).

As a result of this work, and other research now in progress, the process of facial reproduction has become somewhat more respectable. There still remains a reservoir of well-considered doubt (Kerley, 1977), and more testing needs to be done. Recently, however, photographs of a facial reproduction

357

were admitted in court as evidence. The circumstances are summarized herein.

On September 11, 1977, two men discovered a decomposed and mostly skeletonized body partially buried under weeds, clothing, and discards in a dump south of Belen, New Mexico. The report of death addressed the rather suspicious circumstances thus: "A .38 calibre revolver was found in the same vicinity as the victim. Victim is very badly decomposed. Foul play is a definite suspect" (OMI, 1977b).

The body was promptly removed by the Valencia County sheriff, who then notified the New Mexico State Office of the Medical Investigator (OMI). An osteology student from the University of New Mexico Anthropology Department was requested to accompany the investigator to ascertain whether any material had been overlooked.

The autopsy was performed the following day, and the report begins, "Submitted in a plastic body bag is a somewhat disarticulated but largely intact male adult human skeleton" (OMI 1977a). A description of the clothing follows, and then the description of the remains. The body was unremarkable in most aspects; there was a healed fracture of the left zygomatic arch, and two left ribs "not representing ribs 1, 2, 11 or 12" were irregularly fractured. One right rib, similarly identified, was also fractured. The dental examination, done the same day, showed 15 teeth missing ante mortem, 5 teeth missing post mortem, and one amalgam restoration in the remaining teeth. To facilitate a thorough anthropology exam, the skeleton was then prepared.

IDENTIFICATION

The remains were presumed to be those of a 74-year-old Hispanic man, weighing 130 pounds and measuring 5 feet 4 inches in stature. According to a flyer offering a reward by the family, he had brown hair and eyes and a light complexion. The anthropological determination of a white male over 50 years old and 5 feet 6 inches tall was within acceptable limits. Such an agreement is not a sufficient basis on which to establish a positive identification, however. A hospital known to have treated the man named on the flyer was contacted, and ante mortem x-rays were procured for comparison. The x-rays did not match the ante mortem rib fractures noted on the skeletal remains. Further search of the hospital records located x-rays of a second individual with the same name. As he was only 3 years old, he was immediately disqualified. A third person with the same name was also too young.

THE FACIAL REPRODUCTION

All of this investigation had consumed several days, and the family became restive. They were quite convinced, despite the existence of only circumstantial evidence, that these remains were indeed those of their grandfather. To ascertain whether we were moving in an entirely incorrect investigatory direction, we decided to attempt a facial reproduction. Using our rapid method of building up the face with large blocks of clay rather than small strips, we completed the face and returned it to the medical investigator the same afternoon. The face was reproduced "blind"; that is, before the photograph was viewed.

At this time, we were still using a red clay and were experimenting with achieving a more lifelike appearance by modelling clay hair and painting the completed face with poster paint. We spent a great deal of time mixing red and white together, but the various shades of purple thus produced were quite unsatisfactory. In the end, we elected to use an unmixed white, despite its cadaverous effect. Since then, we have mixed clays to achieve a flesh tone, used artificial eyes, and added makeup and wigs for a more natural appearance.

The face was placed in front of a TV camera and the black and white image projected into the conference room where the family was assembled.

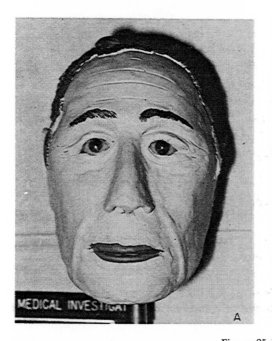 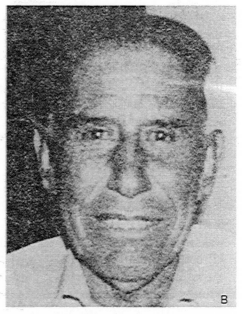

Figure 25-1 A & B.

The protracted silence was finally broken when one of the relatives tersely observed, "The hair is too short." We interpreted this as a favorable reaction. The family then decided that since we were expending a great deal of effort to make a positive ID, they would allow us to pursue whatever path was necessary to make the identification solid. They placated the gathering relatives and postponed the funeral. The very next day, however, the hospital produced yet another set of x-rays bearing the name of the missing man. In these radiographs, the positions of the rib fractures precisely matched those ante mortem fractures seen in the skeleton.

The remains had been recovered on September 11th, the autopsy performed on the 12th, the dentition examined on the 12th, and the anthropology exam performed on the 15th. The first set of x-rays was viewed on the 15th, the facial reproduction was done on the 18th, and the final set of x-rays was seen on the 22nd. That same day the remains were released to the family. Thus, in only 11 days, the body had been recovered, there had been a search of the scene for additional material, and an autopsy, a dental exam, cleaning of the skeleton, an anthropology exam, and a facial reproduction had been completed. In addition, consultation over four sets of x-rays had been accomplished by both anthropology and radiology. A considerable amount of telephoning and investigation, both by the Albuquerque Police Department and the lay investigators of the Office of the Medical Investigator had facilitated the identification. The death certificate was issued the next day, the 23rd.

Neither the forensic autopsy nor the anthropological examination had uncovered a cause of death. A pistol had been recovered from the vicinity of the body, but the minimal remaining soft tissue showed no trace of a gunshot wound—no obvious entrance, exit, bullet track, or radiopaque fragments in the x-ray. Nor were there any indications of stabbing on the bones. Although the cause of death could not be ascertained, the circumstances were sufficiently suspicious that the prosecution elected to tender a murder charge against the deceased man's young wife and her boyfriend.

IN COURT

Without defense objection, the OMI consultant in forensic anthropology was qualified in quick succession as an expert witness in (1) anthropology, (2) osteology, (3) forensic anthropology, (4) pathology, (5) radiology. It is quite unusual for a forensic anthropologist to be qualified as an expert witness in the latter two areas. The extra qualifications in this instance arose from a joint (academic) appointment in pathology and the need to establish identity from an x-ray. Indeed, prudence should require that such gratuitous qualification normally be eschewed in the interest of authenticity of the "expert witness" as a specialist.

The chain of evidence, an important consideration in medicolegal investigation, was accepted on the basis of a deputy's recollection of the clothing and the photographs of the body at OMI showing that clothing. Identification was accepted on the basis of the general agreement between the anthropological description and the description of the missing man, on agreement of the radiographs of the ribs, and on the facial reproduction. It should be emphasized, however, that any facial reproduction is principally useful in stimulating investigative leads and in demonstrating essential agreement or disagreement with a presumed identity. By itself, facial reproduction can *never* be used to establish a positive identification.

As a background for admission of the facial reproduction, the prosecutor elicited a summary of the history of the process, a synopsis of the experience of our lab in performing this sort of work, and our collection of facial tissue thicknesses designed to make the process more accurate and reliable. Our experience with blind testing of the method on known skulls was also noted. This was a fairly long sequence of testimony, running to more than 30 minutes. The defense, quite unprepared for this line of evidence, asked only a few questions. There was no objection to the line of questioning, the projection of slides of the facial reproduction to the jury, or the admission of the slides of the facial reproduction into evidence. The defense council had seen the slides but seemed to have no idea of their intended use and no knowledge of the subject. For the record, the case citation is State of New Mexico, Sandoval County, Docket #1978-3-20.

DISPOSITION OF THE CASE

Investigation by the Albuquerque Police disclosed that the dead man had a considerable quantity of money on his person at the time of his disappearance. He had intended to undertake the cash purchase of a pickup truck on the day he vanished. His young wife and her boyfriend fell immediately under suspicion.

She steadfastly denied any wrongdoing. The prosecution apparently believed, however, that they could not only arrange a confession from her boyfriend but also convince him to implicate the wife. Although convicted, he refused to involve her, and she was freed.

The subject of this paper has now been reinterred, in a more traditional manner, and the boyfriend has taken up a new residence in the hills south of Santa Fe. This is an exclusive suburb, the exclusion being intensified by the fences and guards that are such an integral part of life in the New Mexico State Penitentiary.

REFERENCES

Birkby, Walter H. (1981). Fifty Years in a Dinghy. Paper presented at American Academy of Forensic Sciences meeting.

Brues, Alice M. (1958). Identification of skeletal remains. *J Crim Law, Criminology, and Pol Sci,* 8:551–563.

Charney, Michael, Clyde C. Snow, and Stanley Rhine (1978). The Three Faces of Cindy M. Paper presented at American Academy of Forensic Sciences meeting.

Heglar, Rodger (1978). Bulletin of Sheriff of San Luis Obispo County. California, August 3, 1978.

His, Wilhelm (1895). Anatomische Forschungen uber Johann Sebastian Bach's Gebeine und Antlitz nebst Bemerkungen uber dessen Bilder. Bandes der Abhandlungen der Mathematisch-physischen Classe der Konigl. *Sachsischen Gesellschaft der Wissenschaften, Des XXII, Nr. V:* 380–420.

Ilan, E. (1964). Identifying skeletal remains. *Internat Crim Pol Rev,* 175:42–45.

Kerley, Ellis R. (1977). Forensic anthropology in forensic medicine. Vol. II, *Physical Trauma,* C. D. Tedeschi, W. G. Eckert, and L. G. Tedeschi, Eds. W. B. Saunders Co., Philadelphia.

Kollmann, J. and W. Büchly (1898). Die Persistenz der Rassen und die Reconstruction der Physiognomie prähistorischer Schadel. *Arch f Anth, 25:* 329–359.

Moore, C. Elliott (1980). Facial Tissue Thicknesses of Modern Caucasoids. Paper presented at American Academy of Forensic Sciences meeting.

Office of the Medical Investigator (1977a) Autopsy Report, #7040-77-13V. School of Medicine, University of New Mexico, Albuquerque.

(1977b). Report of Death, #7040-77-13V. School of Medicine, University of New Mexico, Abuquerque.

Rhine, J. Stanley and Homer R. Campbell (1980). Thickness of Facial Tissues in American blacks. *J Forensic Sci, 25:* 847–858.

Snow, Clyde C. (1977). Victim Identification Through Facial Restoration. Paper presented at American Academy of Forensic Sciences meeting.

Snow, Clyde C., Betty P. Gatliff, and Kenneth R. McWilliams (1970). Reconstruction of Facial Features from the Skull: An Evaluation of its Usefulness in Forensic Anthropology. *Am J Phys Anthropol 33:* 221–228.

Suk, V. (1935). Fallacies of Anthropological Identifications and Reconstructions. *Publications de la Faculté des Sciences de l'Université Masaryk, 207:* 3–18.

Welcker, H. (1883). *Schiller's Schadel und Todtenmaske, nebst Mittheilungen uber Schadel und To tenmaske Kants.* Braunschweig.

―――― (1888). Zur Kritik des Schillersschadels. *Arch f Anth, 17:*19–60.

Wilder, Harris Hawthorne (1912). The physiognomy of the Indians of Southern New England. *Am Anthropol, 14:*415–435.

Chapter 26

THE IDENTIFYING PATHOLOGY

WILLIAM R. MAPLES

Most identification techniques used by physical anthropologists place skeletal remains into classes (sex, race, age range, stature range, etc.). Such description, even when extremely accurate, can seldom establish legal identification of the deceased. Forensic anthropologists often see cases where final identification is delayed or even denied because the next of kin refuses to accept the death of his or her relative. In such instances, any particular individual characteristics, such as pathology, can become crucial. The case in reference serves as an excellent example of the value of pathology as a means of establishing identity in forensic identification.

CASE HISTORY

On the last day of March, 1972, a virtually complete skeleton was found in a boggy area near a major highway in the Florida panhandle. The skeletal remains, much of it still in blocks of peat, were turned over to me for identification. I was told at that time that the skeleton was suspected to be the remains of a "90-year-old man."

As the peat was cleared away from the pelvis, light reddish pubic hairs were found in the plant debris. The lower left leg and foot were still covered by a partially decomposed sock, but no tissue remained.

The age of the individual was obviously advanced. All endocranial sutures were fused and obliterated except the anterior portion of the squamous suture, as defined by Todd and Lyon (1924). A root growing through the left squamous suture, separating the temporal bone from the parietal bone, had broken the fused portion and forced the temporal bone laterally. Before that damage, the fusion of that suture was almost but not quite complete. The same was true for the anterior squamous suture on the right side of the skull. The pubic symphysis was clearly beyond the useful range of the McKern and Stewart (1957) technique, although the presence of osteophytes around the margin of the symphysis could have easily been confused for a well-marked rim. Because of the closure of such sutures as the masto-occipital 1 and 2, the parietomastoid, and the posterior portion of the squamous and the near completion of the anterior squamous, the center of the estimated range was in the ninth decade (Todd and Lyon, 1924). The jaws indicated that the deceased had long been edentulous, so there was no possibility of establishing age based on dental histology. No attempts were made at the time to estimate the age based on the histology of bones.

The sex was clearly male based on the morphology of the pubis bone, the auricular surface, and the sciatic notch. The skull was rugged and robust as well. The skull was typically Caucasoid, particularly the narrow nasal aperature and high nasal bridge. Mean estimated stature was 173.4 cm ±3.62 cm standard error (Trotter and Gleser 1958).

Except for the unusual extreme age of the deceased estimated by the notoriously inconsistent cranial sutures (Todd and Lyon, 1924; McKern and Stewart, 1957), nothing in the above would have been particularly useful in establishing identity. The skeletal pathology was far more definitive.

Old healed fractures of the left 4th metatarsal and a proximal foot phalanx were noted, as was wedging of the 12th thoracic vertebra. Such old injuries are seldom useful for identification, as they were not in this case.

Many degenerative pathologies consistent with the extreme age of the deceased were apparent, especially ossification of many of the costal cartilages, with several fused to the sternum. Similarly, both of the first ribs were fused to the manubrium. Osteophytes were present on the head of the right fibula, the fibular facet of the right tibia, and the vertebral skeleton. Bony transformation of the longitudinal ligaments (Fig. 26-1) resulted in fusion of a number of thoracic vertebrae (T3 through T7 and T7 through T11). The sacroiliac joints were not fused. Marked kyphosis was present in the mid-thoracic spine. The pathology of the spine was in keeping with senile ankylosing hyperostosis (Aegerter and Kirkpatrick, 1963).

The one pathological area that was truly distinctive about this individual was the right temporal bone (Fig. 26-2). The external auditory meatus was replaced by a much larger opening with smooth margins. This opening (Fig. 26-3) led to a large excavated space replacing the structures of the middle ear and mastoid air cells. The canal for the facial nerve remained intact. Anteriorly, the disease perforated the tympanic plate into the temporomandibular joint. Superiorly, it had penetrated the tegmen tympani into the cranial vault. The destruction followed the characteristics of cholesteatoma.

Forensic science is characterized by close cooperation of many scientists. The forensic anthropologist must work closely with pathologists and others. Much more can be realized by working together than could be accomplished individually. Without this cooperation, all of us lose some of our effectiveness.

In this case, the skull was referred to Rene Echevarria, M.D., then Associate Professor of Pathology at the J. Hillis Miller Health Center, the medical

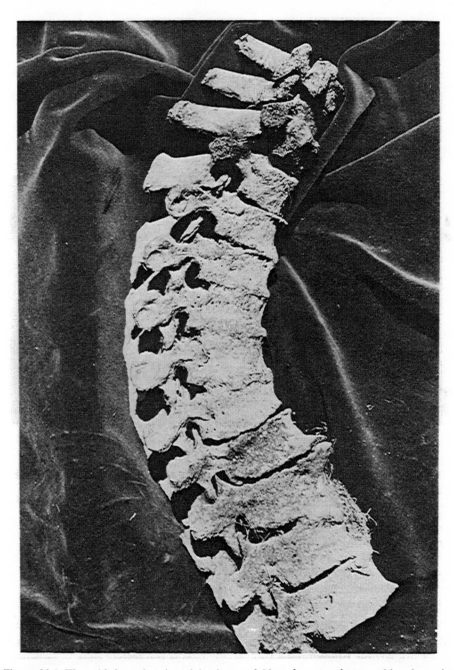

Figure 26-1. The mid-thoracic spine of the deceased. Note the osteophytes and fused vertebrae.

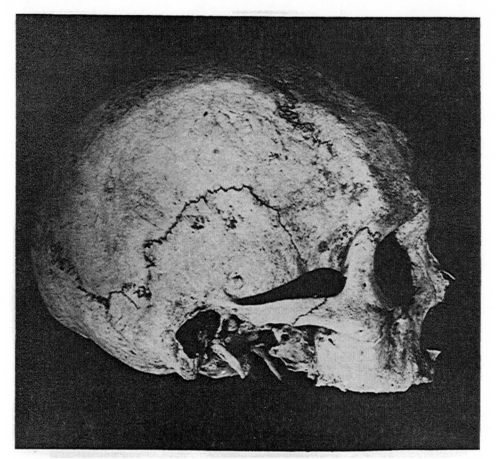

Figure 26-2. The cranium, showing the destruction to the temporal bone.

school of the University of Florida. After consultation with Dr. Franklin Black in the ENT Department, Dr. Echevarria reported that

> the bone defect in the area of the middle ear and mastoid are typical of a cholesteatoma. There is a destruction of the tegmen tympani so the possibility of the patient having had a brain abscess on that side is a very clear one. All the bony loss can be attributed to the expansile growth of the cholesteatoma and there is no evidence that surgery had been done. The bony defect does not correspond to any of the standard mastoidectomies. The possibility of neoplasm is a more remote one. (Personal communication)

It is pointed out in *Scott-Brown's Diseases of the Ear, Nose and Throat* that "cholesteatoma is a misnomer in that it is neither a tumour nor does it contain cholesterin" (Thorburn, 1971). Gray (1964) defines it simply as "skin in the wrong place." The theory of Tumarkin (1961) that is gaining wide acceptance by otologists, according to Thorburn (1971), is that the cholesteatoma is caused by the immigration of the epithelium of the external auditory meatus and the surface of the tympanic membrane after a

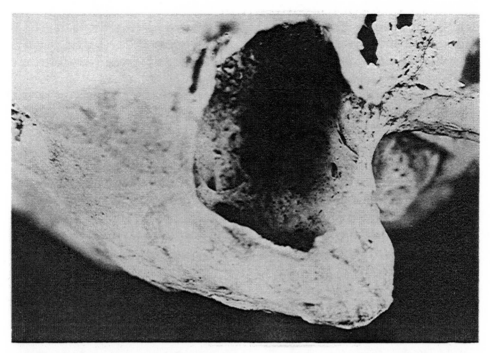

Figure 26-3. A closeup of the affected area of the temporal bone, showing the excavation of the air cells of the mastoid process and the total loss of the auditory meatus.

history of upper respiratory infections "associated with eustachian obstruction and in intratympanic vacuum." The two most consistent symptoms of the disorder are loss of hearing and a foul-smelling drainage. Since the loss of hearing is unilateral and extremely gradual in onset, many victims fail to seek treatment. Even after intracranial invasion, as demonstrated in this case, the symptoms may remain relatively slight. Headache caused by increased intracranial pressure associated with the resultant extradural or subdural abscess, meningitis, or many other resulting complications may be noted. Untreated, the course of the complications resulting from intracranial invasion may be "rapidly fatal, progress at variable speed, or may become so localized as to cause the patient little trouble for years, before resuming a rapid and possibly fatal progress" (Dawes, 1971). It is possible, therefore, that no symptoms were apparent.

In my identification report to the sheriff's office, the summary contained the following:

> His medical history might contain . . . a chronic infection of the right ear, leading to deafness in that ear, with a growth (cholesteatoma) in the region of the ear. This probably was accompanied by a thick drainage, probably of foul odor. He may have suffered a period of loss of balance and vertigo. Later, central nervous system symptoms may have occurred.

When the skeletal remains were returned to the sheriff's office in the Florida panhandle along with the report, I requested word of the final disposition of the case. Since I heard nothing more of the case, I stopped at the sheriff's office in late 1975 as I happened to pass through the town and requested to review the file.

The sheriff's office had identified the missing person as an 85 year old, toothless white male, with sandy hair. His height was estimated between 175 and 179 cm (5'9" to 5'10"). Few medical records were available on him, since the physicians reported (in the records of county social workers) to have treated the missing man had either left the area or denied any record of treatment. Since he lived alone until his disappearance, most of the information concerning his health came from the records of county social workers who had maintained a file on him for 20 years.

In 1952, he told them that he was a little deaf because of x-ray therapy to his right ear for removal of skin cancer. His ear was misshapen at that time but completely healed.

In 1959, he had "a place" in front of his right ear that needed treatment. In 1966, he said his hearing was very bad in his right ear because it was x-rayed at one time. He said that a hearing aid was of little value. In January of 1967, he said he had a light stroke and was dragging his left leg, and his left arm was stiff. The doctor he said treated him denies having seen him. Seven months later, the symptoms were gone. Four days before he disappeared on June 23rd, 1970, he was in a confused state.

One deputy sheriff told me that acquaintances of the missing man reported he had a drainage from his right ear and "he smelled so bad that people didn't like to be around him" (personal communication).

His only known relatives were also of advanced years and senile, according to the law enforcement officers. These relatives did not believe the missing man to be dead.

A coroner's jury found on the basis of reports prepared by "Department of Anthropology, University of Florida, the State Crime Laboratory, and the ... sheriff's office" that the remains were those of the missing person and that he "met his death from unknown, but natural causes" (Washington County Coroner's Jury, 1972).

The remains were refused by relatives of the missing person. The final disposition of the skeleton was not recorded in the file.

DISCUSSION

This case emphasizes two important points: (1) the importance of pathology in a forensic identification report and (2) the significance of medical interpretation in forensic reports. Few practicing physicians and even forensic pathologists are able to convert the characteristics observed on bare bone to disorders of the living. The forensic anthropologist is familiar with the range of normal variation of human bones and their anomalies as well as the pathology of the skeleton. Such information is important in the proper evaluation of human skeletal remains.

Many of the persons who are found in decomposed condition have a life-style that offers little evidence of past medical treatment and diagnosis. In the present case, had the deceased sought medical attention, it might have been possible to get the surgeon who performed the necessary resection of the temporal to identify his or her own work. Since this case and many others involve untreated pathological conditions, we must consult with the proper medical specialists so that we may describe the symptoms that might have been apparent to surviving friends and associates.

Spencer Rogers (1966) wrote:

> If the anthropologist limits his efforts to careful descriptions of evidences as undiagnosed physical states seen in bones, he will avoid the confusion of uncertain disease definition and the errors of attempted diagnosis without the aid of extended laboratory techniques which usually are not at his disposal. . . . It is here urged that physical anthropologists impose on themselves a restraint in assigning premature diagnoses of bone pathologies and at the same time apply themselves to the problem of devising more accurate and better standardized nomenclature of description.

The forensic anthropologist should go beyond that. It is his or her responsibility to go beyond description and, whenever possible, describe the condition as it would likely be observed in a living person. It is essential that description of the skeletal defects be clearly separated from any interpretation of their meaning or significance. In most cases, the anthropologist should not attempt to make these interpretations alone. Most of us have resources available to us that will assist in such difficult and sometimes specialized circumstances. I have an excellent medical school with a cooperative faculty and outstanding medical library a few minutes' walk from my laboratory. I would not make all interpretations without assistance by other specialists, but it is the responsibility of the forensic anthropologist to exhaust all possible information presented in the remains under investigation. It should be done carefully and with discretion, but that is a charge that we must always assume in our role of forensic identification. It further points out the importance of establishing centers of identification where necessary resources exist.

REFERENCES

Aegerter, Ernest, and John A. Kirkpatrick, Jr. (1963). *Orthopedic Diseases*, 2nd ed. Philadelphia and London: W. B. Saunders Co.

Dawes, J. D. K. (1971). Complications of infections of the middle ear. In *Scott-Brown's Diseases of the Ear, Nose, and Throat*, vol. 2: The Ear. John Ballantyne and John Groves, Eds., pp. 205–281. Philadelphia: J. B. Lippincott.

Gray, J. Duncan (1964). The treatment of cholesteatoma in children. *Proc R Soc Med,* 57:769–771.

McKern, T. W., and T. D. Stewart (1957). Skeletal Age Changes in Young American Males. Technical Report EP-45 of the Headquarters Quartermaster and Developmental Command, Natick, Mass.

Rogers, Spencer L. (1966). The need for a better means of recording bone proliferation in joint areas. *Am J Phys Anthropol,* 25:171–176.

Thorburn, Ian B. (1971). Chronic suppurative otitis media – assessment. In *Scott-Brown's Diseases of the Ear, Nose, and Throat*, vol. 2: The Ear. John Ballantyne and John Groves, Eds., pp. 143–163. Philadelphia: J. B. Lippincott.

Todd, T. W., and D. W. Lyon, Jr. (1924). Endocranial suture closure, part I: Adult males of the white stock. *Am J Phys Anthropol, 7(O.S.)*:325–384.

Trotter, M., and G. C. Gleser (1958). A reevaluation of estimation of stature taken during life and of long bones after death. *Am J Phys Anthropol,* 16:79–123.

Tumarkin, A. (1961). Pre-epidermosis. *J Laryngol and Otol,* 75:487–500.

Washington County Coroner's Jury (1972). Report of the Coroner's Jury. May 10, Chipley, Florida.

Chapter 27

THE LIFE AND AFTERLIFE OF ELMER J. MCCURDY*
A Melodrama in Two Acts

CLYDE C. SNOW AND THEODORE A. REYMAN

PROLOGUE

Time: From the Sixth Century AD to the Present.

Early in 1974, the Paleopathology Association received an intriguing letter from Dr. R. Boyer of the Institut d' Archeologie Mediterranéenne in Draguignan. He said:

> Our laboratory is studying two corpses with their clothes and jewels, found in Vth and VIth century AD sarcophagi in Marseilles. In the neighboring sarcophagi, badly preserved skeletons were found: indeed, these sarcophagi were well closed and the place was—and is still—very damp; such conditions are unfavorable to preservation. However, organic remains were partially preserved. From our results with the chemical analysis of these remains, I must mention that the levels of arsenic in the bodies seem too high. It was 0.13% in one body and 3.14% in the other. In these cases, arsenic does not come from the outside (surrounding ground), and it is difficult to admit a poisoning in both cases! Do you think that arsenic may have been used at that time (Vth and VIth centuries AD) to preserve corpses? Do you know of any literature on the subject? If you do, I shall be very happy to get precise references.

This appeal was published in the June 1974 *Newsletter*, but no one came forward with any answers.

However, in April, 1977, an opportunity to study the preserving qualities of arsenic arose from a most unexpected quarter. Drs. Thomas Noguchi and Clyde Snow telephoned from Los Angeles to say that they were about to autopsy a body from 1911 that had been preserved this way, and would we be interested in examining specimens. Six samples were requested and were examined in Detroit with interesting results.

Ralph Smith performed arsenic analyses on the tissues to corroborate that this was indeed the method that had been used for embalming. He obtained the following values:

---

*Reprinted with permission from Paleopathology Association, Special Supplement, Eve Cockburn, Ed., September 1977.

371

	mg As/gm tissue
Lung	0:270
Skeletal muscle	0.080
Skin	0.390
Heart	0.270
Brain	0.700
Bone	0.659
(muscle and skin attached)	

These values are several hundred times those that we had found in Egyptian mummies. Samples from the mummies ranged from zero to 6.2 ppm (0.006 mg As/gm), using similar methodology.

During the processing of the tissue for histologic examination, we noted that the skin taken from the leg was an intense yellow orange. We wondered if the high arsenic content was reacting in some way with the chemicals to produce this color. However, this was presumably because the skin had been painted sometime in the past, perhaps to disguise the body as a dummy.

The most startling discovery was yet to come. When we viewed the finished sections with the microscope, the preservation of the tissue was almost unbelievable. The heart was nearly perfectly preserved, and the individual myocardial fibers were observed to have not only intact cross-striations but also nuclei and lipochrome pigment at the nuclear caps. The coronary arteries were quite normal. Red and white blood cells were easily recognized. The organ appeared normal. Sections from skin, skeletal muscle, and bone were also in an excellent state of preservation. All connective tissue and muscle and epithelial tissue components were easily identified, and blood cells were commonly found intact.

Sections of the brain included both cerebellum and cerebrum. Most of the neurons were intact and recognizable. The Purkinje cell layer of the cerebellum was quite well preserved. The various layers of the cerebral cortex were still identifiable, with good differentiation of glial and neuronal elements. These portions of the brain also appeared normal.

The only part of the tissue that did not appear normal grossly was the lung. The typical spongelike appearance had been lost, and the tissue was heavy and appeared consolidated, not unlike liver. The sections showed an organizing lobar pneumonia with both red and white blood cells, larger mononuclear cells, and proliferating fibrous connective tissue within alveolar spaces. The pleura and bronchioles and vessels appeared normal, but within the vascular spaces, numerous red and white blood cells could be seen. Polymorphonuclear leucocytes were easily identified. Some cells appeared to be eosinophils.

The tissue examination has perhaps given further historical insight into the death of this man. Although most organs appeared normal, the lungs indicated that he had significant disease when he died. The organizing nature of the process indicated also that he had had it for some time before his death. Possibilities would include tuberculosis, though the tissue preservation was so good that granulomas would probably be recognizable, and there were none to be seen. He may have had pneumonia at the time he was shot and killed. A third possibility is that he was shot but did not die immediately, lingering on, perhaps aspirating food or gastric contents into his lungs. This latter clinical picture is not uncommon with severely ill patients and seems to be a logical explanation for the findings in the lungs.

The play begins . . .

Although the name Elmer J. McCurdy is hardly a household word in the annals of either show business or crime, it does deserve some minor mention in both. His career as an outlaw and later as a trouper spanned seven decades and may be conveniently divided into two phases, antemortem and postmortem.

ACT I: ANTEMORTEM

The antemortem, or criminal, period of Elmer's career is still dim. We have not yet determined his birthplace, although there is some indication that it was either Kansas or Colorado. As a young man, he may have served an enlistment in the United States Army. By the early 1900s he had drifted to Oklahoma, where he worked both as a miner and a plumber. Sometime during this period he also served a term in the Oklahoma Territorial Penitentiary. In the spring of 1911 he was part of a gang that robbed a Missouri Pacific train near Coffeyville, Kansas. Emboldened by this success, Elmer recruited two companions to rob a Missouri, Kansas and Texas (Katy) train. The intended target, one of two daily Katy trains southbound from Kansas into Oklahoma, was carrying several thousand dollars in Indian tribal payments. McCurdy and his gang struck on the night of 6 October 1911, stopping the train on an isolated stretch near Okesa, Oklahoma. Boarding the engine, they overpowered the crew, detached the engine and baggage car carrying the cash box, and leaving the passenger cars stranded, moved them several miles down the track, where they could leisurely collect the loot. At this point, the operation, which until then had been carried out with commandolike precision, began to unravel. Perhaps, as many another traveler before and since, Elmer had difficulty reading railroad timetables, because at this time the robbers discovered they had hit the wrong train—the cash box on this one contained only $46.00. However, as a consolation, they discovered that the baggage car contained a shipment of liquor. While still on board, they drank several bottles of beer, and on their departure Elmer grabbed two demijohns of whiskey.

Two nights later, with a posse on his trail, Elmer showed up at the Revard Ranch in the Osage Hills, an area described as one in which

> escaped criminals are able to disappear for days at a time, regardless of the advanced civilization made during the past two or three years. Ranches have been converted into farms in nearly every section of the new state (Oklahoma) with the exception of Osage County, where that district outside of the developed oil belt contains every element of wildness that it did in the old territory days. (Bartlesville, Oklahoma, *Daily Enterprise*, October 8, 1911)

The same paper described the final hours of Elmer's antemortem career. When he arrived at the ranch, he

> had one of the jugs of whiskey taken from the train by the robbers and had been drinking heavily. He told the man at the ranch that he was Frank Amos (an alias) and that the whiskey had come off that train which was held up down below Okesa. After drinking with the ranch employees for an hour he asked for a place to sleep and was shown to the hay mow. He had been asleep only a few minutes when the three members of the posse who had been trailing him for two days arrived. They took their stations about the barn and waited for daylight. Bob Fenton (one of the posse members) telephoned the *Enterprise* this morning about the fight. "It began just about 7 o'clock," he said. "We were standing around waiting for him to come out when the first shot was fired at me. It missed me and he then turned his attention to my brother, Stringer Fenton. He shot three times at Stringer and when my brother got under cover he turned his attention to Dick Wallace. He kept shooting at all of us for about an hour. We fired back every time we could. We do not know who killed him . . . [on the trail] we found one of the jugs of whiskey which was taken from the train. It was about empty. He was pretty drunk when he rode up to the ranch last night."

Later that day, Elmer's body was taken to the Johnson Funeral Establishment in nearby Pawhuska, Oklahoma, where it was formally identified. Examination of the body revealed that he had been struck by a single bullet entering the right upper thorax and traveling downward and to the left to lodge in the lower abdominal region. The bullet track was explained by Elmer's lying in the hayloft, firing from a prone position when he was struck. Authorities were puzzled about Elmer's refusal to surrender peaceably once he found he was surrounded. However, it seems evident that anyone who had spent a cold night in a hayloft after consuming the better part of two jugs of whiskey might be in an exceptionally quarrelsome mood if aroused at seven in the morning.

ACT II: POSTMORTEM

On 10 December 1976, a Universal Studio television crew was filming an episode of American television's *Six Million Dollar Man* on location at the Nu-Pike Amusement Park in Long Beach, California. The scene to be filmed involved a chase through an establishment known as the "Laugh in the Dark Funhouse." In a darkened area of the funhouse there was a "dummy" hanging from a gallows. The dummy was painted with a phosphorescent red paint that glowed in the dark when a nearby ultraviolet light was switched on. The cameraman, seeking a better shot, asked a technician to move the dummy. As he did so, its arm fell off, revealing a bone. Police were summoned, and they questioned the manager of the funhouse, who was rather disconcerted to find that his dummy was, in fact, a mummy.

The mummy was transported to the Los Angeles County Coroner's Office, where it was autopsied by Joseph H. Choi, M.D., Deputy Medical Examiner. Dr. Choi found that the mummy was that of an adult Caucasoid male. There was a modified Y-shaped incision of the anterior thorax and abdomen and bilateral inguinal embalming incisions. The abdominal and thoracic viscera and the brain were hardened to a stonelike consistency. There was a gunshot entrance wound located on the right anterior thorax 4 inches to the right of the midline. The path of the bullet was downward and to the left, penetrating the right sixth rib, right lung, diaphragm, liver, and intestine. A bullet was not found, but a copper bullet jacket, or gas check, was found embedded in the musculature of the pelvis. Ballistic examination of the bullet jacket revealed that it was from a .32-20 caliber bullet with six-right rifling. Manufacture of such bullets was discontinued before World War II; gas checks were introduced around 1905. SEM/EDX examination of tissue samples from the mummy indicated a high arsenic content, apparently the result of embalming with arsenic, a practice discontinued in the United States early in this century.

Meanwhile, the Long Beach Police Department continued their questioning of the funhouse manager, whose consternation at learning his exhibit was an actual human body turned to utter dismay when he was informed it was also a possible homicide victim. He told the investigators that the dummy had, until 1971, been displayed in a coffin in the Hollywood Wax Museum, another concession in the amusement park. He took over the mummy (which he thought was made of papier-mâché) when the wax museum operators defaulted on their rent.

Once on the trail, the Long Beach detectives proved to be as dogged in pursuit as the Oklahoma posse that tracked Elmer through the Osage Hills in 1911. Within a few days, it was established that the mummy had been a starring attraction in a number of traveling shows and exhibits such as "Louie Sonney's Museum of Crime" and "Craft's Carnival Circus." At one point it had been scheduled for permanent exhibit in an establishment called the Haunted House near Mount Rushmore, South Dakota, but was rejected as not being sufficiently lifelike!

The trail finally ended in Pawhuska, Oklahoma, where we left Elmer at the Johnson Funeral Establishment. Its proprietor was apparently a believer in H. L. Mencken's observation that nobody ever lost money by under-estimating the taste of the American public. Finding that Elmer had no known next of kin, he embalmed him heavily in arsenic and, instead of burying him, kept him in a back room of the funeral parlor for several years. For a nickel, local curiosity seekers were allowed to view Elmer, billed by now as the "bandit who wouldn't give up." Before condemning such a barbaric exhibition, one should recall that displays of this kind were not so unusual in the American hinterlands a generation or two ago. Our rural forefathers did not have the advantage, as we do today, of being able to view violence and its aftermath in the comfort of their living rooms.

Elmer was thus launched on his postmortem career in show business. His local engagement in Pawhuska ended about 1916 when a stranger came to town and paid his nickel to see Elmer. He emerged pale and shaking. Elmer, he claimed, was his long-lost brother. He tearfully demanded that the body be released to him so that he might bury it in the old family graveyard up in Kansas. The undertaker, probably fearing legal action, complied. By the time it was learned that the "brother" was actually a carnival operator, Elmer was well launched on his long engagement, touring the western states in sideshows for many years before winding up in the Laugh in the Dark Funhouse in 1976. Thus, like his more famous Oklahoma contemporaries, Will Rogers, Tom Mix, Gene Autry, and Woody Guthrie, he followed the sawdust trail to movieland, hanging around Hollywood for a few years before getting his big chance. Unlike them, however, when his moment finally came—a guest appearance in the *Six Million Dollar Man*—Elmer blew in and literally went to pieces on the set.

The salient facts of Elmer's odyssey emerged within a few weeks after his autopsy. A strong chain of evidence, based on old documents and interviews with his former owners, linked the mummy and the Oklahoma outlaw. Lacking, however, was any antemortem physical description on which a positive identification could be based. Without this, and in the absence of any next of kin, Elmer faced consignment to a crematorium under his official L.A. County Coroner's case number: 76 14 812, Doe, John 255. Fortunately word of his predicament had spread to Oklahoma. Now Oklahomans are a rather peculiar breed. Traditionally, they have dealt rather harshly with local lawbreakers while they are still alive but become uncommonly sentimental about them fifty years after they are dead. Also, many still remember those dark dustbowl days of the 1930s, dramatically documented in Nobel laureate Steinbeck's *Grapes of Wrath*, when "Okie" migrants to California were treated shabbily on the West Coast, and sentiment favored bringing Elmer back home.

Aware of the difficulty, local historians combed the newspaper and court records of the period. Among other items they found Elmer's physical description and mug shots made at the time he entered the Oklahoma Territorial Prison. According to this, he was about 31 years old and 5 feet 8 inches in height. Of course, dental records and fingerprints were not available from this early period. Also found in the University of Oklahoma's Western History Collection were two photographs of Elmer taken in Pawhuska after his death. The first, a full-length frontal pose, shows him before the embalming. He is still wearing the same clothing as when he was shot. The second, taken after embalming, is a profile view, showing Elmer dressed in a black suit, laid out on a bier. Both photographs are clearly labeled with Elmer's name, that of the photographer, and the date. Apparently, they were used not only to help identify Elmer formally, so that the deputies could obtain their reward, but were also passed out (or perhaps sold) as souvenirs of the occasion.

Armed with this information, a committee of prominent Oklahomans contacted Dr. Thomas T. Noguchi, the Los Angeles City/County Coroner, concerning the possible release of the body for burial in Oklahoma. Dr. Noguchi graciously agreed that this could be done, provided that a review of the available descriptive data by a team of experts could convincingly establish the identity of the mummy as that of Elmer J. McCurdy and that, if returned to Oklahoma, Elmer would be given a decent and dignified burial.

At the request of the Oklahoma committee, the author went to Los Angeles on 9 April 1977. The examination was conducted in consultation with Dr. Noguchi and his staff. Dr. Judy Suchey of California State College in Fullerton, who is Dr. Noguchi's consultant in forensic anthropology, and the author spent two days reviewing the available documentary evidence and examining the mummy itself.

On the basis of our examination, which will be detailed in a more formal report, we were able to conclude that the mummy was that of a slightly built Caucasoid male about 30 ± 3 years with an antemortem stature of 170.5 ± 6.54 cm (67.1 ± 2.4 in). The few remaining patches of scalp hair were light brown in color. In Elmer's prison description, a note was included that he had a "scar two inches long on the back of the right wrist." Although difficult to discern due to postmortem shrinkage and wrinkling of the skin, the mummy also had a slender scar running obliquely across the dorsum of the right wrist.

We also compared the facial profile of the mummy with the post-embalming profile photograph taken of Elmer shortly after his death. This was done by a modification of the superimposition technique long used in forensic medicine to compare unidentified skulls with antemortem photographs of possible decedents. In the author's laboratory, we have improved this method by substituting videotape equipment for the still camera ordinarily employed.

In Elmer's case, we used two small Hitachi videocameras circuited through a special effects generator into a single monitor. One camera was trained on an enlargement of Elmer's profile in the 1911 photograph, the other was targeted on the mummy. With both displayed on the same monitor, it was immediately evident that Elmer's profile and that of the mummy were remarkably coincident. While such a superimposition cannot by itself be used to establish positive identification, it strongly supports the other evidence.

The best indication of the date of death was provided by the 32.20 bullet jacket and the embalming technique. As noted previously, such bullet jackets were not manufactured until about 1905, and arsenic embalming was outlawed in most states by about 1920. Finally, the location of the entrance wound and track of the bullet established by Dr. Choi in his autopsy of the mummy matches the description of Elmer's fatal wound.

In addition to the physical findings of our examination, we had the testimony of the several carnival and amusement park entrepreneurs who, at one time or another over the years, had exhibited the mummy. When pieced together, it provided a virtually complete documentation of Elmer's six-decade odyssey, which took him from the funeral parlor in Pawhuska to the Funhouse in Long Beach. Considering both the physical and documentary evidence, we were able to conclude beyond reasonable doubt that the mummy was indeed the late Elmer J. McCurdy. On this basis, Dr. Noguchi was able to sign a California death certificate, clearing the way for Elmer's return to Oklahoma.

Before he left California, the old trouper finally got his chance for the big time. As the case had attracted considerable attention throughout the country, correspondent Leslie Stahl taped a brief update on the story for NBC's evening news using Elmer as her backdrop. All agreed that he put on a stellar performance.

Elmer arrived by jet in Oklahoma City on 14 April 1977. He was met by a delegation from the Oklahoma State Medical Examiner's Office and taken to the morgue until final arrangements could be made for his funeral. The expenses of his funeral, including a moderately priced wooden casket and tombstone, were undertaken jointly by the Indian Territorial Posse of Westerners, an organization of prominent Oklahomans interested in the state's colorful history, and by the Oklahoma Historical Society.

The following week, on a rainy Friday morning, Elmer was buried in the Summit View Cemetery at Guthrie, the old Territorial capital of Oklahoma. This cemetery, one of the oldest in the state, contains the graves of several other notorious outlaws and many prominent earlyday pioneers, ranchers, and politicians, a circumstance prompting one wag (whose name will not be disgraced by mentioning it) to propose the following epitaph:

Rest in peace, dear Elmer
Beneath this Okie sky.
Where many an outlaw slumbers
And politicians lie.

The coffin was carried to the site in an old-fashioned horse-drawn hearse with glass sides and velvet curtains, and he was attended by a mounted escort of the Oklahoma Territorial Posse. At the insistence of the State Medical Examiner, Dr. Jay Chapman, two cubic yards of concrete were poured over the coffin before the grave was closed to ensure that the restless Elmer would wander no more.

The authors wish to thank Ralph G. Smith, Professor of Environmental and Industrial Medicine, University of Michigan, Ann Arbor, for his contributions in the preparation of this chapter.

Chapter 28

FORENSIC ANALYSIS OF OSSEUS MATERIAL EXCAVATED AT THE JAMES SITE, CLAY COUNTY, MISSOURI

MICHAEL FINNEGAN

INTRODUCTION

On the afternoon of 18 November 1978, the Osteology Laboratory at Kansas State University received a package shipped via United States Postal Service that contained six packets of hair, bone, and dental materials. These materials had been submitted for forensic analysis by Dr. Milton F. Perry, Superintendent of Historic Sites, Smithville, Missouri. Assuming them to be human, Perry requested a determination of age, sex, stature, race, anomalies, and pathologies to aid in the investigation of identity and possible cause of death. Dr. Perry had directed the excavation of these materials from a grave in Clay County, Missouri, during 12–14 October, 1978.

MATERIALS PRESENT

1. *A piece of nonhuman long bone with greatest cortical thickness 74.05 mm by 14.85 mm by 3.70 mm.* I determined this to be a portion of long bone from an animal, based on size, gross morphology, fine morphology, texture, and differential erosion of the edges and osteogenic layer of the periosteum.

2. *One human atlas (first cervical) vertebra, normal in every respect.* There is a very slight surface erosion of the left and right superior articular processes at the posterior and lateral edges without the loss of much gross morphology. The left transverse process shows some erosion, which extends into the left transverse foramen. Maximum transverse diameter is 76.15 mm, while the maximum A–P diameter is 45.05 mm. The maximum height of the vertebra is 20.70 mm. Relative height index (height × 100/A–P diameter) equals 45.95

I should like to thank Drs. Heglar, Guffy, Riordan, and Hinshaw and Mr. Knight for their assistance with various aspects of this analysis and particularly Dr. Milton F. Perry for his historic research, necessary in providing identification for the skeletal material analyzed. Thanks also goes to K. Wapp, M. Duell, and F. Brennan for typing various drafts of this paper. — Michael Finnegan

380

(see Ossenfort, 1926). None of the standard nonmetric traits were observed as present (Finnegan, 1978; Allen, 1879). Additionally, no pathology is seen on the atlas vertebra.

3. *One piece of nonhuman cancellous bone measuring 17.71 mm by 15.30 mm by 10.38 mm thick.* Adherant to this cancellous bone is a patch of cortical bone measuring 2.50 mm. The morphology of the external surface of the cortical bone does not match the morphology of the body or centrum of the vertebra. Rather, I would suspect this material to have originated in the proximal or distal end of a long bone, based on the thickness of the cortical bone and the alignment of the bony trabeculae underneath. This alignment suggests that this might have been one of the weight-bearing structural bones, although positive identification as such cannot be made at this time. Additionally, the texture of the outer cortical bone is not like that in number 1 above, nor is it similar to any human material from our comparative collection. I cannot tell at the present time if this particular material is human or not, but I assume not.

4. *Three proximal phalanges of a human right foot: representing the first, second and third toe.* The maximum oblique lengths are 41.15 mm, 31.31 mm, and 31.42 mm, respectively. The proximal maximum diameters are 21.65 mm, 12.94 mm, and 12.20 mm. Some bits of soft tissue and a few hairs still adhere to the first phalanx. We often find soft tissue adhering to foot bones because of the tanning action of fluids leached from the boots or shoes or from the protection that these artifacts offer to the underlying anatomical structures. There are no apparent anomalies or pathologies on any of these phalanges.

5. *Three teeth, one of which is human.* The first nonhuman tooth is a right mandibular PM3 of the domestic pig (*Sus scrofa*, comparative sample O.L. 704). The second nonhuman tooth has a maximum length of 38.08 mm, a mesial–distal diameter of 14.52 mm, and a buccal–lingual diameter of 7.91 mm. The tooth shows fused roots, which may represent twinning or possibly a unique formation of a single root, and the crown surface is greatly worn and polished diagonally from the upper buccal surface to the lower lingual surface. The tooth is large and probably comes from a relatively large animal. Not enough crown morphology remains on this tooth for positive identification. It may be a portion of one of the first or second premolars from the mandible of a cow (*Bos taurus*) or a buffalo (*Bison bison*). It is certainly not human.

The third tooth is a human right maxillary canine measuring 27.12 mm in length with a maximum crown diameter of 7.62 mm and a maximum root diameter of 7.75 mm. Dental hypoplasia is seen in the enamel of the crown at a location representing a developmental age of five years (Sopher 1976, Brothwell 1972). Some pathological destruction (carious lesion?) is seen on the labial surface of the root, beginning 1.65 mm below the enamel crown and extending 3.50 mm inferiorly. The maximum mesial–distal cord of this lesion is 5.70 mm. Dental attrition is observable macroscopically on the occlusal surface.

6. *Two portions of flat cranial bone.* One portion is made up of two pieces of bone divided roughly in half by a cranial suture. The maximum diameter of these joined pieces is 39.05 mm, while the lesser diameter is 32.10 mm. Maximum thickness of this bone at the suture line is 7.75 mm. This portion is apparently made up of the parietal bone and mastoid portion of the temporal bone including the parietomastoid suture. Additionally (and if this is the right side) one piece displays an edge of the occipitomastoid suture. Side identification of these pieces as portions of the right mastoid and parietal is problematic, as they lack sufficient objective fine morphology for a definitive identification.

The smaller portion of bone has a maximum diameter of 19.77 mm, while the minor axis is 12.25 mm and maximum thickness is 3.80 mm. It is a portion of the base of the occiput, apparently from the right side, between the foramen magnum and the occipitomastoid suture as determined by the differential thickness of the bone and the slight muscle markings. It would be desirable to have more material of the cranium to be absolutely positive of the location of the "parietal" fragment. While the piece is definitely part of the occipital, there might be some question as to exact location. These pieces were compared with three sectioned cadaver crania, two forensic cases, and 18 portions of crania from our comparative collection to determine location and side.

7. *Hair imbedded in dirt.* This material was forwarded to the Kansas Bureau of Investigation laboratory in Topeka for species identification and, if human, racial type.

ANALYSIS

The bone and dental material described above are in excellent condition and, with the exception of the right maxillary canine, no gross pathological condition was noted. Dental hypoplasias are thought to be due to either a high fever over an extended period of time or some mineral or metabolic deprivation suffered during the developmental years (Sweeney, Carera, Urrutia and Mata, 1969; Sweeney and Guzman, 1966). No gross anomaly was found in the remains, and all morphological structures appear to be well within normal variation for human material. The only possible evidence of trauma present, by gross morphological inspection, is seen in the two portions of cranial bone. Though microscopic examination of the edges of these bones was inconclusive, it is possible that this breakage occurred at the time of death. Alternatively, it may reflect postmortem damage.

With the help of Dr. Mark Guffy, Department of Surgery and Medicine, Kansas State University, an x-ray was taken of the cranial fragments (parietal-mastoid portion and occipital portion). The exposure value of the x-ray was 64KV, 150MA, .005 Sec. In reading this x-ray I find no anomalous conditions and no lead or heavy metal fragmentation that would suggest a gunshot wound.

Achieving great accuracy for skeletal age, sex, stature, and race is sometimes difficult with complete skeletal material. This difficulty is increased when the amount of material to be analyzed is severely limited. Reliable determination of age, sex, race, and stature is nearly impossible when only a few fragments are present. When these conditions are encountered, it is necessary to use all possible methodologies to extract reliable information and to achieve a definitive result. Our clients should realize both the potential and the limitations of anthropological analysis (Finnegan, 1980a).

The sex criteria used in this case were the maximum length of the canine tooth and Baudoin's sexual index of the atlas vertebra (Comas, 1960). The canine tooth, which is relatively long, is not long enough for a precise diagnosis as male. Baudoin's sexual index shows that the breadth of the atlas is greater in males, but suggests that this is due to an increase of the transverse diameter of the vertebra rather than an increased transverse diameter of the vertebral foramen. A discriminate function was set up based on known male and female atlas vertebrae from our comparative collection. When the sectioning point was determined for this sample, the unknown atlas vertebra was found to be in the intermediate range, although closer to the mean for male individuals. As with the maximum length of the canine tooth, this sexual index for the atlas vertebra did not facilitate precise sex diagnosis. Although some hair bulbs were present, sex determination could not be made due to the deteriorated condition of the sample (see Ishizu et al., 1973). Therefore the sex of this material, although it appears to be male, remained in question.

Age of this individual was determined on the basis of the Gustafson (1950) method. In preparation for this, the tooth was imbedded in bio-plastic and sectioned following the methodologies of Burns and Maples (1976) and Kilian (1975). A buccal-lingual section was cut, polished, and etched, and an acetate peel was made of the section. Another section was subsequently taken, allowing a thin section 200 microns to be mounted on a glass slide. The block section, the micro section, and the peel were read using a hand lens for the first reading and a steromicroscope for the second reading. I followed the methodology of Gustafson (1947, 1950) without the modification of Vlcek and Mrklas (1975) and Maples (1978). A standard rating of these materials produced an age, based on the Gustafson (1950) criteria, of 38

± 3.6 years at the time of death. Although the Gustafson technique has been criticized (Maples and Rice, 1979) and modifications suggested (Vlček and Kilian, 1975), my own work supports the general methodology when the standard error is expanded to ± 9.0 years (Finnegan, 1981a, 1981b).

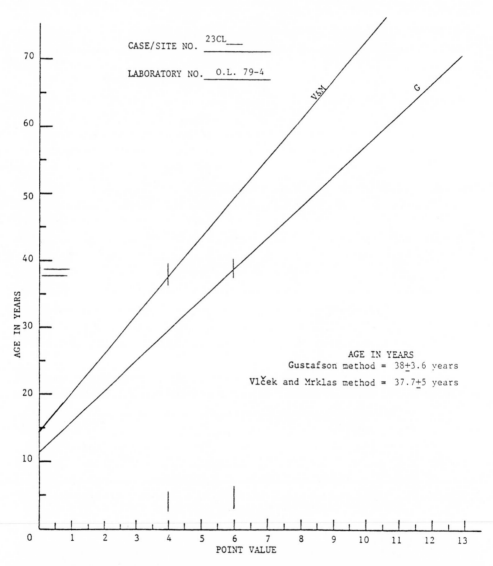

Figure 28-1. Relationship between age and point value for archaeological samples, based on Vlček and Mrklas (1975) (upper diagonal) and the Gustafson method (1950) (lower diagonal). The Vlček and Mrklas method is based on 4 traits, while the Gustafson method is based on 6 traits.

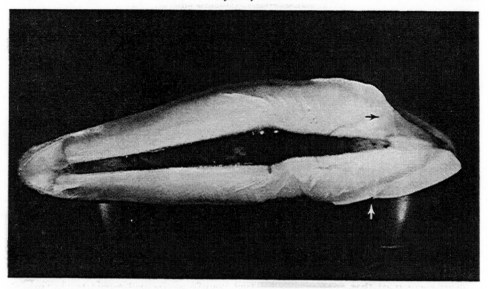

Figure 28-2. Lingual-buccal slab section of the right maxillary canine from which age was estimated. The arrow indicates the location of enamel hypoplasia on the lingual aspect of the tooth. The following scores were determined for the six attributes appropriate to the Gustafson method of age assessment through dental histology: attrition = 2; secondary dentine = 1; paradontosis = 1; cementum = 0.5; root resorption = 0.5; transparency = 1.0. The total tooth length is 27.12 mm.

The bone material supplied gives no indication of race. Based on the structural analysis of the hair samples, however, the individual appears to be Caucasoid (see hair analysis to follow).

The material presented for study does not, at the present time, lend itself to a reconstruction estimate for stature. However, recent work by Musgrave and Harneja (1978) has generated equations for the ascertainment of adult stature from metacarpal bone length. In the future the possibility is good that stature determination can be achieved by measurements of various phalanges of the hands and/or foot.

For a rough estimation of the time since death, the proximal phalanx of the right first toe was sectioned and subjected to irradiation by ultraviolet light (2537 Å) with subsequent observation of the fluorescence of the cross section of cortical bone, following the methodology of Knight and Lauder (1967, 1969) and Knight (1969). The result of this test showed a fluorescence of yellow to yellow green in color with a slight bluish cast (reflected visible light from the ultraviolet source) around the periosteum and the medullary cavity endosteum. The amount and intensity of yellow to yellow green fluorescence across the cortical bone suggests that this individual has been dead for about 100 years. Although the Knight and Lauder methodology has recently been criticized by Stewart (1979), it has been supported in recent prehistoric, historic, and forensic cases (Finnegan, 1980b).

The piece of animal long bone (#1 above) was also subjected to irradiation by ultraviolet light (2537 A) before and after immersion in a 0.05% aqueous uranium nitrate solution to enhance the fluorescence. After drying, the bone showed a perceivable color change with respect to the fluorescence before enhancement and with respect to the right first proximal phalanx, which further suggests that this bone is not human and quite possibly was intrusive in the site at a later time (McKern, 1958; Eyman, 1965; Finnegan, 1976).

The first proximal phalanx of the right foot, which had been sectioned for ultraviolet light irradiation, and soil samples taken from the site were subsequently sent to Dr. Rodger Heglar, Department of Anthropology, San Francisco State University, for analysis of paleoserology to identify the blood group of this material. The purpose of testing these samples was the ascertainment of the presence of ABO(H) antigenicity indicating the ABO blood group of this material. The test results show antigenicity A and H, which indicates blood group A. His test sequence was as follows:

1. Phalanx reduced to bone powder.
2. Powder added to known-titered anti-A, -B, -H antisera. (Control titer against RBC at 1:64)
3. Refrigeration and aggitation of above for 6 hr. and 24 hr. incubation times.
4. Re-titering of bone powder-exposed antisera;
    6 hr. Run = Anti-A 1:32, Anti-B 1:64, Anti-H 1:16 (=A)
    24 hr. Run = Anti-A 1:16, Anti-B 1:64, Anti-H 1:4 (=A)
5. A "control" for contamination was run by testing the dirt sample in the above manner. There was an A and H response similar to the bone on a 6 hr. run. This can be argued as caused by the neighboring body and hair chemistry, where we are seeing an influence in the soil from the body. If there was general environmental contamination, the titers of all antisera usually "drop" in strength, not specifically A *and* H. (Heglar, 1979)

The above testing and documentation support a blood type of A for this material. Reference for the methodology is found in Heglar (1972).

Point number 5 above is of the greatest importance to the overall blood grouping methodology. Chemical or bacterial transfer from bone to soil, or conversely from soil to bone, may invalidate the test results or inhibit the ability of the researcher to get any results on a particular test. This not only is important for blood typing, but also holds for trace element analysis, chemical studies, and dating by ultraviolet fluorescence and other nuclear dating methods. With the range of qualitative and quantitative chemical analyses that is now available (and the list will surely grow), it becomes increasingly important to sample the soils in and surrounding the skeletal remains. This may be accomplished by taking an array of soil samples; the exact array is somewhat dependent on the analyses to be run. As a general principle soils should be sampled above, directly under, and at some distance below the bones (see also Chapter 4). I routinely take a matrix of five samples above the skeletal remains, five samples intrusive in the remains, and another five samples 10 to 20 cm below the remains. These samples are deployed such that I have samples above and below both heavy cortical bone and cancellous bone. Additionally, a sample is taken some 2 to 3 m from the remains (above and below) with respect to the slope of the land. In each soil sample taken, the provenience is critical, and when a skeleton is found intrusive in to more than one identifiable strata, more samples are necessary.

For similar reasons, the skeletal material should be dry brushed (not washed), and preservatives should not be used. If, for some reason, preservatives are used, a sample of the skeletal remains should be withheld so the preservative does not hinder further chemical analyses.

Microscopic analysis of the hair was conducted with the assistance of Mr. Ken Knight of the Forensic Laboratory, Kansas Bureau of Investigation, Topeka, Kansas. The hair is in a good state of preservation considering the "assumed" ground/soil conditions (pH slightly acidic) of the area in which the material was retrieved. The hair displayed a brownish color (although obvious leaching had occurred). Race of this individual is based on the structure and color of the hair: It is definitely not Negroid and probably not Mongoloid. The probability is good that the hair is Caucasoid, although some destruction of the hair structure limits the racial assessment. The hair is therefore probably Caucasoid. Here, as in blood typing, the soil samples are of value in assessing color and structural changes.

Under further microscopic examination the presence of nits was observed. These are identified as the eggs of the louse and for human hair samples are probably those of the common head louse, *Pediculus humanus capitis.*

Mineral analysis of the hair and bone was performed by the Bio Center Laboratory, Wichita, Kansas under the direction of Drs. Hugh D. Riordan and Charles Hinshaw. The resultant profile of the various minerals assayed and the usual range of values with respect to modern clinical cases are presented in Table 28-I. Although this profile is interesting, with respect to the elevation of most elements measured, we are unable to analyze these results with respect to the environment because we cannot process adequate soil samples in and near the area of the bone remains. (Soil samples per se had not been taken at the time of excavation, and the small amount of soil adherent to the bone material was not sufficient to test against the elemental analysis. In this case I thought the blood typing to be more important. This further attests to the necessity of adequate soil sampling.)

TABLE 28-I

RESULTS OF MINERAL ANALYSIS ON HAIR SAMPLE

	Results mcg/gm		*Usual Range of Values* in mcg/gm (p.p.m.)	
P	429	HI		100–170
S	0.64%			0.50%–0.90%
CL	131			40–180
K	208	HI		8–80
CA	190			140–600
TI	71.58		to be established	
V	1.90	HI		0.05–0.6
CR	11.75	HI		0.50–1.7
MN	18.80	HI		0.30–2.0
FE	•••••¹	HI		6–40
NI	7.81	HI		0.30–1.0
CU	323.9	HI		7–30
ZN	4155	HI		100–220
SE	9.95	HI		0.50–1.5
BR	•••••¹		to be established	
HG	•••••¹	HI		0.20–2.0
PB	720	HI		3–20
MG	17			15–130
NA	1300			50–300*
MO	4.62			0.1–0.5*
CO				0.3–1.0*
CD	3.46			0.1–0.2*

*Magnesium levels are calculated by ratio to calcium peak in spectra display.

¹Numerical size exceeds the parameters of the testing equipment and subsequent readout.

RESOLUTION OF THE CASE

On receipt of the forensic osteological report, Dr. Perry telephoned the identity of the individual represented by the dental and osseus material which I had evaluated: "You have just identified Jesse James."

Of course, I had not positively identified Jesse James. However, many of the findings of the osteological report are compatible with what we know about Jesse James from the historical record. According to Perry, Jesse James died April 6, 1882 (at the age of 34 years, 6 months), as a result of gunshot wounds. He was buried at the James homestead near the village of Kearney, Missouri, but in 1902 his body was exhumed and removed for reburial in the family plot at the Kearney cemetery. During the exhumation the bottom was separated from the casket and the skull (and obviously some other material) dropped into the grave pit where the October excavations occurred. The skeletal age at death (38 years), as determined by the Gustafson

(1950) method, is amazingly close to the 34.5 years of Jesse James. Racial analysis of the hair, and to a lesser extent the color of the hair, are also compatible with written reports of Jesse James. Although sex could not be definitively established on the basis of the material supplied for examination, the suggestion of a male individual was given. The presence of dental hypoplasia and the suggested age of 5 years for the occurrence of the hypoplasia fits rather well with one historically documented illness of Jesse James. Paper filed with the Probate Court of Clay County (1854) after the death, intestate, of the Reverand Robert S. James, father of Jesse, who died in 1850, lists the bills paid by the widow for the children. In October, 1853, when Jesse was 6 years old, Dr. F. A. Rice of Kansas City was paid a total of $8.85 "for medical services for Jesse W. James." Jesse was so seriously ill from an abscess in the right thigh that the attending physician (Rice) called on Dr. Joseph W. Woods for consultation. Both doctors visited him at the home of an aunt in a suburb of Kansas City. Thirty years later, Dr. Wood remembered the fiery temper of Jesse's mother for the outlandish medical fee. The scar from the abscess was also noted in the autopsy performed in 1882.

However, the best proof of identity may come from a number painted on the bottom of the casket (11/1256), which corresponds to the number 11S on the casket provided by a St. Joseph, Missouri undertaker for the James burial (Croy, 1949; 193). Further documentation of the artifacts and reference to the history of Jesse James can be found in Settle (1977), Hale (1980), Kansas City *Daily Journal*, April 6 and 7, 1882.

SUMMARY

In this case study, a few bones, bone fragments, and other remains were used in attempting to determine the age, sex, race, and time of death, as well as pathological and anomalous conditions. Although I could not supply a positive individual identity of these few remains, my data were certainly compatible with those provided by the comprehensive search of historical documents, as well as archaeologically recovered information. Had there been no prior knowledge of individual identity, my analysis could have served as a basis for a search of missing person records or other forms of historic documentation. Thus, this study is quite similar to more recent forensic cases where the skeletal remains are frequently identified on the basis of a thorough investigation, excellent crime scene searches, and analysis of physical remains associated with these skeletal materials.

Although the osteological analysis fits well with what is known of Jesse James, the intent of this case report is to show the extent and types of methodologies that can be used on just a few or fragmented bones.

Additionally, the presence of hair and its analysis and the modern techniques that allow us to determine the ABH´blood group are techniques that should not be overlooked by forensic anthropologists. Certainly the paleoserological techniques and the mineral analysis of bone and hair are superfluous in this case, as these techniques had not been developed during the life of Jesse James. However, in a modern forensic situation, these types of analyses may provide the necessary data in a differential diagnoses for either positive identity or as criteria for the exclusion of a number of individuals, each of which may fit the osteological profile. As we continue to use and refine these techniques, we will certainly profit by an increased understanding and "practice the application of our science to the purpose of the law."

REFERENCES

Allen, W. (1879). On the varieties of the atlas in the human subject, and the homologies of the transverse processes. *J Anat, 14*:18–28.

Brothwell, D. R. (1972). *Digging Up Bones*, 2nd ed. London: The British Museum (Natural History).

Burns, K. R., and Maples, W. R. (1976). Estimation of age from individual adult teeth. *J Forensic Sci, 21(2)*: 343–356.

Comas, J. (1960). *Manual of Physical Anthropology*. Charles C Thomas: Springfield.

Croy, H. (1949). *Jesse James was my Neighbor*. Duell, Sloan and Pearle: New York.

Eyman, C. E. (1965). Ultraviolet fluorescence as a means of skeletal identification *Am Antiq, 31 (1)*:109–112.

Finnegan, M. (1976). Walnut Creek Massacre: Identification and Analysis. *Am J Phys Anthropol, 45(3)*:737–742.

———— (1978). Non-metric variation of the infracranial skeleton. *J Anat, 125(1)*:23–37.

———— (1980a). Forensic Anthropology: What to expect from a forensic anthropology report. *Identification News, 30(2)*:5–8.

———— (1980b). Osteological examination and possible historical record from site 14BT478, near Fort Zarah, Barton County, Kansas, *Journal of the Kansas Anthropological Association, 1(2–3)*:42–63.

———— (1981a). An Analysis of Age Determination by a Modified Gustafson Method. Paper presented at the 33rd annual meeting of the American Academy of Forensic Sciences, 17–20 February 1981, Los Angeles.

———— (1981b). The Use of Dental Histology for Age Estimations on Adult Teeth from Archaeological Remains. Paper presented at the 50th Annual Meeting of the American Association of Physical Anthropologists, Detroit, Michigan, 22–25 April 1981.

Gustafson, G. (1947). Microscopic examination of teeth as a means of identification in forensic medicine. *J Am Dent Assoc, 35(10)*: 720–724.

———— (1950). Age determination on teeth. *J Am Dent Assoc, 41(July)*:45–54.

Hale, D. R. (1980). The Resurrection of Jesse James. *Quarterly of the National Association and Center for Outlaw and Lawmen History, 5(3)*: 2–7.

Heglar, R. (1972). Paleoserology techniques applied to skeletal identification. *J Forensic Sci, 17(3)*: 358–363.

———— (1979). ABO Blood tests on bone and soil. Analysis received 9 April 1979.

Ishizu, H., Ando, K., Seno, M., Nobuhara, M., and Mikami, Y. (1973). Sex identification with a minimal sample by combining the Y-chromatin identification and the X-chromatin detection method. *Jpn J Legal Med, 27*(5):287–294.

Kilian, J. (1975). Age determination on teeth by means of Gustafson's method *Scripta medica, 48*(3–4):197–201.

Knight, B. (1969). Methods of dating skeletal remains. *Med Sci Law,* 9:247–252.

Knight, B. and Lauder, I. (1967). Proceedings of the British Assoc. in Forensic Medicine. Practical methods of dating skeletal remains: A Preliminary Study. *Med Sci Law,* 7:205–208.

———— (1969). Methods of dating skeletal remains. *Hum Biol, 41*(3):322–341.

Maples, W. R. (1978). An improved technique using dental histology for estimation of adult age. *J Forensic Sci, 23*(4):764–770.

Maples, W. R., and Rice P. M. (1979). Some difficulties in the Gustafson age estimations. *J Forensic Sci, 24*(1):168–172.

McKern, T. W. (1958). The use of short wave ultra-violet rays for the segregation of commingled skeletal remains. Tech. Report EP-98, U.S. Army Quartermaster Research and Engineering Center, Natick, Mass.

Musgrave, J. H. and Harneja, N. K. (1978). The estimation of adult stature from metacarpal bone length. *Am J Phys Anthropol, 48*(1): 113–120.

Ossenfort, W. F. (1926). The atlas in whites and Negroes. *Am J Phys Anthropol, 9*(4):439–443.

Settle, W. A., Jr. (1977). *Jesse James Was His Name.* University of Nebraska Press: Lincoln.

Sopher, I. M. (1976). *Forensic Dentistry.* Charles C Thomas: Springfield.

Stewart, T. D. (1979). *Essentials of Forensic Anthropology.* Charles C Thomas: Springfield.

Sweeney, E. A., Cabrera, J., Urrutia, J., and Mata, L. J. (1969). Factors associated with linear hypoplasia of human deciduous incisors. *J Dent Res,* 48:1275–1279.

Sweeney, E. A., and Guzman, M. (1966). Oral conditions in children from three highland villages in Guatemala. *Arch Oral Biol,* 11:687–698.

Vlček, E. and Kilian, J. (1975). Age determination of a prince from the Premyslide Dynasty buried in tomb No. 89 in the St. George's Basilica according to preserved teeth on the basis of the modified Gustafson method. *Scripta medica, 48*(3–4):209–214.

Vlček, E. and Mrklas, L. (1975). Modification of the Gustafson method of determination of age according to teeth on prehistorical and historical osteological material. *Scripta medica. 48*(3–4):203–208.

Section V
PRESENTING EVIDENCE

Court appearances as an expert witness are relatively rare for forensic physical anthropologists when compared to the other forensic sciences. Snow (1982) attributes our typical court testimony rate of perhaps once or twice a year to a number of factors. Even with our best efforts, the remains may not be identified due to a lack of association made between the remains and medical or dental records. In those cases where identity is established but no ascertainable cause of death is indicated or evidence is insufficient to build a case against a homicide suspect, the case may not be prosecuted in court. Finally, the identification evidence may be presented by a forensic pathologist or the other consultants such as the forensic odontologist or radiologist, or the lawyers may possibly stipulate or concede the identification issue.

In most instances, the forensic physical anthropologist's legal competence is limited to identification, and we are not considered medically qualified to give an opinion on cause or manner of death. As mentioned in several previous cases, however, evidence suggesting cause and manner of death detected during anthropological analysis should be passed on to the forensic pathologist. This aspect is included in the examples presented by Sauer, Angel and Caldwell, and Snyder et al. in the cause of death portion of Section II. Besides the important discussion of the distinction between cause and manner of death, Sauer illustrated the importance of osteological evidence in supporting other testimony on these important issues. Although the ability of Angel to suggest cause of death was questioned in court, establishing anatomical and physical evidence with the commonsense links established probabilities that led to a jury conviction. Angel and Caldwell rightly stress that we need to stay within our areas of expertise. It is indeed unusual for a forensic physical anthropologist to be qualified by the court as an expert in the diverse, but related, areas involved in the testimony phase of the facial reproduction example given by Rhine in Section IV.

Even though court appearances may be relatively rare for most forensic physical anthropologists, each consultation and analysis should be conducted with the possibility of eventual testimony in mind. Crime scene investigators, for example, are frequently taught to handle each case as if a court appearance will ensue. As Sundick indicates in the example in this section, extensive notation and documentation should be maintained even if the report is brief or limited. Besides the importance of the findings or the opinion, particular attention should be given to documentation of the chain of evidence possession.

As Sundick suggests, the increase in forensic anthropological consultations will likely increase the rate of court appearances. Although individual experiences at testifying are often related anecdotally, little formal attention has been given to being an effective witness in the professional anthropological literature. An important contribution of Stewart's forensic anthropology textbook is the chapter on the role of the expert witness (Stewart, 1979). The general procedures with specific examples should be reviewed as part of a witness's preparation. Court procedures share many characteristics, but as with each forensic consultation, the specifics will be unique, and the witness will be part of a cooperative effort.

Since many forensic anthropologists have had little experience in testifying, close collaboration with the court officials and extensive consultation with the attorneys are recommended. A number of the legal aspects of forensic science in reference to the expert witness have been reviewed by Kuzmack (1982). Joling (1963) and Cook (1964) have examined the legal implications and the role and rights of the expert witness. Of particular significance is the realization that the expert witness must be impartial and that the results of the case do not concern us as scientists, regardless of our personal feelings of the merits of the case being tried. The ultimate decision as to the facts or the truth resides with the jury. Scientific impartiality is essential to establish even though we may have been subpoenaed or paid a fee for testifying by one of the parties in the adversary court proceedings. Our major responsibility to the court, as well as to the investigative team, is to present our findings and opinions as clearly and effectively as possible.

The clarity and effectiveness of court testimony will likely depend upon the depth and extent of pretrial preparation. Once the witness has been notified regarding a pending court proceeding, thorough review of the case from the reports, files, and notes is suggested. Sundick stresses the significance of records of contacts as well as the procedures, conditions of the materials, and analytical tests conducted with the evidence. Since considerable time may pass between the conclusion of a forensic analysis and a court appearance, thorough review of all materials can be very important.

Experienced witnesses strongly recommend a pretrial conference with the consulting attorney. This should be routine, but it is especially important for the witness and the attorney who may have never met and have little idea of what to expect from each other. Besides the general procedures to be followed, the pretrial conference is the time to discuss the degree of legal certainty derived from the analysis (see Conrad, 1964, for a good review), clarification of issues in the case, mutual expectations of the participants, scheduling, the preparation of exhibits or illustrative materials, and fees for testifying. Only rarely will the actual remains be admitted into the court, and even notes as well as any illustrative materials may be retained as part of the court records. Duplicate copies of all materials should be made. Credentials and experience of the witness should be discussed to expedite the subsequent qualifying of the witness by the court. This process usually reflects the education, training, and experience (including other court appearances) of the witness. Certification by the American Board of Forensic Anthropology should be a definite asset.

The general format of court proceedings for an individual witness usually follows this sequence: swearing in, qualifying the witness by the court, direct examination by the attorney calling the witness, cross-examination by the opposing attorney, a redirect examination, and finally dismissal by the judge. It is during the direct examination that the evidence, other pertinent information, what was learned from various tests, and exhibits are presented. The cross-examination period frequently can be trying for the witness, since the opposing attorney, in trying to present the best case for the client, may question the witness closely to try to minimize possibly damaging testimony or establish doubt with the jury. Impartial, truthful, and unemotional responses by the witness during this time are the most appropriate and effective strategy. This point is well illustrated in the cases presented by Angel and by Sundick. The redirect examination by the retaining attorney allows for clarification and restatement of any questions developed during the cross-examination. Stewart (1979) provides several examples and recommendations from his experiences.

Although Sundick suggests that forensic physical anthropologists should be effective testimony presenters from experience in the classroom, important suggestions and analysis of the court situation have been developed by other forensic scientists. Miller (1963) discusses some of the problems with forensic scientist encounters in court and recommends manners of resolution. Wilber (1974), Kogan (1978) and Burke (1975) also provide good guides to courtroom behavior and preparation. These recommendations are general and may be modified for specific cases and witnesses. The perception of credibility of the witness by the jury has also received attention by Tuchler (1963), and Tanton (1979) has documented the effects of dress and demeanor of the witness.

The concluding case in this volume reflects the usual end of the involvement of a physical anthropologist in a forensic case. A number of themes seen in the cases in this volume come together in the presentation of evidence. The contribution by a forensic physical anthropologist will be enhanced by early involvement in the case, collaborative research and analysis, systematic collection and analysis of data, extensive notation, thorough preparation, clearly stated reports of findings and opinions, and increased recognition of our expertise developed through academic research.

REFERENCES

Burke, J. J. (1975). Testifying in court. *FBI Law Enforcement Bulletin*, September, pp. 8–13.

Conrad, E. C. (1964). The expert and legal certainty. *J Forensic Sci, 9(4)*:445–455.

Cook, C. M. (1964). The role and rights of the expert witness. *J Forensic Sci, 9(4)*:457–460.

Joling, R. J. (1963). Legal commentaries on the forensic scientist in court. *J Forensic Sci, 8(3)*:339–354.

Kogan, J. D. (1978). On being a good expert witness in a criminal case. *J Forensic Sci, 23(1)*:190–200.

Kuzmack, N. T. (1982). Legal aspects of forensic science. In R. Saferstein (Ed.), *Forensic Science Handbook*. Englewood Cliffs, New Jersey: Prentice-Hall, pp. 1–27.

Miller, F. M. (1963). The forensic scientist in court. *J Forensic Sci, 8(3)*:315–324.

Snow, C. C. (1982). Forensic anthropology. *Annu Rev Anthropol, 11*:97–131.

Stewart, T. D. (1979). *Essentials of Forensic Anthropology*. Springfield: Charles C Thomas, pp. 18–29.

Tanton, R. L. (1979). Jury preconceptions and their effect on expert scientific testimony. *J Forensic Sci, 24(3)*:681–691.

Tuchler, M. I. (1963). Credibility of a witness. *J Forensic Sci, 8(3)*:325–338.

Wilber, C. G. (1974). The art of testimony. Appendix C In *Forensic Biology for the Law Enforcement Officer*. Springfield: Charles C Thomas, pp. 347–355.

Chapter 29

POSITIVE IDENTIFICATION FROM THE RADIOGRAPHIC COMPARISON OF FRONTAL SINUS PATTERNS

Douglas H. Ubelaker

Since 1978 I have followed a long Smithsonian Institution tradition in serving as the consulting forensic anthropologist for the FBI laboratories in Washington. In this role, I offer opinions on all skeletonized remains thought to be human that have been submitted to the Bureau from investigative authorities throughout the United States. Of the 136 cases I have reported on to date, nine have been nonhuman, 32 archeological in origin, and 95 from recently deceased individuals. Of these 95, 22 have shown evidence of foul play, and only three resulted in my testifying at murder trials. Although most cases are "routine" in nature, occasionally they call for an appearance in court and for additional research as well.

THE CULT MURDER OF KAREN MARSDEN

On April 25, 1980, FBI agents brought to my laboratory a well-preserved human adult calvarium with considerable dried soft tissue still present. The calvaria skull showed no sign of injury other than the absence of bones of the face and cranial base. Morphology of the mastoid processes and supraorbital ridges suggested female sex. Lack of union of the vault sutures suggested that age at death was in the younger adult range, but a more exact estimate was not possible. The calvarium had been found on April 13, 1980 in the Westport area of Massachusetts, and the presence of dried blood and soft tissue on the remains suggested a relatively short time since death.

Authorities believed that the calvarium was that of Karen Marsden from Fall River, Massachusetts, who belonged to a group of prostitutes led by Mr. Carl Drew. Authorities also had information that Mr. Drew used satanism as a method of group control. According to later testimony, Marsden had previously witnessed the murder of another prostitute by Drew and others, and Drew feared she was providing information to authorities. On February 8, 1980, she was supposedly murdered by Drew and others, who somehow disposed of all of the body except the calvarium.

An important aspect of the case centered on proving that the recovered calvarium was that of Marsden. Of course, positive identification was not possible from my examination of the fragmentary skull alone. A photograph of Marsden was obtained, but since facial bones and teeth were lacking, identification was not forthcoming. Following the submission of my report, a search was made at local hospitals for any cranial radiographs of Marsden. It was discovered that shortly before her death Karen Marsden had entered a local hospital for treatment of a severe headache. At that time frontal and lateral radiographs had been taken and were located for the authorities by hospital personnel. Subsequently, radiographs of the recovered calvarium were taken at about the same angle by William Sturner, Chief Medical Examiner for the State of Rhode Island, and his staff and were available for comparison with the original radiographs taken during life. Comparison of the lateral view radiographs (Fig. 29-1) revealed exact similarity in the shape of the lower frontal area and especially in the size and shape of the sella turcica. Comparison of the frontal views (Fig. 29-2) revealed an exact match of details of the orbits and vault and of the size and pattern of the frontal sinus. Morphological details, especially those of the frontal sinus, matched so closely that both Dr. Sturner and I testified that both sets of radiographs were from the same individual. The Court permitted this expert testimony on the question of identity of the calvarium to be heard and evaluated by the jury. The jury later convicted Carl H. Drew of the murder of Karen Marsden.

During preparation for testimony and cross-examination two important questions arose: "What is the precedent for making positive identification from radiographic comparison?" and "What are the chances that two different individuals would happen to have identical frontal sinus patterns?" To answer these significant questions, the forensic and medical literature review and my research project involving uniqueness of frontal sinus patterns are summarized below.

POSITIVE IDENTIFICATION FROM RADIOGRAPHIC COMPARISON

As early as 1921 Schuller recommended comparative radiography, especially of the frontal sinuses, for purposes of making positive identification from skeletonized human remains. Over the years the importance of radiographic comparison has been established in positive identification in mass disasters (Brown et al., 1952; Singleton, 1951; Stevens, 1966); in the location of bones, bullets, or other radiodense materials in burned or matrix cases (Morgan and Harris, 1953; Fatteh and Mann, 1969); and in identification of skeletonized homicide victims (Kade et al., 1967) or other missing persons (Dutra, 1944; Murphy and Gantner, 1982; Murphy et al., 1980; Sanders et al.,

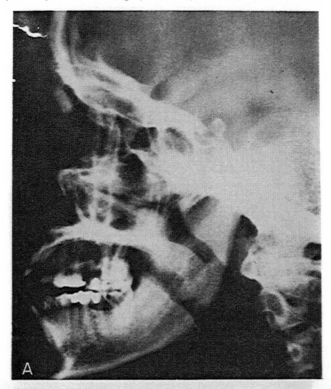

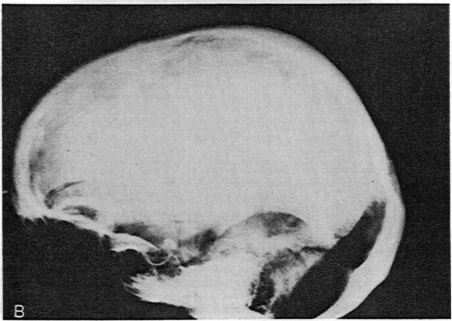

Figure 29-1. Comparison of lateral cranial radiographs of (A) Karen Marsden during life and (B) the recovered calvaria skull.

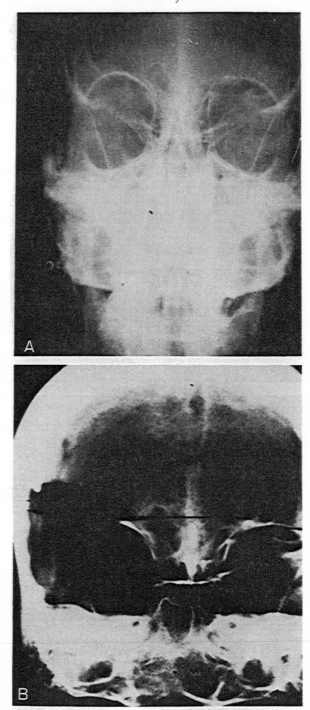

Figure 29-2. Comparison of frontal cranial radiographs of (A) Karen Marsden during life and (B) the recovered calvaria skull.

1972). According to Murphy et al. (1980), radiographic comparison is routinely used for positive identification at the City of St. Louis, Missouri, Office of the Medical Examiner where between April, 1978, and July, 1979, 30 of the 50 identifications were made from radiographs.

Martel et al. (1977) report on a partly burned, mutilated body, positively identified through comparison of chest radiographs. They found that the size and shape of the ribs, as well as the pattern of costal cartilage, proved important. As an experiment on the accuracy of radiographic identification, they obtained 25 male and 25 female radiographs from the University of Michigan hospital. They then obtained nine additional radiographs of individuals represented in the first sample of 50. These additional nine radiographs had been taken from one to eight years before the others. Two radiologists working independently correctly matched the nine "unknowns" with their counterparts in the sample of 50. Martel et al. (1977:683) conclude that "errors can be made, but are not likely if the observer is experienced, and meticulous attention is paid to detail." Sassouni (1958) reached similar conclusions using his method of comparing 24 measurements of cranial radiographs.

SELLA TURCICA COMPARISON

The considerable variability in the morphology of the sella turcica area of the sphenoid has been documented in early studies by Camp (1923, 1924) and Royster and Moriarty (1930). Dillon and Gourevitch (1936) examined the appearance and dimensions of the sella turcica in 24 pairs of twins, 11 monozygotic and 13 dizygotic. They found greater similarity between identical twins than between fraternal twins, although many differences were apparent in both categories. Francis (1948) noted that adult dimensions of the pituitary fossa were attained at about 18 years, and Haas (1954) proposed a method for measurement.

Voluter (1959) found radiographic comparison of the pituitary fossa area very useful in identifying victims of the *Noronic* disaster. The steamship *Noronic* burned while tied up at the pier in Toronto, Canada on September 17, 1949. The fire resulted in 119 deaths, 107 burned beyond recognition. Radiographs, especially those of the sella turcica area, provided the most important evidence for identifying 19 individuals. Voluter classified the pituitary fossa into types and provided statistics on size and shape, commenting, "We could never find two identical sella turcica, complete identity existing only among identical twins" (Voluter, 1959:13).

Finally, Ravina (1960) stressed the utility of sella turcica comparison for identification purposes because of its durability and individual variability. Like Voluter, Ravina stressed the form and volume of the fossa, but also the angle it forms with the basilar and with the anterior cranial fossa, and the morphology of the clinoid apophyses.

FRONTAL SINUS COMPARISON

The literature on the use of frontal sinus comparison for identification purposes has its roots in Turner's 1901 study of 578 crania representing several different populations. Turner provided anatomical descriptions of the frontal sinuses and noted that (1) they are not present at birth; (2) they commence development at the end of the first or beginning of the second year; (3) large supraorbital ridges do not correlate well with large frontal sinuses; and (4) they display great variation in size and symmetry. Turner found no correlation between the size and shape of the sinuses and the size and shape of the entire skull. Generally he observed that males had larger sinuses than females and that frontal sinuses were visually absent in about 27 percent of the crania examined.

Development and variation of the frontal sinus was then documented in detail by Cryer (1907) and in a series of articles by Schaeffer (1910a, 1910b, 1910c, 1912, 1916a, 1916b, 1916c). Schaeffer's work established that the "frontal sinus develops variously by a direct extension of the frontal recess or from one or more of the ventral ethmoidal cells which have their point of origin in frontal furrows. In many instances the frontal sinus is, embryologically speaking, a ventral ethmoidal cell which has grown sufficiently far into the frontal region to be topographically a frontal sinus" (Schaeffer, 1916b:238–239). He noted also that a sinus may appear to be absent, but actually is only very diminutive; true "agenesis of the frontal sinus is very unusual" (Schaeffer, 1916a:667). In 1918 Davis dissected 160 crania of children aged birth to 16 years and concluded that on the average "the sinus begins its ascent into the vertical portion of the frontal bone during the second year, and at three years is 3.8 millimeters above the level of nasion, and continues its vertical advance at an average rate of approximately 1.5 millimeter per year until the fifteenth year" (Davis, 1918:942). These observations were later confirmed by Maresh (1940), who found that although anatomically they appear as early as one year, they are not clearly visible in radiographs until seven to nine years.

Schuller (1921) appears to be the first to recognize the utility of frontal sinus comparison for identification purposes and strongly recommended its use. Four years later Culbert and Law applied this technique for the first time in identifying a former patient of theirs. In January of 1920 Culbert had operated on the patient for mastoiditis on the left side. The patient subsequently disappeared in June of 1925 in the Indus River in India. Culbert and Law later identified a body found in the river as their former patient through radiographic comparison of the frontal sinuses as well as other accessory sinuses, the sella turcica, and the mastoid process with its air cells (Culbert and Law, 1927). Law (1934) later emphasized the importance of frontal sinuses for identification purposes and agreed with Carmody (1929) and later Schuller (1943) that in adults the sinuses can be altered only by trauma, tumors, surgery, or infection.

In 1935 Mayer again emphasized the importance of frontal sinuses for identification, citing the work of Dr. Thomas A. Poole of the Washington, D.C. area. According to Mayer, Poole was establishing a "library of sinus prints" to aid in identification, although I have been unable to locate any published results of Poole's work.

Twin studies focusing on the frontal sinus (Turpin et al., 1942; Schuller, 1943; Asherson, 1965; Dillon and Gourevitch, 1936) clearly demonstrate that although the frontal sinus shows greater similarity between pairs of monozygotic twins than between dizygotic twins, even the former show at least minimal differences. The Turpin et al. study suggested that the differences increase with age, at least until adulthood. Asherson's (1965) important summary article found that each of 74 pairs of twins all showed different frontal sinus patterns. Asherson also proposed a system of classification of frontal sinuses in this article and noted that he had never observed identical frontal sinus patterns in over 2000 cases.

OTHER CASE REPORTS IN THE FORENSIC LITERATURE

In addition to the Culbert and Law (1927) identification discussed earlier, at least five other identifications made from frontal sinus comparison are documented in the forensic literature. Camps (1969) compared radiographs of frontal sinus patterns to associate a skull with a previously identified torso found at sea. Cheevers and Ascencio (1977) reported that a Canadian missing since 1969 was found in 1976. Dental records were not available, but identification was made from comparison of the frontal sinus pattern in the skull with that in cranial radiographs taken in 1968. Atkins and Potsaid (1978) used frontal sinus comparison along with other approaches positively to identify a skull found in Boston Harbor on July 6, 1977, as a man who was lost when a boat overturned nearby on April 30, 1977. Stewart (1979) described a 1976 Florida case where a frontal sinus comparison was used positively to identify a skeleton as that of a missing hospital patient. Finally, Murphy and Gantner (1982) reported that a skeleton found in 1980 in the St. Louis, Missouri area was positively identified from the radiographic comparison of frontal sinus patterns and other details.

The above discussion drawn from the literature documents the precedent for positive identification from frontal sinus comparison as well as the available information on the development and variability of that anatomical area. The question remains, however, "What are the chances that two individuals would happen to have identical frontal sinus patterns?" Asherson (1965), Camps (1969), Schuller (1943), Mayer (1935), and others have suggested that expression of the frontal sinuses is unique to each individual and thus can be used for positive identification. None of the studies, however, present data on the probability of uniqueness of the feature in any one individual.

MATERIALS AND METHODS

Thirty-five frontal radiographs of American Indian and Eskimo crania were randomly selected from those on file in the Department of Anthropology, National Museum of Natural History/National Museum of Man. Each radiograph was compared to each other radiograph in the sample to assess the number of differences in the frontal sinus itself and in its relationship to the surrounding skeletal structures. The area studied is outlined in Figure 29-3. A difference was defined as any detail of the frontal sinus, orbits, frontal crest, or related structure within the area shown in Figure 29-3 that was present on one radiograph and not on the other. In complicated sinuses with intersecting borders, a difference constituted a line (usually curved) defined from the points where it intersected with another line or shifted in direction. This system is conservative, since each line is composed of an infinite number of points that all may be unique to an individual.

All of the 595 individual comparisons showed at least three differences. The number of differences in each comparison ranged from three to fifteen with an average of eight (S.D. 2). The numbers of comparisons found to yield each number of differences are as follows: 2-3, 11-4, 63-5, 82-6, 102-7, 10-8, 81-9, 72-10, 36-11, 27-12, 8-13, 6-14, and 2-15.

The degree of variation is illustrated in Figures 29-4 and 29-5. The comparison illustrated in Figure 29-4 revealed fifteen differences in the area of the frontal sinuses and documents the increased number of differences that occur when both sinuses in the comparison are large and complicated. In contrast, the comparison shown in Figure 29-5 revealed only three differences and represents one of the closest matches in the frontal sinus area found in the study.

SUMMARY

The forensic literature documents that at least six positive identifications of human remains have been made from radiographic comparison of frontal sinus patterns. To my knowledge, however, the Drew case described above represents the first instance where this procedure has been used to establish positive identity of the victim in a murder trial. The published literature on

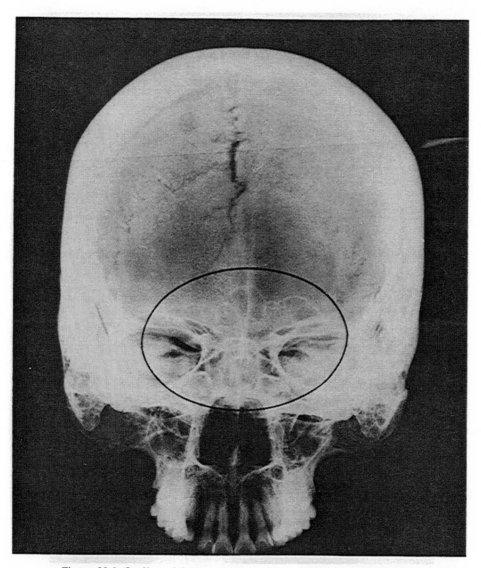

Figure 29-3. Outline of the area examined in radiographic comparison.

the development and variability of the frontal sinus and the new research reported here all argue strongly for the validity of this procedure. There is no doubt that an exact match of details of frontal radiographs, especially in the frontal sinus area, is sufficient basis for positive identification. Practitioners of this procedure should be aware, however, that (1) radiographs must be taken at the same angle and distance to allow meaningful comparison; (2) skeletal features are likely to be more clearly defined in the radiographs taken of the skeletonized remains than in those taken during life because of

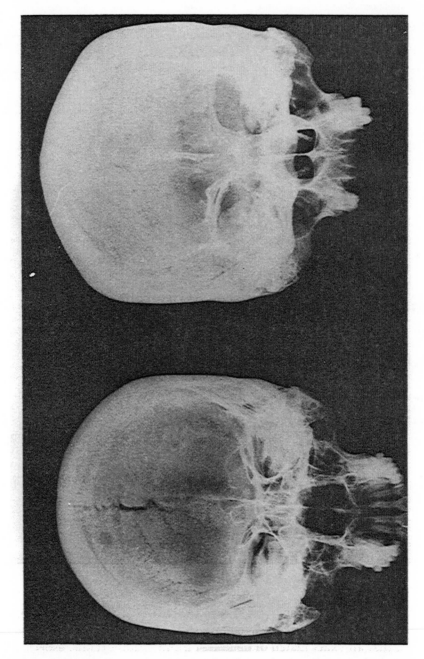

Figure 29-4. Comparison of two frontal cranial radiographs showing many differences in the frontal sinus area.

the presence of soft tissue in the latter; (3) some artificial differences may appear in the comparison due to postmortem trauma to the skull, artificial

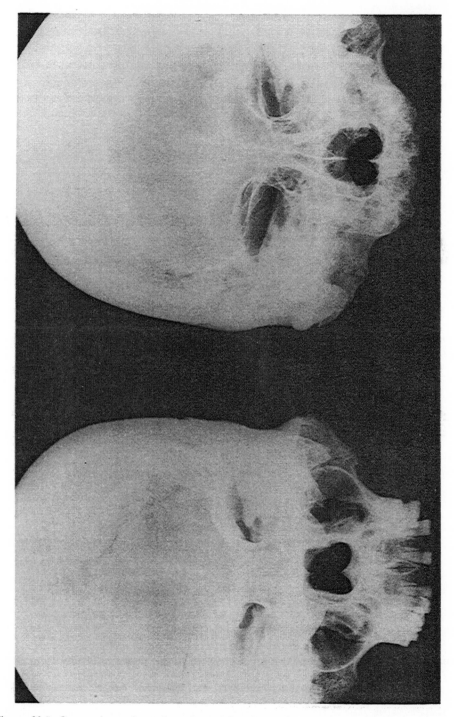

Figure 29-5. Comparison of two frontal cranial radiographs showing few differences in the frontal sinus area.

inclusions in the skull, or alterations of the frontal sinus area made during life but after radiographs were taken. These alterations in the living could be produced by trauma, surgery, infection, or other disease processes affecting that area; (4) caution should be used in comparing radiographs of the frontal sinus taken from individuals younger than 18 years, since some normal growth changes may have occurred between the dates the radiographs were taken.

REFERENCES

Asherson, N. (1965). Identification by Frontal Sinus Prints. London: H. K. Lewis.

Atkins, L., and Potsaid, M. S. (1978). Roentgenographic identification of human remains. *JAMA, 240*:2307–2308.

Brown, T. C., Delaney, R. J., and Robinson, W. L. (1952). Medical identification in the "Noronic" disaster. *JAMA, 148*:621–627.

Camp, J. D. (1923). The normal and pathologic anatomy of the sella turcica as revealed at necropsy. *Radiology, 1*:1–9.

———— (1924). The normal and pathologic anatomy of the sella turcica as revealed by roentgenograms. *Am J Roentgenol, 2*:143–156.

Camps, F. E. (1969). Radiology and its forensic application. In F. E. Camps (Ed.), *Recent Advances in Forensic Pathology.* London: Churchill, pp. 149–160.

Carmody, T. E. (1929). The development of the sinuses after birth. *Ann Otol Rhinol Laryngol, 38*:130–134.

Cheevers, L. S., and Ascencio, R. (1977). Identification by skull superimposition. *Int J Forensic Dent, 13*:14–16.

Cryer, M. H. (1907). Some variations in the frontal sinuses. *JAMA, 48*:284–289.

Culbert, W. L. and Law, F. M. (1927) Identification by comparison of roentgenograms of nasal accessory sinuses and mastoid processes. *JAMA, 88*:1634–1636.

Davis, W. B. (1918). Anatomy of the nasal accessory sinuses in infancy and childhood. *Ann Otol Rhinol Laryngol, 27*:940–967.

Dillon, I. G., and Gourevitch, I. B. (1936). Research on the pneumatization of the nasal accessory sinuses and of the mastoid processes and on the shape and dimensions of the sella turcica in twins. *Am J Roentgenol, 35*:782–785.

Dutra, F. R. (1944). Identification of person and determination of cause of death from skeletal remains. *Arch Pathol, 38*:339–349.

Fatteh, A. V., and Mann, G. T. (1969). The role of radiology in forensic pathology. *Med Sci Law, 9*:27–30.

Francis, C. C. (1948). Growth of the human pituitary fossa. *Hum Biol, 20*:1–20.

Haas, L. L. (1954). The size of the sella turcica by age and sex. *Am J Roentgenol Rad Ther Nucl Med, 72*:754–761.

Kade, H., Meyers, H., and Wahlke, J. E. (1967). Identification of skeletonized remains by x-ray comparison. *J Crim Law, Criminol, Police Sci, 58*:261–264.

Law, F. M. (1934). Roentgenograms as a means of identification. *Am J Surg, 26*:195–198.

Maresh, M. M. (1940). Paranasal sinuses from birth to late adolescence. *Am J Dis Child, 60*:55–78.

Martel, W., Wicks, J. D., and Hendrix, R. C. (1977). The accuracy of radiologic identification of humans using skeletal landmarks. *Radiology, 124*:681–684.

Mayer, J. (1935). Identification by sinus prints. *Vir Med Monthly, 62*:517–519.

Morgan, T. A., and Harris, M. C. (1953). The use of x-rays as an aid to medico-legal investigation. *J Forensic Med, 1*:28–38.

Murphy, W A, and Gantner, G E (1982) Radiologic examination of anatomic parts and skeletonized remains. *J Forensic Sci, 27(1)*:9–18.

Murphy, W. A., Spruill, F. G., and Gantner, G. E. (1980). Radiologic identification of unknown human remains. *J Forensic Sci, 25*:727–735.

Ravina, A. (1960). L'identification des corps par le v-test. *La Presse Medicale, 68*:178.

Royster, L. T., and Moriarty, M. E. (1930). A study of the size of the sella turcica in white and colored males and females between the eighth and ninth years. *Am J Physiol Anthropol. 14*:451–458.

Sanders, L., Waesner, M. E., Ferguson, R. A., and Noguchi, T. T. (1972). A new application of forensic radiology: identification of deceased from a single clavicle. *Am J Roentgenol 115*:619–622.

Sassouni, V. (1958). Physical individuality and the problem of identification. *Temple Univ Law Q, 31*:341–351.

Schaeffer, J. P. (1910a). On the genesis of air cells in the conchae nasales. *Anat Rec 4*:167–180.

———— (1910b). The lateral wall of the cavum nasi in man, with especial reference to the various developmental stages. *J Morphol, 21*:614–707.

———— (1910c). The sinus maxillaries and its relations in the embryo, child and adult man. *Am J Anat, 10*:313–368.

———— (1912) An unusual sinus frontalis. *Ann Surg, Sept*:397–400.

———— (1916a). Further observations on the anatomy of the sinus frontalis in man. *Ann Surg, Dec*:665–671.

———— (1916b). The embryology and anatomy of the nasofrontal region in man. *Anat Rec, 10*:238–241.

———— (1916c). The genesis, development and adult anatomy of the nasofrontal region in man. *Am J Anat, 2*:125–145.

Schuller, A. (1921). Das rontgenogramm der stirnhole-ein hilfsmitte fur die identitatsbestimmung von schadeln. *Monatsschrift Fur Ohrenhbilkunde 55*:1617–1620.

———— (1943). A note on the identification of skulls by x-ray pictures of the frontal sinuses. *Med J Australia, June*:554–556.

Singleton, A. C. (1951). The roentgenological identification of victims of the "Noronic" disaster. *Am J Roentgenol, 66*:375–384.

Stevens, P. J. (1966). Identification of a body by unusual means. *Med Sci Law, 6*:160–161.

Stewart, T. D. (1979). *Essentials of Forensic Anthropology.* Springfield: Charles C Thomas.

Turner, A. L. (1901). *The Accessory Sinuses of the Nose.* Edinburgh: William Green and Sons.

Turpin, R., Tisserand, M., Bernyer, G., and Caspar-Formarty, M. (1942). *Comptes Rendus, 136*:203–205.

Voluter, G. (1959). The v-test. *Radiologia Clinica, 28*:7–17.

I thank Elizabeth Beard and Stephanie Damadio of the Department of Anthropology, Smithsonian Institution for their assistance in the preparation of this manuscript. Illustrations were provided by the Office of Photo Services, Smithsonian Institution and the Federal Bureau of Investigation. Information on the Drew trail was provided by the District Attorney for the Bristol District of the Commonwealth of Massachusetts, Ronald A. Pina and his staff. I also acknowledge the work of Dr. William Sturner, Chief Medical Examiner for the State of Rhode Island, and his staff in the preparation and interpretation of the Marsden radiographs.

Chapter 30

ASHES TO ASHES, DUST TO DUST OR WHERE DID THE SKELETON GO?

Robert I. Sundick

T he number of physical anthropologists interested in forensic anthropology has been growing steadily over the past decade, as can be seen by an examination of the membership roles of the American Academy of Forensic Sciences, physical anthropology section, and by the list of Diplomates of the American Board of Forensic Anthropology. Rhine (Chapter 3) documents dramatic increases in case loads in the American Southwest. As more of us become involved in this new and developing field, the likelihood of our appearing in court as an expert witness multiplies. It is therefore important that we understand the significance of our role as an expert witness and how to operate within the American legal system. As noted by Stewart (1979), this is especially true of forensic anthropologists whose training has traditionally been in the academic area of anthropology and not in criminal justice. With the expanding use of expert witnesses from all fields of science, there is an increasing number of articles appearing on the role of expert witnesses in the legal system (Kogan, 1978; Philipps 1977) and special seminars at the annual Academy meetings.

The types of cases in which physical anthropologists can be involved may be quite varied. I have been asked to testify on such things as the percentage of black males in the United States who have blue eyes and on the importance of the thumb to modern day humans, in addition to the more traditional requests of identification of skeletal remains. In the former case I was contacted by the defense attorney representing a black male who had been accused of murder. The sole witness to the crime was only able to say that the assailant was a black male with blue eyes, and thus it was important for the defendant's case to know what percentage of black males also had blue eyes. In the second case a prosecutor requested my testimony in a case where an individual was being tried for an assault upon a female police officer during which he nearly bit off her thumb. More traditionally, I have identified the skeletal remains of murder victims, possible missing persons, and skeletal remains that were recovered from grave-robbing incidents.

Because we, as forensic anthropologists, are most often involved in the identification of skeletal remains, more often than not initial contact comes from police departments or prosecutor's offices rather than from defense attorneys. From the time that contact is first made, each of us should be aware of what might be expected of us and what legal responsibilities we have in the administration of justice. Each case is unique, but general principles and procedures apply.

I. INITIAL CONTACT

It has been my experience that contact generally has been made by a local police department or a prosecutor's office asking if I would be willing to examine some bones for them. They usually do this because they want to learn whether the bones are human or nonhuman. If human, the question then is whether they are recent or over 100 years old. If the bones are nonhuman or very obviously over 100 years old, then the forensic aspect of the incident will be over. If, however, the bones are human and recent, then our responsibilities and duties as an expert become important.

In the very first case in which I became involved I made a number of significant errors, which I have not since repeated. On that occasion I was contacted by a state police officer who asked if I would identify a pile of bones that they had just finished collecting in and near a pine forest. They "knew" the bones were those of a black female who had been reported missing just six weeks earlier, and they showed me a complete skull that had been identified by a local dentist as the missing person. Apparently in the intervening six-week period a pack of dogs had consumed portions of the postcranial skeleton and had scattered the remainder over a tremendous area. The police had scoured the entire area and picked up anything that looked like bone. They brought that assemblage to me and asked if I would quickly examine them and sort out the human bones. I was told that I would not have to do anything else, as the local dentist had already made a positive identification from the skull. I accepted their statements uncritically and made a cursory examination of the remains. There were a number of fragmentary human bones in addition to many cow bones, pig bones, and twigs. I then recorded on a typical skeletal analysis form what bones I had seen and how complete they were, but I did not photograph them or make more complete records, since I was assured by the police that I would never see them again. Those bones were then taken away and shortly thereafter buried, and I believed that the case was then closed, or at least that my involvement in it was then over.

Close to two years later, however, I was contacted by the local district attorney who had charged the missing girl's boyfriend with her murder. He explained to me that the dentist could not say much more than that he had identified a skull as belonging to the missing person. Therefore I would be called as the prosecution's key witness to identify both the skull and the remainder of the skeleton. At that point I wished that I had made a photographic record of everything I had seen and more complete notes so that I would have them to refresh my memory.

Unfortunately, the situation could not be changed at that point, and I was subpoenaed to testify in the case. I had no choice but to testify on the basis of those notes which I did have. Fortunately for me, the notes were adequate to confirm the identification, although not as complete as my notes now are for such situations. The accused boyfriend was, in fact, convicted for the murder of his girl friend. The conviction was based on the suspect's having been seen with the victim at the place where the body was found on the night of her disappearance and also on the discovery of a knotted rope with bloodstains upon it that was found near the body.

Under similar circumstances I would recommend that anyone now becoming involved in a forensic identification case adhere to the following guidelines:

1. Upon being contacted by a law enforcement agency or prosecutors office to identify skeletal remains, agree to do so either in your own laboratory, in their laboratory, or at the scene of the find. In most instances it would be preferable to go to the scene yourself because you, as a trained expert in human skeletal remains, will be better able to find and identify bones, particularly if they are disarticulated and scattered. If there is a choice to be made as to where to examine the skeletal material, it would probably be best to study it in your own laboratory facility where you can work in an unhurried atmosphere with all your equipment and reference and comparative materials available. As noted by Morse and Brooks and Brooks in this volume, context can provide important information in both archaeological and forensic cases.

2. At the time of the initial contact it is appropriate, if other more formal arrangements do not already exist, to inform the individual or agency contacting you that as an expert in the field of forensic anthropology who is willing to go to court to testify, you expect and are entitled to a consultant fee. This is appropriate, as experts in all other fields are compensated for their time and expertise in similar circumstances. The fee can either be a flat rate, say something between $100.00 and $200.00 or more depending on the amount of time involved, or else can be based on an hourly rate. In my area an hourly rate of between $30.00 and $50.00 would be reasonable, but in other communities a greater fee might be appropriate.

3. Keep a careful account of everybody who contacts you in regard to the case, the date, and under what circumstances such contact occurred. Detailed

notes should be kept on all conversations that take place. Be aware, however, that any and all of your records can be the subject of subpoena and thus made part of the evidence presented in court.

4. If the bones or any other evidence are turned over to you for examination, you will most likely be asked to sign for the material to establish the chain of evidence. If no one asks you to do so it would probably be best for you to get the signature of the law enforcement officer in charge attesting that certain bones or pieces of information were turned over to you for examination.

5. Carefully note the condition of all material submitted to you. Photographs of the material as well as written notes are essential for review prior to testimony and as evidence if remains are not available at the time of trial. One of my colleagues videotapes all investigations, which seems to be a useful technique. Forensic squads for some law enforcement agencies routinely use videotape to supplement traditional photography. Individual courts rule on the admissibility of these materials.

6. Take careful notes of all that you observe and record all tests that you perform. For example, if you section the bone to determine a histological age, this should be clearly recorded.

7. After completing the examination of the material, note what condition it is in when it leaves your laboratory, and make sure that whoever takes it from you signs for it so that the chain of custody can be documented.

8. Be careful to mark all pieces of the evidence so that you can identify it at a later date.

9. After completion of your analysis, you should prepare a written report of your findings. Be certain to present all important observations, as well as your conclusions. This detail can be invaluable later. Reference standards should also be noted.

10. Be patient and wait to see if you are contacted again about the case.

II. PREPARATION FOR COURTROOM APPEARANCE

According to Kogan (1978), a report written for a federal court can be examined by the defense attorney before the trial. This is also true of some state courts. You should therefore be prepared to defend on the stand all information presented in the report.

Shortly before an actual trial date, it is probable that you will be contacted by the district attorney's office, if they first contacted you, or by the defense attorney, if he or she was the one who contacted you. In my experience this first contact is generally made to ascertain whether a particular trial date and time is convenient, as some leeway is generally available in the scheduling of witnesses. If the time or date is not convenient, you should mention this and perhaps a change could be made in the schedule.

At the time when you are contacted you should definitely try to schedule a pretrial conference with the attorney. You want to discuss with the attorney those credentials which establish your credibility as an expert witness. Second, you want to consider the nature of your testimony so the attorney will know exactly what questions to ask of you and so that all the pertinent information is established in the direct examination. Angel and Caldwell (Chapter 14), Sauer (Chapter 15), and Rhine (Chapter 25) illustrate some of these aspects.

In the very first case in which I testified, the district attorney suggested that we have a pretrial conference, and it was then that we discussed my credentials and the nature of my testimony. In most subsequent cases the attorneys did not indicate the need for a pretrial conference; however, one was agreed to at my suggestion. These conferences are important because they ensure that proper credentials are presented and that the appropriate questions are asked during direct examination. In this discussion you should also carefully define forensic anthropology and the specialized expertise of a certified forensic anthropologist. This is necessary because few attorneys today have worked with forensic anthropologists or are familiar with the literature in forensic anthropology. During this time you could indicate that forensic anthropologists with expertise in skeletal identification are capable of making identifications in regard to age, sex, race, unique identifying characteristics, etc. This might also prevent the embarrassing situation in court where your own attorney might ask you some unanswerable question such as, "What color eyes did the individual have?" or "Can you tell me from your examination of the skull how much the individual weighed?" While both of these questions can be answered by saying "No, we can't determine the color of eyes, nor can we determine the weight of an individual by examination of the skull," it might be misleading to a judge or jury who could draw the erroneous conclusion that the entire science of skeletal identification is an inexact one and that little of the testimony is to be believed.

Courtroom Appearance

Even the most impressive credentials can be enhanced by the appearance and general demeanor of an expert witness. The individual should be well dressed and should convey the feeling of confidence and self-assurance. Kogan (1978) indicates that demeanor includes

> such factors as the tone of voice in which a witness' statement is made, the hesitation or readiness with which his answers are given, the look of the witness, his carriage, his evidences of surprise, his gestures, his zeal, his being, his expression, his yawns, the use

of his eyes, his furtive or meaning glances, or his shrugs, the pitch of his voice, his self-possession or embarrassment, his air of candor or seeming levity.

In addition, the expert should be able to communicate effectively with judge and jury. He or she should speak in terms that are understandable to a lay audience. Scientific terminology may be too technical for the individuals who should be listening, and if this is the case they will just stop listening and possibly ignore some very important testimony. This ability to communicate with individuals, i.e. in a language that is understandable to them and in a manner where you establish eye contact with your audience, is crucial and can be improved with practice. Since most forensic anthropologists come from the academic area, where we are constantly communicating with students, we already should have developed these important skills.

While testifying it may sometimes be necessary to refer to written notes. This is permissible, but it should be realized that if notes are referred to at all while on the witness stand then the opposing attorney generally has the right to examine them. If there are inconsistencies in these notes or even irrelevant information, such data can then be used to damage the credibility of the witness. In addition, any illustrative devices, such as charts or slides, may be entered as evidence and be retained by the court during the trial and all through the appeal process. Duplicate copies are advisable.

Establishing the Qualifications of the Expert Witness

On the day of the trial the attorney with whom you are working will generally tell you what time you might expect to be called to the witness stand and what time you should arrive at the courthouse. Although you may be allowed to hear other testimony, it is more common for all witnesses to be excluded from the trial. Despite all efforts and consideration by attorneys and the court, you may not be called to the stand on schedule. Be prepared to be patient.

The expert witness must always be sworn in. Stewart (1979) mentions that in one trial, through an oversight, he testified but was never sworn in and did not realize it until he had left the courthouse. At that point he returned to the courthouse, where arrangements were made for him to be sworn in after the fact. Failure to have done this may have been grounds for a mistrial.

The purpose of qualifying a witness is to indicate to the judge and jury that the expert is, in fact, knowledgeable in his or her field and is qualified to state his opinion in regard to the particular evidence. This qualification includes the expert's educational background, experience, publications in the field, memberships in professional organizations, and certifications by established certifying agencies. In regard to forensic anthropology, certification as a Diplomate of the American Board of Forensic Anthropology is important. Angel and Caldwell (Chapter 14) as well as Rhine (Chapter 25) also caution us to stay within our areas of expertise and experience. Qualification also includes whether or not the expert has previously qualified as an expert in other courts. If you have previously qualified as an expert, you should be prepared with a list of those courts which previously accepted your credentials, and you should know whether they were Circuit Courts, District Courts, or Federal Courts. If all of this information is given to the attorney who has subpoenaed you at a pretrial conference, then he or she can ask you point by point what your qualifications are. Kogan (1978) indicates that the presentation of an expert's qualifications may be half the battle in court, since greater emphasis may be put on the testimony of a well-qualified expert as opposed to that given to a less qualified expert.

In some situations, although probably not often, an opposing attorney may indicate when the expert takes the stand that he or she is willing to stipulate as to the credentials of the expert. This means that the opposing attorney is willing to admit that the expert is, in fact, knowledgeable in his or her field and does not want the qualifications to be discussed in front of the jury. If the attorney does so stipulate and the judge approves it, then the expert will not need to document credentials.

Direct Examination

During direct examination the expert is given the opportunity to present the evidence to the court, which includes what was studied, what tests were performed on the materials, and what was learned. If the expert and attorney have previously considered this, then the attorney can carefully phrase questions that will bring out all the pertinent information in a clear, logical, and understandable manner. All answers should be given in language that is understandable to a lay jury and judge. It may be possible to present pictures, charts, or diagrams of the evidence, but before this is done it should be discussed with the attorney. If pictures or other illustrative materials are presented, they should be of professional quality, as poor photographs or diagrams may detract from the importance of the testimony.

According to Goldstein (1935) if the witness is being compensated for his or her testimony then the attorney should bring this out in the direct testimony, so that the opposing attorney cannot bring it out in cross-examination and in doing so insinuate that the testimony may be somewhat biased to insure payment of a fee.

Cross-Examination

During cross-examination, the opposing attorney has the opportunity to question the expert to see if there is anything that can be elicited that would be beneficial to his or her client's case. This can be done in a number of ways. The attorney may attempt to point out possible inconsistencies in the testimony of the expert. If it can be established that the expert's testimony differed from information presented in a previous trial, pretrial hearing, published report, deposition, or the expert's own notes, then the credibility of the witness may be damaged, and the remainder of the testimony may not be accepted by the judge or jury. If this should happen, try to explain any inconsistencies that exist. For example, if you did make a mistake and stated something incorrectly or misidentified a bone, then calmly indicate on the stand the nature of your mistake rather than becoming confused or maintaining the veracity of a previously given incorrect answer.

It is also possible that the opposing attorney may bring books or articles by other experts and ask why others might interpret similar information in different ways. If you are confronted with this type of examination, ask to see the reference so as to establish the context of the attorney's information. If you don't think that the reference is a valid one, you should indicate that and explain why the reference is inappropriate or inaccurate.

It is common for the opposing attorney to rephrase prior testimony and then ask the expert if the rephrased statement is correct. In response you should be certain that you understand absolutely everything that is said. If not, feel free to ask the attorney to explain those words or parts which you do not understand. You want to ensure that no words are incorrectly attributed to you.

You should realize that the opposing attorney is not trying to attack you per se, but is really trying to get you to say something that may be beneficial to his or her own client's case. Once the cross-examination is over, there is a final opportunity for your own attorney to question you during redirected examination. At this time points that you made during cross-examination can be clarified further.

Case History

The following case report illustrates a trial in which I testified as an expert witness.

In the Fall of 1979 the caretaker of a small cemetery in southwestern Michigan was requested to prepare a grave in a family plot for a recently deceased individual. At the time that the gravesite was being prepared, the caretaker was aware that two infant burials were already interred in that family plot. One of the infants had died on January 30, 1923, and the second on May 8, 1928. Both had initially been buried at another gravesite and moved to this family plot when it was purchased in 1953. The two infants were allegedly placed in a single burial container and interred on March 25, 1953. In 1979 when this gravesite was being prepared for the father, no clear marker existed to indicate exactly where the infant burials were located. Burial of the father took place on September 4, 1979 with no indication that any problem had occurred in the preparation of the gravesite.

Three months later, one of the two cemetery workers who had prepared the gravesite went to authorities with the following story. He claimed that during the excavation of the grave with their backhoe they came across the top of some type of metal container. Upon reaching the container they supposedly went to the cemetery office to ask for further direction. The worker claimed he was told by the caretaker's secretary in the office that he should dispose of the container. Later the caretaker allegedly went to the gravesite and told the workers that there were babies in the container and that they should dig it up and dispose of everything. To substantiate this story, the worker turned over to the police a bent-up piece of galvanized sheet metal, which he claimed was the remains of the container, which he had taken home and kept there for the past few months.

A short time after this information came to light, authorities arrested the caretaker and charged him with disinterring human remains without a permit. He pled no contest to the charge and was released on his own recognizance until sentencing at a later date. On the date that he was to be sentenced, he contacted an attorney for the first time and asked the attorney if he would represent him and change the plea to not guilty. The attorney agreed to represent the caretaker, and shortly thereafter I was contacted by the defendant's attorney to see if I could give any advice as an expert in forensic anthropology, specifically in the identification of infant human skeletal remains. Since my major research interest lies in the study of human skeletal growth from birth up to 30 years and I have personally examined the skeletal remains of thousands of individuals in this age range, I felt that I was well qualified to participate in the case.

Although I indicated to the attorney my willingness to consult on the case for the defendant, I carefully pointed out to him that if any bones were available for study and if I were able to identify them as human remains, I would have to testify to that effect. I was quite confident that I would be able to identify any newborn human remains, if indeed that was what they were.

As it turned out, there were no bones for me to study, but the attorney wanted me in court to listen to the testimony of the graveyard workers and then to testify as to what bones may or may not look like after more than fifty years in the ground. Other testimony indicated that the soil was neither very acidic nor alkaline and as such there should have been good preservation of bone. I have examined the skeletons of newborn individuals who were in the ground for over 5,000 years and found the skeletons to be completely intact. Preservation of skeletons in the ground or in graves depends upon many factors, some of which are discussed by Bass (Chapter 11). Another interesting aspect of this case was that the prosecuting attorney had also retained his own forensic anthropologist to testify at the trial. To the best of my knowledge, this was the first time in the State of Michigan that forensic anthropologists were employed by both the defense and the prosecution.

On the day of the trial the defense attorney asked me to arrive early because he wanted me to listen to the testimony of the graveyard workers and to give advice during cross-examination. I was nearly unable to do this because one of the first motions made by the prosecutor was that all witnesses should be excluded from the courtroom. The defense attorney then argued that he had no objection to excluding all witnesses with the exception of the forensic anthropologists. He argued that the main evidence against his client was the testimony of the two graveyard workers in which they would claim that they had recovered the remains of two newborn infants. Since those alleged bones were not available for us to study, the only evidence was their description of the remains. He also pointed out that the graveyard workers were not qualified as experts in the identification of human skeletal remains while both I and the other forensic anthropologist previously had been accepted by other courts as experts in the identification of such remains. The prosecuting attorney objected to this argument primarily because he had not asked his expert to arrive until some time later in the day, and he felt that the defense would have an advantage having a forensic anthropologist in court while he did not. The judge ruled in favor of the defense, and thus, I was allowed to sit in court during the course of the trial.

Among the first witnesses to testify were the two graveyard workers, who offered nearly identical descriptions of the "remains." They continually referred to the remains as either small pieces of dust or ashes and little pieces of black material. At my suggestion, the defense asked during cross-examination whether anything like feet, hands, or skulls were found and how large the so-called pieces of dust or ashes were. The response was that nothing that looked like skulls, feet, or hands had been seen and that they had observed only little balls of dust or ashes. They assumed that these were the remains of the infants.

I pointed out to the defense attorney that their description was nothing like what one would expect to see of newborn remains after fifty years in the ground under conditions that they described and that from the description it was impossible to say that human remains had been disinterred. I went on further to say that from their description I got the impression that they had no idea what excavated or skeletonized human remains should look like and that they were basing their description of the bones on that oft repeated statement, "earth to earth, ashes to ashes, dust to dust" (*Book of Common Prayer*). In this particular disinterrment, I am personally convinced that the grave diggers did not see any human bones and that their description of ashes and dust most likely came from the above mentioned prayer.

After the testimony of the grave diggers and a number of other witnesses, the prosecutor's forensic anthropologist was called to the stand. He was asked if infant remains might consist of small dark pieces. He then described how teeth develop and pointed out that if they fall out of the alveoli of the mandible or maxilla, they could be small dark pieces. He was technically correct in his description, but since he had not heard the testimony of the grave diggers, he could not have known that their description of the remains did not match what he so carefully described. I pointed this out to the defense attorney and suggested that he could bring this discrepancy out in my direct examination. Neither the judge nor the prosecuting attorney gave any indication that they realized that the grave digger's ashes and dust were something other than these teeth that were described.

After the prosecution rested its case, the defense attorney asked for a directed verdict of not guilty for a number of technical reasons. The judge denied this motion and then called for a recess before calling the defense to present its case. I was to be the first to testify.

For some reason that was never explained to me, the defendant decided during the recess to change his not guilty plea to no contest. The judge accepted his no contest plea and thus ended the trial. This no contest plea is considered to be the same as a conviction in criminal matters but cannot be used as an admission of guilt in later civil actions. At a later sentencing, the defendant was ordered to pay a small fine plus court costs and thus ended an interesting trial in which the defendant was fined, probably for disinterring nothing more than small pieces of dirt.

This trial illustrates that most people have some conception of what they believe human bones should look like. This conception probably stems from their previous experience of having seen skeletons or pictures of them at Halloween or in mystery shows on television or the movies. Some people also believe in the biblical concept that we are made of ashes or dust and that upon our death we will return to ashes and dust. Given this popular image, many individuals would likely be able to identify a complete articulated human skeleton if they ever came upon one. Similarly, most individuals would probably be able to identify a complete human skull because of its obvious humanlike appearance. However, I seriously doubt that many people would be able to identify disarticulated human adult bones simply because they are difficult to distinguish from animal bones or, under many circumstances, roots or twigs. When it comes to the identification of subadult bones, I would guess that even fewer people would be able to identify them because they are so much smaller. Skulls of younger individuals fall apart because the bones are not yet united at the sutures. Thus, identification of human skeletal material should be left to the knowledgeable experts, i.e. forensic anthropologists.

REFERENCES

Goldstein, I. (1935). *Trial Technique*. Callaghan and Company, Chicago, Illinois.

Kogan, J. D. (1978). On being a good expert witness in a criminal case. *J Forensic Sci,* *23(1)*:190–200.

Philipps, K. A. (1977). The "nuts and bolts" of testifying as a forensic scientist. *J Forensic Sci,* *22(2)*:457–463.

Stewart, T. D. (1979). *Essentials of Forensic Anthropology: Especially as Developed in the United States*. Charles C Thomas, Springfield, Illinois.

The order for the burial of the dead, *The Book of Common Prayer*, the Church of England.

AUTHOR INDEX

425

SUBJECT INDEX